Run for Life

Run for Life

The Breakthrough Plan for Fast Times, Fewer Injuries, and Spectacular Lifelong Fitness

Roy M. Wallack

Skyhorse Publishing

Skyhorse Publishing books may be purchased in bulk at special discounts for sales promotion, corporate gifts, fund-raising, or educational purposes. Special editions can also be created to specifications. For details, contact the Special Sales Department, Skyhorse Publishing, 555 Eighth Avenue, Suite 903, New York, NY 10018 or info@skyhorsepublishing.com.

www.skyhorsepublishing.com

10 9 8 7 6 5 4 3 2

Library of Congress Cataloging-in-Publication Data
Wallack, Roy M.

Run for life : The breakthrough plan for fast times, fewer injuries, and spectacular lifelong fitness / by Roy M. Wallack.
    p. cm.
    ISBN 978-1-60239-344-8 (pbk. : alk. paper)
    1. Running for older people. 2. Running—Training.
    3. Running—Health aspects. I. Title.
    GV1061.18.A35W35 2008
    613.7'1720844—dc22
    2008038008

Printed in Canada

To Elsa and Joey, my running mates.

Contents

RUN FOR LIFE

RUN FOR LIFE

Introduction

Run for Life's agenda is simple: Run to 100. Not just live to 100 and shuffle along when you get there, but do what few, if any, have ever done: Actually run on your 100th birthday—fast enough and far enough to feel the wind on your face, the exhilaration of speed, the endorphin high, and maybe even a 10k or marathon finisher's medal around your neck. Wouldn't that be cool, to run pretty much like you do now, 40, 50, or 60 years from now, long after the average running career ends?

An oxygen-debt delusion, you say—a "forever young" fantasy? Not anymore. Whether you grew to adulthood with the running boom or got your athletic epiphany later in life, the idea of running and fitness as lifelong pursuits—and not just for kids— gets more realistic every day.

After all, one out of every 10,000 Americans already lives to 100, and the numbers will explode in the coming years as we build more bionic body parts (marathon-worthy hips are here now; see Chapter 23), grow new ones from stem cells, and painlessly zap cancer with radio waves (I saw it on *60 Minutes* in February, 2008). But while medical miracles and genetic luck may get tens of thousands of us to triple digits, hitting the tape in real running shape is entirely in your hands (and feet).

Enter *Run for Life*, a blueprint for using running as the linchpin of a superfit longevity program. Using information from some of the world's most innovative coaches and trainers, reviews of the latest scientific studies, and in-depth, oral history interviews with some superfit pioneers of the sport, including Frank Shorter, Bill Rodgers, Rod Dixon, Dr. Kenneth Cooper, Bobbi Gibb, and others, it will show that genuine fitness and vigorous, exhilarating quality of life is not only possible at all ages, but also can be achieved in as little as 20 serious minutes a day. *Run for Life* is a paradigm-changer. It will give millions of Gen-X and baby-boomer runners an eye-opening, commonsense plan for staying in (or returning to) the sport they love—long after the common wisdom would have them switching to cycling, swimming, shuffleboard, or the rocking chair.

Run for Life starts with the premise that running is well-suited to lifelong fitness, with its terrific cardio endurance, unbeatable calorie burn, and superb side benefits: the body confidence, the compliments from your spouse's friends, and the convenience of doing it anytime, anywhere. Its health and longevity powers are increasingly documented: A 2008 Stanford study that compared 538 runners to a similar group of healthy non-runners over 21 years found that the runners had less than half their peers' death rate (15 to 34%) and saw the onset of disabilities like osteoarthritis and knee replacements delayed by 12 to 16 years.

But like any sport, running's not perfect: It doesn't stop the alarming deterioration in muscle mass, power, and reaction time that starts in your 30s and accelerates after 50 and 60—even, surprisingly, in your legs. And while its weight-bearing g-forces cue leg and hip bones to stay strong and thick (unlike non-impact sports like cycling), it suffers a high injury rate, ranging from temporary maladies like tendonitis and plantar fasciitis to chronic knee, hip, and lower-back pain. Statistics say half of all runners are injured at any one time. Ultimately, running can break you down as it builds you up. Maybe that's why participation plummets after age 50, with legions of hobbled, aging ex-runners moving on to cycling, swimming, rowing, or the living room couch.

Bottom line: *If all you do is run, you will not run to 100.* You might not even run to 80—or 60.

Run for Life is out to change that attrition rate—by changing how you approach the sport. Think of it in the way you do a long-term business plan or financial planning for retirement. Instead of focusing on short-term training to make you fast right now and short-term fixes to patch up nagging injuries, it focuses on a long-term, multi-pronged strategy that restructures your form and posture to cut the damage of running, restricts your cumulative impact time with cross-training activi-

RUN FOR LIFE

ties that can actually make you a faster runner, and rebuilds your declining muscle mass and $V0_2$ max—the dual scourges of aging—with powerful, high-octane weight training and intervals the likes of which you've never seen before. Special stretches, a runner-specific yoga program, and a unique runner's posture plan complete the realignment that readies you to run into the future.

• RUN SOFT • RUN LESS • RUN STRONGER • RUN FLEXIBLE • RUN STRAIGHTER • RUN FASTER

In a nutshell, that's the *Run for Life* plan. Combining innovations from cutting-edge coaches and inventors, academic sports science research, and real world examples, it'll work for runners of any age and ability. While raw speed is not the book's main goal, the beauty of its strength- and safety-focused program is that you'll probably get faster, too. The combination of a rebuilt body and the reduced injury downtime will maintain or improve your current speed. And if it doesn't, you'll still move up in your age-group as you outlast (and outlive) your peers.

Taking the *Run for Life* medicine won't be easy. To "run young" as you age, you won't have to work out any longer, in terms of total hours, but you do have to change the way you run, add training alternatives you may find odd, and run less. The hardest part may be mental: combating a

pervasive anti-technique mentality that says "mileage is everything." It isn't. Millions of ex-runners are proof of that.

Proudly, *Run for Life* takes a fresh look at running form and breaks ground on a variety of subjects:

• **Soft running:** Learn a classic 5-step running-form overhaul that is proven in laboratory tests to reduce knee-joint pounding and pain by 50%.

• **A call to arms:** Learn why a vertical arm swing is a key element in overall running speed and health, and how a small, inexpensive tool will automatically give you a perfect pendulum on every stride.

• **High-intensity strength training to revive power, reaction time, and balance:** Runners often hate weight training, but you absolutely will not be running at 100 without it, given the relentless decline in muscle mass and power as you age that occurs if you do nothing to stop it. To minimize gym time and maximize the benefits, follow the example of pro athletes: use explosive, rapid-contraction lifting, which resuscitates the invaluable fast-twitch fibers you need to accelerate, swerve to avoid obstacles, safely descend dirt trails, stay functional—and stay alive. A bonus: doing so restores youthful bulges to age-flattened muscles, burns fat like crazy, and will increase oxygen-processing capacity. Included are exercises to build key running muscles that are underdeveloped, like the glutes, and special quadriceps

RUN FOR LIFE

and spinae-erector exercises to rearmor vulnerable areas that deteriorate due to running, like knees, hips, and lower back.

- **Super-intensity, HGH-producing "Ultra-intervals":** Conventional interval training builds up your oxygen capacity but can put joints and connective tissue at risk. *Run for Life* cuts the injury risk, builds muscle, and bumps your VO_2 max up even higher by using all-out, lung-searing efforts as short as 20 seconds to jack up your own body's natural spurt of human growth hormone. You'll dread them—and love the results and time savings. A cross-training bonus: you can do them in any aerobic sport, getting real run-specific benefits in the hills, on the bike, and in the pool.

- **High-tech water running:** H_2O isn't just for rehab anymore. Runners have set world records after training in the pool with joint-saving, body-blasting water-resistance devices.

- **Run-specific yoga:** An exclusive 10-position, 8-minute yoga warm-up routine designed just for runners by renowned high-performance yogi and multisport champion Steve Ilg.

- **Perfect, no-back-pain posture:** An exclusive runner's plan from Symmetry, a leader in postural therapy, that eliminates long-term structural imbalances and locks in correct running form.

- **Bionic body parts:** Direct from the operating room, *Run for Life* reports on the new ultra-advanced hip prosthetics, just approved in the U.S., that are giving hobbled, broken-down runners the joints—and race times—of their 30-year-old selves.

- **Secrets of the Kenyans:** Ever wonder how Kenyan runners got so good? Join *Run for Life* on a trip out to the Rift Valley to run with the Kenyans and get tips from Dr. Gabriele Rosa, the mastermind behind their success.

- **The overtraining checklist:** Famed aerobics researcher Dr. Kenneth Cooper teaches you not to let the endorphin high brainwash you into ignoring debilitating injuries and compromising your immune system.

- **50-plus motivation secrets:** Read case studies of how racing, rivalry, crazy events, giving back, and joining organizations like the one-of-a-kind "65-plus New England Runners' Club" can keep you off the couch.

In addition, *Run for Life* features in-depth, oral history interviews with some of the most influential personalities in running history: Four-time New York and Boston Marathon winner Bill Rodgers; Olympic gold medalist Frank Shorter; mile-to-marathon champion Rod Dixon; Dr. Kenneth Cooper, who laid the intellectual foundation of the running boom with his bestsellers *Aerobics* and *Anti-Oxidant Revolution*; Bobbi Gibb, the first woman to run the Boston Marathon; Laszlo Tabori, the third man to run a 4-minute mile, and more. All of them are long past 50 and still deeply involved with running and fitness. The amazing journeys and lessons they are still learning about training and lifelong running will inspire, inform, and help fire your own motivation.

As for me, in case you're wondering, I am a longtime health-and-fitness journalist and an earnest-but-unremarkable runner whose motivation probably isn't much different from the stars'—and yours: I don't want to stop. I began my own Run for Life as a college wrestler, running around the track at midnight in a plastic sweatsuit in order to boil out enough beer to make my weigh-in the next morning. I became an official runner the day after I graduated from Whittier College in June, 1978, with a 5-mile run intended to make a personal statement: "I will stay fit for the rest of my life." It worked.

For three decades since, sports and fitness have been the main threads of my journalism career and life, and running has provided some of my greatest personal memories: competing not-so-spectacularly in the Badwater Ultramarathon (see Chapter 16); finishing the Boston Marathon on five days of training (see Chapter 1); taking a 90-minute run in San Juan, Puerto Rico, on my first honeymoon and a 2-hour run through Rome on my second; doing a 10-miler to the beach and back the day my son was born; running in Kenya with some of the greatest runners in the world (see Chapter 25); and scoring a first-place finish in the 2000 Human Race 10k in downtown L.A.

The latter proves a point I constantly make: We can all be great; you just need to find a tiny, first-time race no one's heard of yet.

Although my editors at the *L.A. Times* and various magazines may think of me as more of a cyclist (I've bike-toured around the globe, done some of the world's toughest multi-day endurance rides, edited several bike and triathlon magazines, and in 2005 coauthored the book *Bike for Life: How to Ride to 100*, which naturally led to *Run for Life*) running is what I've always used for daily fitness and to gauge the progress of my lifelong fitness plan. And, I must say, having interviewed dozens of experts over the years and gradually evolved the strategy laid out in this book, the plan's working out. As I write this, I'm 52, feel about 30, and have no trouble hanging with people half my age. And I'm not slowing down much.

Of course, I was never that fast to begin with. But that's okay, because fit aging is not about how fast you are, but how effectively you slow the deterioration. That's the number-one goal of this book—*slowing the deterioration*. Do that, and the speed takes care of itself. Example: While I never cracked 40 minutes in a 10k in my 20s and 30s, I haven't slowed much as my anti-aging running plan has taken shape over the last decade. In October 2007, I ran a 44:20 at the Manhattan Beach 10k, good for 17th in my 50–54 age-group out of 135. That's in the top 15%, my best finish in a big race.

While nothing spectacular now, that trajectory puts me right on pace to set an age-group national record when I'm 94. You may laugh, but after all, the goal here is to run to age 100. Fact: If I can keep my 10k deterioration down to 90 seconds a year from this point, I will break the 10k mark of 1:47:28 set by 94-year-old Paul Spangler of San Luis Obispo, California, in 1994. And if I don't, no big deal. There are no records at all after age 94. That means all I have to do is stay alive and walk a 10k when I'm 95 or 100.

Of course, in keeping with the theme of this book, you can bet I will run it.

Please try out a few things you read about in these pages. Because it'll be a lot more fun with competition.

—**Roy M. Wallack**
Age 52
October 2008

The Cheat Sheet

Everything you need to know, right now

As a journalist and average athlete—not a coach—my goal with *Run for Life* was to produce an objective synthesis of the best of what's out there. However, there are a lot of pages here; that may mean that a lot of good information lies buried in them, unseen. I want this book to have an impact now, the day you read this. Hence, this cheat sheet—the whole book, boiled down to a few pages.

The upshot here is that there are eight key athletic actions you can take to extend your running life and overall athletic health *at any age*. A side effect of these steps is that they will also make you faster. You may have heard of some of these eight, but I think this will be the first time they have been put together in one plan. Note that you don't have to do all of them to benefit. Each one will work on its own to extend your running life. But two of them will work better than one, and three better than two. Do you have time to do all eight? I prefer to think of it in this way: If you want to run deep into old age, do you have time not to? Here's the logic:

1. If you don't RUN SOFT—i.e., lessen your impact with a short-length stride and shock-absorbing forefoot landing—you won't run to 100, because you'll wear out your knees, hips, and lower back. Studies prove you can cut impact forces to the knee by 50%. Step one: don't heel-strike. Step two: don't overstride. Step three: Get rid of shoes with a big heel cushion. Run in flat, light shoes. To understand the concept, RUN BAREFOOT around the block. It is impossible to heel strike. A pair of individual-toed Vibram

FiveFingers will change your life. And, of course, run on dirt, grass, and trails as often as possible.

2. If you don't RUN STRONG—i.e., STRENGTH-TRAIN—you won't run to 100 because you'll fall over while vacuuming the floor at 80 and break your hip. Normal distance running does little to stop the inexorable decline in muscle mass and power (1% a year, more after 50 or 60) that starts at 35; after 60, even leg muscles wither precipitously, and they are a key to functionality as you enter old age. But weights do stop the slide if done right—meaning *fast, heavy, rapid-contraction, all-body weight lifting*. The body, alarmed by this stress, sends out a signal for the brain to send human growth hormone to strengthen you fast with more muscle.

Since every muscle of the body deteriorates, try to hit as many of them as possible while at the gym, twice a week. Don't waste time; use no-rest circuit training with as many freeweight and natural body-weight exercises as possible safely and efficiently. Move between opposing muscle groups (for example, a chest press and a seated row or lat pull down) and alternate between upper/lower exercises (a biceps curl following a squat). Go to "failure" (the point at which you can do no more) on each set of exercises, raising the weight and the reps as you get stronger. Don't forget to hit often-ignored muscles like the calf, hamstring, and butt, and build the interior portion of the quadriceps to enhance knee stability. Figure 45 minutes for a workout—any longer and you're going too slowly. Try to follow with easy aerobics to cut soreness, and immediately eat some protein afterward to rebuild muscles.

Do not socialize while lifting weights. If you have limited time that day, choose weights over aerobics. Without strong muscles, you get old fast.

3. If you don't RUN STRAIGHT—i.e., have GOOD POSTURE—you won't run to 100 because you will develop imbalances that will cause long-term bone, joint, and muscle damage and chronic pain. Ask yourself: Why do some people only wear out one hip, and not the other? The key is a VERTICAL ARM SWING. A subset of Run Soft, a vertical arm swing forces you to run straight with little side-to-side wasted energy and less wear and tear on hips and knees. Do posture drills religiously to fight the slouching imposed by sitting at a desk 8 hours a day.

4. If you don't RUN LESS you won't run to 100. Even if you run soft, years of pounding by running's *g* forces will take their toll. You must cut cumulative running miles. Do that by never running more than three or four days a week and two days in a row (to allow full recovery) and by utilizing cross-training.

5. CROSS-TRAIN. Other sports—aerobic and non-aerobic—can provide an endorphin fix on your off-days and give

running muscles a chance to heal. Special cross-training drills, such as STANDING BIKE INTERVALS and WATER RUNNING, can actually improve your running without the impact. Use the elliptical machine with and without arms. Use convenient and effective WATER RESIST-ANCE DEVICES, like AQx shoes and Speedo Hydro-Boxers (the former helped Lornah Kiplagat set a half-marathon record in 2007). In addition, sports that involve twisting and multiplanal movement, like tennis, racquetball, basketball, boxing, and soccer are valuable balance-enhancers and core-strengtheners for "linear" athletes like runners.

6. If you don't RUN FASTER—with ULTRA-INTERVALS—you won't make it to 100. Short, all-out-intense intervals of 20 to 30 seconds expose you to less cumulative repetitive-motion pounding than long 5k-pace intervals that last for minutes. They actually force you to run with good forefoot-landing form and deliver a potent jolt of fountain-of-youth hormones, including HGH. In fact, the effect is very similar to rapid-contraction weight lifting; all high-intensity work cues HGH production, but going all-out (out of breath, gasping, lung-heaving) gets you the most, building up your speed, stamina, and VO_2 max. In an ultra-interval, anything longer than 30 seconds probably means that you're not trying hard enough and thereby limiting the hormone surge, says Phil Campbell,

the inventor of the Sprint 8 program that partially inspired this chapter.

Ultra-intervals are hard, but the benefits are huge: muscle growth, fat burning, and much-reduced workout time. Think of it like this: what rapid-contraction weights are to muscles, intervals are to lungs, veins, and metabolism; your body quickly responds to the extreme stress. Twenty minutes is plenty of time to do 8 intervals. One study showed similar benefits in a 4-minute workout comprised of eight 20-second intervals separated by 10 seconds of rest. Warning: Strengthen your connective tissue and warm-up before blasting off, and use hills, water running, and standing cycling to do joint-safe intervals. Research has shown that brief, intense exercise is the best way to obtain a healthy, long-lasting body.

7. If you don't RUN FLEXIBLE you get old before your time. The first thing you notice about "old" people is how stiffly they move. Stiff muscles and connective tissue not only make you look bad, they hinder athletic performance. If you don't take a few minutes a day to stay loose and supple with some of the relaxing stretching and run-specific yoga exercises outlined here, you build cumulative stiffness that increasingly sabotages the other elements of your longevity fitness plan.

8. If you don't RUN MOTIVATED, you might not leave the couch. Studies show that aging accelerates when you do it alone. Make running social by getting

a rival, going to races, joining clubs like the Los Angeles Trail Runners Club or the New England 65-Plus Runners Club, and running regularly with a pal. Volunteer to do something good with your running, like training kids. And of course, keep yourself excited once in a while by pushing the envelope with challenges outside your comfort zone.

9. FINALLY, A WORD ABOUT DIET: Although I have written a lot about food over the years, this book does not delve much into diet. Here's why: The story on supplements seems to change day by day; many swear by glucosamine and chondroitin for joints, but some recent studies say it's merely a placebo. Resveratrol, the wonder nutrient found in red wine, will extend the life of rats—if they have the equivalent of 1,000 glasses of wine a day. Save money and snack on red grapes. Even Dr. Cooper's vaunted "anti-oxidant cocktail" of vitamins C, E, and beta-carotene has come under fire. As for food, it is common knowledge at this point that fruits and vegetables, lean meats and fish (although take it easy on mercury-heavy tuna and swordfish), and complex carbs constitute a healthy diet. Find convenient healthy foods and keep the fridge stocked with them. I graze all day on bell peppers, grapes, raw green beans, and apples.

While high-calorie-burning athletes can get away with ingesting simple sugars and even terrible man-altered creations like high-fructose corn syrup and hydrogenated oils, it makes sense to put the most pure, natural, high-octane fuel into your body. Carbs fuel muscular movement, so put in good ones—whole grains. And since building and maintaining muscle is key to staying long and strong, do not short yourself on protein. Vegetarians: go heavy on the nuts and other nonmeat protein sources; beware piles of pasta. Preceding and following a weight workout with protein is a necessity. A hamburger on a whole-grain bun within a 30- or 45-minute window after a weight workout or an interval session (which has similar muscle-building effects as weights) is a good idea.

Lastly, what about calorie restriction, the rage among academics who consider restocking their bookshelves to be athletic exercise? Cutting your calorie intake by 50% won't be fun or logical for runners, who need more calories than average people to support their endorphin high. Just do your best to make sure that they are high-quality calories.

RUN SOFT

Why you need a new, impact-reducing running form that can save your knees

According to the London-based *Sports Injury Bulletin*, 60 to 65% of all runners are injured each year. According to a 2006 survey of 510 runners, cyclists, and triathletes by Active.com, 90% suffered an injury in the previous year, with half sidelined for two weeks or more.

Those stats are why this chapter is a crucial first step for running longevity. They drive home the key concept of preserving your body—particularly your joints and connective tissue—against the injuries and irreparable deterioration caused by running itself. After all, you can rebuild age-shriveled muscle and power with weights, as you'll see in Section 2, but you can't rebuild worn-out cartilage, at least until some dazzling futuristic technology comes along. While the bionic hip may be upon us now (see Section 8), bionic knees aren't there yet and wrecked lower backs aren't even a glint in an engineer's eye yet. When the materials that coat, cushion, and separate bone from bone disappear, you have osteoarthritis. And your days of running—or at least running without pain—are over, period.

Fortunately, you can reduce the damage of running substantially—as much as 50%, according to one study—with a change in form that literally causes you to run "softer." Not surprisingly, it's known here in *Run for Life* as "Soft Running."

If Soft Running instantly makes you think of lower-impact activities like trail running and water running, that wouldn't be wrong. Both are key elements in a damage-control plan, and discussed at length in Chapter 6 and Chapter 14. But the lion's share of day-in, day-out Soft Running refers not to soft venues, but to a specific Soft Running form that reduces impact on all surfaces, especially asphalt, where we run most of the time.

This injury-reducing, soft running form is universal, meaning it applies to all runners of all ages. And that means that you are going to have to do something you may not have considered before: Learn how to run. Not learn how to train—that's something different. I mean literally learn how to run, as you would learn a skill, like golf.

If you believe running is a God-given activity that is individual to everyone and not to be messed with, you're among the vast majority who will find advocacy of a standard running form odd, to say the least. After all, while form is obsessively analyzed in swimming, cycling, and other endurance sports, it has long been ignored in the running world. *The Lore of Running*, Dr. Timothy Noakes's beloved opus on all things running, has 930 pages—just 2½ of them about running mechanics. Talk to coaches and search "proper running form" on Google and you get bits and pieces—some agreement about the benefits of shorter strides and rapid turnover, some random, often incompatible tips about posture (run tall or lean), arm swing (push elbows backward or let flop naturally), and knee lift (high, medium, or shuffle).

Even the Kenyans, often labeled as having "perfect form," say that there is no form in running. When I went to Kenya in 2004 and posed the question of form to past and present champions including Kip Keino, the 1968 Olympic 1500 winner, and Paul Tergat, the world champion marathoner, the answer was always the same: "Running is natural, individual, not to be messed with. Our success is due to training, nothing else." (For the details of their comments, check the sidebar in Chapter 2.)

Fine. But keep in mind that the primary purpose of this book is not speed (although that will be a side effect), but to help you stay fit and healthy enough run to age 100. I believe that running longevity makes a logical case for a universal soft-running form, especially if you consider that running for fitness is a very recent phenomenon.

Before the mid-1970s, few people ran daily. Even competitive runners stopped running once college or the Olympics was over. Thirty-, 40-, 50-, and 60-year-olds doing 25 to 50 miles a week is an anomaly in human history, and therefore calls for special protective measures.

"Homo erectus was not designed for the type of running we do today," explains William R. Leonard, Ph.D., chairman of the Anthropology Department at Northwestern University, a runner and one of the world's leading experts on nutrition and energetics among contemporary and prehistoric populations. "Running is an inefficient use of calories. Early man only used it in short bursts—to catch an animal, or run away from one. To cover long distances, we employed striding—fast walking. Humans are much more economical (energy-efficient) than quadrupeds at fast walking rate." He told me that this might indicate that humans have to learn how to run long distances.

On the flip side, a 2005 study in the scientific journal *Nature* argued that evolution made the human body a long-distance machine for running. Our torsos are longer than other primates', so we have more skin to keep us cool on longer runs. Our heel bones are bigger, to help cushion the blow of constant foot pounding, and we have shorter toes for improved push-off. As proof, many like to point to Phidippides, the Greek messenger who ran 26.2 miles from Marathon to Athens in three hours (after running 280 miles back and forth from Athens to Sparta the previous three days) to warn of a Persian naval invasion as proof that ancient humans were capable of running long distances. The fact that he died from exhaustion when he got to Athens may indicate that we weren't designed to do it very often.

Ultimately, whether we were or weren't meant to run long distances is irrelevant. The fact is that doing so for many years is wearing most of us out. And as for form, the claim that we don't need to learn anything about technique doesn't wash with increasing numbers of coaches. "In any other sport, it'd be ridiculous to say form can't be learned. You can always be made more efficient," says Ken Mierke, coach and author of *Training for Triathlon Running*. "Training only goes so far. As you get older, all you can do is get more economical and eat better."

Learning how to do the Soft Running advocated here in *Run for Life* is not necessarily difficult, because it's logical, lab-certified, instinctive, and natural—and has thousands of anecdotal success stories. The Pose Method, started by Russian sports scientist Nicholas Romanov in the early eighties, and the similar Chi Running, begun by American Danny Dreyer in 1999, have converted untold thousands to Soft Running already, but few did it overnight. Changing your form will take some time, and can be frustrating because it will initially stress certain muscles more than they are used to (particularly calves and hamstrings) and entail unlearning many long-engrained habits, like heel striking and elbows-out/cross-chest arm swing. But as you get into it, it'll start to feel right. You'll see that it's actually the correct way to run for efficiency and speed, whether you care about preserving your body or not.

The real hurdle of Soft Running will be getting religion before your joints are too far gone. If you're lucky, you'll get your epiphany while you still have cartilage to save. I got mine at age 43 at the Boston Marathon during one of the craziest athletic challenges of my life, and it changed my perspective so much that it ultimately led to this book. So, as a preface to the nitty-gritty instructional overview and tutorial of Soft Running mechanics found in Chapter 2, the first chapter of this Run Soft section is a real-life story that provides a clear black-and-white/before-and-after look at the technique's benefits. It's a real-time petri dish, a science experiment run amok that I think of as The Boston Revelation.

RUN FOR LIFE

CHAPTER 1

THE BOSTON REVELATION

What better way to learn to run soft than in the world's most famous race?

"Short strides. Rapid turnover. Landing under your center of gravity. Forget these three things, and you will be destroyed." I was desperate, so I listened closely as my friend Robert Forster, a physical therapist who runs Phase IV, a high-performance training center in Santa Monica, explained that my only hope of finishing the Boston Marathon was to completely change my running form. *Right now.*

After all, it was April 5, 1999. Boston was 14 days away. I had a non-refundable frequent-flyer ticket in hand, but I had not run in four months due to a shoulder wrecked in a bike crash and intense, searing pain in my left hip whenever I jogged a step. A doctor had just told me I'd developed Paget's Syndrome—excess calcium buildup in the joint. He said it was caused by years of running, which he recommended I never do again.

So I had no choice. "Your only hope of survival is to baby your muscles and connective tissue by minimizing impact and running softly," explained Forster, who got his start in physical therapy by readying and rehabbing two famous athletes—world-record 100- and 200-meter runner Florence Griffith "FloJo" Joyner and her world-record-setting heptathlete sister-in-law, 3-time Olympian Jackie Joyner Kersee. "Running softly means no heel-striking," he said, "just short, fast strides that keep your foot strike right under your body mass, your center of gravity—not out in front. The smaller steps take the workload and distribute it over more foot strikes, reducing the forces at each one. If you allow your strides to lengthen, you'll fly through the air further and crash down harder,

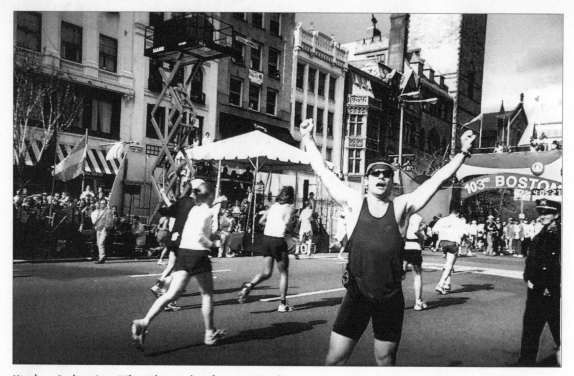

Miracle on Boylston Street? The author ran the soft-running gauntlet.

naturally heel-striking, and putting more leverage and stress on your muscles and tendons.

"To picture it, think of the Road Runner," he added. "His legs go in a little circle, and barely touch the ground. They go so fast they blur. You are going to shoot for a cadence of 180 strides per minute. You're going to spin your legs like the Road Runner."

As Forster finished his lecture, Steve Tamaribuchi, a Shiatsu massage therapist visiting from Sacramento, handed me a strange pair of purple-colored plastic handgrips he had invented called the e3

Grips. They looked like what's left over after you squeeze your hand around a lump of clay.

"You say you've got hip pain?" said Tamaribuchi. "Hold these as you run and it'll straighten out your arm swing, which will reduce the excessive sway of your hips. I bet the pain will disappear."

Right, I thought, rolling my eyes. *I'm going to run with tiny little steps for 26 miles holding these funky purple handgrips.*

An hour later, however, I was pinching myself. After leaving Forster's office, I'd gone right to the gym and run 5 miles on the treadmill—with no pain. Facing a mirror, I could clearly see that my arms were swinging vertically, not crossing over my chest at an angle, just as like Tamaribuchi had said.

As a test, I'd occasionally put the grips aside. Each time I ran without them, my hip would hurt again. Then, when I regripped, the pain would instantly disappear.

I was amazed. And I knew right then that the 103rd Boston Marathon would be one of the most interesting experiences of my life.

AFRAID *NOT* TO RUN SOFT

During the next 10 days, I alternated short-stride, rapid-turnover running with the elliptical machine, logged 34 total miles in 5 runs, and topped out with a 14-miler before beginning my "taper" and flying east. In the past, ramping up the mileage so quickly would have left me with pulled muscles, shin splints, and tendonitis. But now, on my most accelerated schedule ever, I simply felt great. Connective tissue, muscles, and hips were all perfectly pain-free.

Still, 26.2 miles seemed nuts to my friends, who had a tradition of flying in from all over the country every year to meet in Boston to run the marathon as "bandits"—people who hadn't met the qualifying times to officially run the race. They were amused by my little strides, weird grips, and lack of training. On an easy three-mile out-and-back to Jamaica Pond the day before the marathon, they

placed bets on the mile I'd quit, break down, or permanently injure myself at. I'd been thinking of this as a neat experiment; they thought it was suicide. I started to worry.

By the time we arrived in Hopkinton the next day about an hour before the 12-noon start, I was scared to the point of paranoia. Clutching my Grips as if holding invisible ski poles, I jogged around the start area mouthing my soft-running mantra over and over: "Short strides, rapid turnover, footfall under the body's mass." People looked at

The Experiment begins

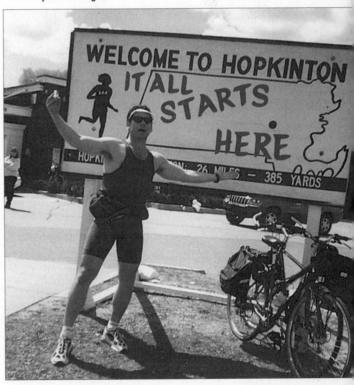

me as if I was a religious fanatic praying for a miracle.

The miracle part was right. All the logical scenarios that played out in my head ended the same way: my muscles imploding 10 miles from the finish, leaving me a scorned, pathetic failure marooned miles from home. I wasn't necessarily worried about being an illegal runner anymore—there were hundreds of numberless bandits openly warming up around me, including a pair of full-suited Blues Brothers imitators, and one guy with a torn-out piece of brown shopping-bag paper pinned to his shirt with the word BANDIT scrawled on it—but not being an official entrant still could be a problem. I'd have no access to the pickup buses that ferry broken-down runners to the finish line in Boston, where my wife and kid would be waiting for hours.

What was I thinking?

When the starting gun sounded, I didn't budge. I jogged in place for eight minutes as the multitudes crossed the start line, then burrowed into the middle of the last pack to find role models—preferably slow ones. Above all, I did not want to push it, and didn't need fast people to tempt me. The plan worked. When we got moving, it was absolutely glacial. The first mile took 13 minutes—a perfect warm-up. Finishing, not speed, was the goal.

Throttling back the engine took all my focus, as the crowd's enthusiasm, even way

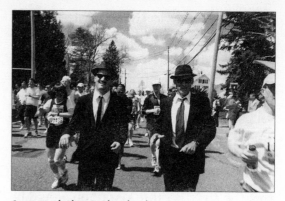
Cruising with Blues Brothers bandits.

out in the suburbs, was unlike anything I'd ever experienced at an athletic event. As my body imperceptibly sped up to easy 10-minute miles, it didn't seem like running as much as riding an energy current of love. From the sidelines came endless slices of oranges and bananas and shouts of "Go Bob!" An hour later I noticed that another bandit running just off my left shoulder was wearing a red T-shirt with "Bob" written on it.

"Short strides, rapid turnover," I repeated, fighting the urge to surge. Even the incredible sight and sound of thousands of crazed, out-of-control women at the deafening Wellesley College "Scream Tunnel" near mile 13 could not distract me. By then I was down to 8-minute miles, my normal pace, but not pushing it—although I wanted to. My body craved speed the way a starving man craves food, but I firmly kept the governor on the engine, well aware it could suddenly blow.

By mile 16, with legs feeling indestructible and body and soul nourished by the adoring crowd, the paranoia began to fade. I was—for lack of a better word—flowing. I was high beyond a runner's high. I had achieved nirvana. I don't think I had ever felt this good in my life. It got even better when I hit Heartbreak Hill—mile 20—at 2 hours 44 minutes. I did the math. At this rate, I'd get my PR by 10 minutes!

Exhilarated, I stopped in front of the "Heartbreak Hill" banner and pulled my disposable camera out of my race belt pocket, only to discover that there was just one shot left, which I was saving for the finish line. No problem. Three different people in the crowd offered to snap a shot of me on their own cameras and mail it to me (which, in fact, a guy named Scot Butcher did two weeks later).

I was already in love with Boston by then, and that cinched it. I posed with arms raised triumphantly, then glided up that famous 300-foot, 1-mile hill with my tiny, pinwheeling, Road Runner stride. I passed Bob. I passed dozens of red faces grimly clumping up the monster as if they were about to be eaten by it. I wasn't running—I was levitating.

At the top of Heartbreak came an astounding revelation: Only five miles to go. No pain. Hey, I thought, I can get my PR by 15 minutes!

A mile into the long gradual downhill into Boston, I blew by Tim Carlson, a

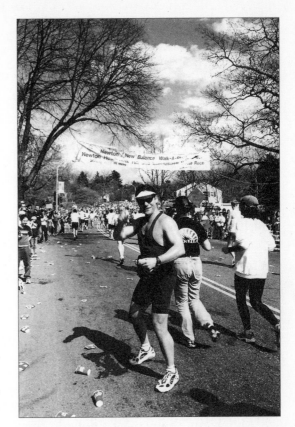

Heading up Heartbreak Hill.

training buddy and fellow *Triathlete* magazine writer from L.A., so fast that his hair would have surely ruffled in my breeze if it wasn't plastered to his skull. Surprised to see him, I slowed and began babbling about my breakthrough with the abbreviated stride and the amazing e3 Grips.

Tim did not share my elation. Although he had actually qualified for Boston, now he couldn't speak and looked wasted, as if he'd already been to hell and was dreading the return trip. He was on his way to a personal worst.

So I waved good-bye. But not before the worst possible thing happened: I got cocky.

In my mind, I'd become invincible, a man of destiny. As the descent continued, I picked up speed, lengthening my strides like a racehorse. Soon, I was no longer running, but galloping, bounding. My footfalls seemed to stretch yards ahead of my body; I was airborne, Olympian, god-like. The pace effortlessly pushed to 7:30, 7:15, 7:00 miles, maybe less. I started seeing myself as a TV movie, a Hollywood tale, *Chariots of Fire* meets *Against All Odds*. Oh, the story I'd have someday for the grandkids: The day old Gramps ran a PR at the Boston Marathon on virtually no training!

Then I hit mile 23.

Boiiiing!

My right hamstring pulled. Just slightly. I immediately shortened my stride and slowed down—but it was too late. I knew I'd screwed up. What a fool!

On mile 24, my right calf blew. Really blew. It knocked me to the ground.

I yelped like a wounded dog as I laid there and stretched for three minutes.

When I got up, I was seriously worried. The last two miles suddenly seemed like 200. Every inch of me was out of control. Painful spasms wracked both forearms from holding the Grips so long. And now every muscle in my left leg—not just the right—felt ready to pop. I felt like I was booby-trapped, a human land mine. One false step and ...

At mile 25, it exploded like a gunshot. My left interior quadriceps muscle—the vastus medialis—balled up into a fist of pain. I went down, screaming "Awwwwwww!" at the top of my lungs. Dozens of heads turned. "I'm a doctor—I'll call for a medical unit," said a red-haired woman who ran over from the sidelines with a cell phone. As I spread my legs wide like a Tibetan yoga master, lowered my face to the ground, and held that stretch for a good minute, moaning and crying, as I frantically tried to massage my shredded quad with shredded arm muscles that could barely control my hands, a drunken fellow ran up and launched a tirade just inches from my nose. I can still feel his spit.

"Get the hell up! Get up, dammit!" he yelled. "You ain't here to lay around, lazy-ass! Get up and finish this thing now or I'll kick you all the way there!"

God, I thought, *I love these people.* The Boston Marathon is run on Patriots' Day, which commemorates the day two centuries ago when the American Revolution started, when the Redcoats marched on Lexington and Concord. So everyone in Boston is officially off work and on the sidelines, drinking, partying, cheering on the river of runners in the city that created the modern marathon. In no other city on Earth would they care this much.

My last mile was 20 minutes of jogging on eggshells, praying for my body not to explode. Making the left turn on to Boylston Street, with only 100 yards to go, I was overcome by a sun-breaks-through-the-clouds moment of joy. I'd broken four! The clock at the finish read 4:04, but since I started eight minutes late, my time was 3:56. Not a PR. But I broke four!

I handed my throwaway camera with the one shot left on it to a woman behind the barrier and posed, bursting with happiness. Then I tip-toed across the line, wrapped myself in a foil blanket, and wandered around in a state of total bliss. *If I was to die at this moment*, I thought to myself, *my life will have been complete.*

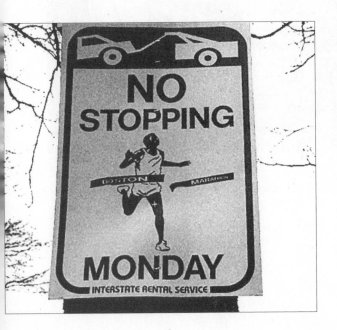

WHY NOT ALL THE TIME?

Like everyone, I've got a nice highlight reel of personal triumphs, but my finish of the 1999 Boston Marathon was off the charts. Of course, I wouldn't recommend anyone doing something like this, but from a pure learning standpoint as an athlete and journalist, the lesson was invaluable: Soft Running and a vertical arm swing work.

If I had stuck with Forster's plan to the very end, instead of reverting to my old long-stride pounding, I'd have pulled it off with a PR.

That's when it hit me: Soft Running shouldn't be used just for undertrained fools like me, but all the time. If it's far easier on the muscles and joints in one marathon, imagine the stress it'll save over a lifetime of running. It could extend your running career by many decades.

From that point on, I began questioning everything about running, especially the long-established maxim that training is everything, technique doesn't matter much, and you don't mess with someone's natural form. Technique does matter. I proved it.

I began researching new running methods and meeting innovative coaches and athletes outside the running mainstream. I talked to successful coaches in the mainstream, too. And I was surprised to find that, when it comes down to it, the two camps actually agree: There is a better way to run—safer as well as faster. And as you get older, that way becomes even more important.

I have been a believer in Soft Running ever since Boston. It was clear to me after that crazy day that there was a lot more to running than simply putting one foot after the other.

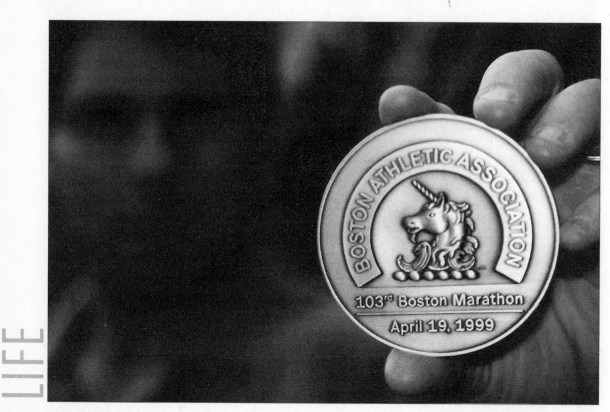

Expo paperweight—and finisher's medal.

THE 50% REVELATION

Learn the form that can cut the shock to your knees by half—in 5 easy drills

In 2003, Dr. Timothy Noakes of the University of Cape Town in South Africa conducted the most important study in running history: he put runners on a tread-mill, hooked electrodes up to their knees, and measured the shock transmitted through them. I call it the most important because Noakes, an esteemed running researcher best known for his 930-page tome *Lore of Running*, confirmed what very few knew: that changing the way you run can reduce shock to your knee by as much as 50%—an amount far more than the shock absorption of the most-cushioned shoes.

Fifty percent. That number has immense implications for injury reduction, both short- and long-term. It has long been accepted that at any one time, half of all runners have injuries severe enough to stop them from running. And that most runners give up the sport altogether not due to age, but to recurrent, accumulated injuries.

Keep in mind that the injuries that result from the shock that travels up your leg every time you pound it with as much as 5 times your body weight on each stride aren't limited to knees. Hips get the shock. Your lower back gets the shock. Your tendons and ligaments get the shock. Your cartilage—the smooth, white, glistening coating at the end of your bones that lets them slide as smoothly as ice on ice on one another as you bend your leg—gets it, eventually fraying and wearing and giving you the painful snap-crackle-pop of osteoarthritis. The shock squishes the spinal discs that separate your vertebrae; do it often enough and they might eventually bulge out to the side or flatten, allowing your backbones to painfully rub directly on one another or on the spinal cord. The shock pounds the meniscus in your knee, often deteriorating it to the point where it no longer provides cushioning between the bottom of the femur and the top of the tibia.

Bottom line: If you reduce this shock, you can run a lot longer. Theoretically, decades longer.

That's why the running world owes a debt of gratitude to Nicholas Romanov, who begged Noakes to do the above study, which ran in the March 2004 issue of the American College of Sports Medicine journal *Medicine & Science in Sports & Medicine*. Romanov, a Russian running and triathlon coach who lives in Miami, is the philosophical founding father of Soft Running, having refined his theory in the late seventies and early eighties. (The similar Chi Running was developed in 1999.) He went to Noakes because he wanted some legitimacy for a controversial running technique

THE BASIC RULES OF GOOD FORM

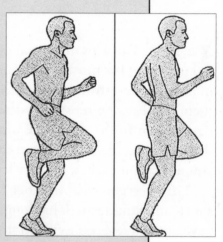

Shorter Stature: Landing with knees slightly bent to absorb shock, you'll run at a height 2 to 3 inches shorter than normal standing.

Short Stride: Your foot should land under the body, not ahead of it, utilizing core balance and reducing stress on muscles and ligaments.

Land on forefoot, not heel: Initially contact the ground on the ball of the foot, avoiding the shock and momentum-killing "braking" effect of a heel strike. The heel then briefly touches the ground.

Rapid Turnover: Cadence should be 180+ strides per minute, probably higher than you're used to. Remember: The longer the foot's on the ground, the more injury potential and momentum lost.

Pull, Not Push: After the heel's brief ground touch, pull it butt-ward by contracting the hamstring. Fight the urge to push off from the toes, using the quads and calves; the backward "pull" makes you "paw" the ground like an animal, providing forward propulsion.

Pendulum Arms: To direct all your momentum forward, swing arms vertically along the side of the body with elbows bent at a 90-degree angle or less. Don't swing them at an angle across the chest, which directs your momentum crossways and places additional compensating forces on hips, shoulders, knees, ankles, and back.

he had invented, the Pose Method (see Chapter 5). And he got it.

While the Pose Method is Soft Running, not all Soft Running is the Pose Method, which has an unusual feature—a forward lean that turns running into "controlled falling"—which makes it complex enough to merit a separate chapter. This chapter will outline the more conventional soft-running basics that work for everyone, partially underlie the Pose, and led to my unlikely Boston Marathon finish in 1999: Short strides, forefoot strike, butt-kick heel lift, and rapid turnover.

The guy who taught me those elements of Soft Running technique, Robert Forster, owner of the Phase IV clinic in Santa Monica, California, learned them himself from running coach Bob Kercee, who taught them to his world-champion heptathlete wife, Jackie Joyner, and his mediagenic Olympic medalist sister-in-law, FloJo. Kercee is a fine coach, but not a genius. Many other notable coaches, like Laszlo Tabori, the third man to break the 4-minute mile (see his interview following Chapter 11) preach nearly the same thing, although they may not call it "Soft Running."

It turns out that most good runners run this way, because it's actually the most efficient way to run.

STRIKE THE HEEL STRIKE

If you remember one thing about Soft Running, it is this: Do not land on your

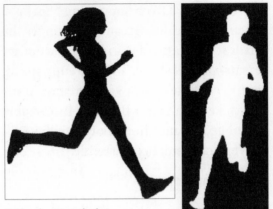

Heel strike: Don't do this

heels, no matter how puffy the air, gel, and foam in your shoes. Heel-striking may seem normal—even the apostrophe of the old *Runner's World* logo (above right) was a heel-striker. But heel-strikers have two strikes against them:

A braking effect: When you thud down onto your heel, it actually slows your momentum momentarily.

A breaking effect: In the long run, a heel landing breaks you down. As Noakes's study showed, heel striking, ironically made possible by the cushioning technology stacked under the heel in the name of safety, doubles the shock you'd normally get from a midfoot or forefoot landing in a non-padded shoe. So whereas great runners with classic midfoot landings wear out their joints because they run 20 miles a day for decades, we slower, heel-striking folk hobble and destroy our running careers on a fraction of the mileage.

RUN FOR LIFE

To stop that from happening, you have to ban long strides. Because the longer the stride is out ahead of your body, the harder it is to *not* heel strike. To keep your speed, you need faster turnover. To stay motivated, keep in mind that you'll probably speed up, because the lack of injuries will let you train more consistently.

BAREFOOTING

Interestingly, in his landmark study, Noakes used "Pose Running" and "barefoot running" interchangeably. That was no surprise; Romanov openly says that the Pose Method is an imitation of running barefoot—in shoes. The benefits of barefoot running go beyond shock reduction, claim its proponents: Strengthened feet with widespread, grippy toes; reborn proprioception, your foot's shoe-dulled sensation of where it is in space; and ultimately, the improved body balance that yields better speed and fewer injuries. That's why barefoot drills have been used for years by many top coaches (see Chapter 4).

As radical as barefoot running sounds, it isn't. Learning how to do it, as I found one day in February 2004, is as simple as taking off your shoes. On grass or concrete, it doesn't matter. Barefooted, you simply will not run with a long stride and a heel strike; it hurts too much. You automatically run slightly crouched and light-footed, your whole body a shock-absorbing spring. With no preparation, I ran three miles barefoot on the bike path at Bolsa Chica Beach in Orange County, California, with barefoot-running guru Ken Saxton (see Chapter 4). I was perfectly comfortable during our run and suffered no ill effect other than a little tenderness.

Fortunately, for those of you still leery of stepping on wayward rocks and twigs *sans* shoes, you can still get barefoot benefits with the Vibram FiveFingers, a "foot glove" with individual toes and a form-fitting 1/8-inch-thick sole. It may be the best of both worlds for those who want to make use of Soft Running, but want to avoid the learning curve that comes with doing it in shoes.

Shoes, by the way, are the root of all evil to barefoot aficionados like Saxton. But it's hard not to conclude that big, cushy air- and gel-filled heels can cause more harm than good, encouraging heel-striking, after seeing the results of Noakes' study. That and endless anecdotal evidence seem to indicate that soft-running techniques plus a cheap, minimalistic shoe with a flat, non-cushioned heel (which would not encourage heel-striking), is the best strategy for the goal of running to 100. And the benefit isn't just due to lack of impact. The improved balance, foot and ankle strengthening, and proprioception brought about by flat shoes will reduce injuries and keep you going in the long run.

THE IMPORTANCE OF ARM SWING

Whether you do your barefoot running in shoes, Vibrams, or bare skin, remember that there is an important variable in the Soft Running tutorial that the Pose Method does not address: A vertical arm swing.

Many coaches don't consider arm swing important and offer no advice on the subject, other than to do what feels natural, whether your hand swings all the way across your chest or pumps precisely up and down like a piston. But logic suggests that the latter, with the bent arm swinging like a pendulum on vertical plane and the elbow brushing the rib cage, plays a key role in running efficiency *and* longevity.

That's because the vertical arm swing reduces side-to-side motion, and therefore stress on your whole body—especially your joints. Running with your hands crossing the midline of your chest and elbows splayed out to the side not only looks bad—as I discovered while watching myself on a computer screen during a video gait analysis at Phase IV—but unnecessarily torques your core and puts lateral stress on leg joints more comfortable with up-and-down motion. Sure, plenty of great runners don't have perfectly vertical arm swing; Paula Radcliff, pictured in Chapter 3 on the cover of *Runner's World*, has the three fastest marathon times in history with a form that looks like Grampa McCoy square dancing at the country hoedown. But this book is about running longevity, not about raw speed, and her form is probably not conducive to running to 100.

Physiology dictates that the excessive swaying that Paula's cross-chest arm swing puts on her hip joint will translate to accelerated wear. Will she be hobbled by age 45? That's what happened to two-time Hawaii Ironman triathlon champion Scott Tinley, a former 100-mile-a-week runner who was limping along with the help of a cane in his late 40s. He was effectively crippled for five years until he got a radical new hip resurfacing operation done at age 49 in December 2007. (See Chapter 23.)

It cost upward of $35,000 for Tinley and other megamilers I interviewed to install the new-fangled bionic hips that restored their running. But straightening your gait out with a vertical arm swing is free—and won't cost you 5 years of your running career. To have your form looking like that of Ryan Hall, the fastest U.S. marathoner in history (2:06:17 in London, 2008) check out the 5-step Phase IV tutorial below. Also, consider shelling out $39.99 for a pair of e3 Grips, the devices described in my Boston Marathon tale in Chapter 1. If you don't mind holding something in your hands as you run, they'll instantly and effortlessly lock you into a vertical arm swing.

RUN FOR LIFE

Keep in mind that swaying hips and twisting torsos wreck more than hip joints. They change the angle of the knee and ankle, force muscular compensations to maintain balance and posture, and exaggerate any natural imperfections you might have, like leg-length discrepancies of more than one-quarter inch. Of course, serious runners may pay the price for bad form more than casual joggers, as the greater mileage and intensity can cause small, otherwise-imperceptible imbalances to mutate into large problems.

THE 5-STEP SOFT-RUNNING TUTORIAL

Before you begin to practice the five technique drills described below, do yourself a big favor: Do a 6th drill. Make a before-and-after videotape of yourself on a treadmill, filmed from the rear, the side, and the front. You'll see how good or bad you really run, and how quickly the five techniques here can work.

First, run with your natural form without any thought to proper technique. Then, after you've practiced the five drills, concentrate on running with short strides, high knee and heel lift, and vertical arm swing. The camera doesn't lie, so it'll be an eye-opener. If you're anything like me, you'll be stunned at how much better you'll look.

I was shocked by how bad my form was on the "before" half of the video.

Elbows out, shoulders rolled forward, and hands flailing across the midline of my chest. My torso was torquing side to side and my hips, to counterbalance, were swinging like a Brazilian conga dancer at Carnival. My strides were long and slow, my feet thumping on the ground, nearly heel-striking, No wonder my obliques often hurt on long runs over the last several years. It seems like I'd almost forgotten everything I'd learned since 1999.

The "after" shot, taken following the 5-step, 10-minute exercise routine laid out below, was a revelation. I looked like I thought I looked: like a real runner again. Efficient, balanced. A vertical arm swing humming like a metronome. Half the hip sway as before. Midfoot landing under my body.

Ironically, for years after Boston, I thought I'd been running soft. Taking the Pose class in 2003 had reinforced it, along with a "barefoot" run in my Vibrams every once in a while. But in regular shoes, it seems, I had slipped back into my old ways. So I dug out Steve Tamaribuchi's e3 Grips, which lay buried in my workout bag for years. And like before, I instantly improved.

Bottom line: Seeing is believing. Even if you aren't convinced that Soft Running will add decades to your running career, watching your form instantly become more efficient and smooth after the 10-minute tune-up below will tug at your vanity. Hey, we all want to look good, right? If it helps you run to 100, so much the better.

To prepare yourself for proper soft-running form, try these five tried-and-true, old-school drills from Phase IV, which come right out of coach Bob Kercee's playbook. As exaggerations of correct form, they improve your range of motion and train your neuromuscular pathways—a.k.a. muscle memory—to fire in the correct speed, angle, and sequence. "During arm swing, for example, your nerves not only tell your anterior deltoid to actively move forward, but tell your posterior deltoid to relax," says Phase IV director Forster. "The drill overexaggerates the motions to really burn it in."

Doable in a few minutes, the drills give your warm-up some purpose and provide an immediate benefit that you can see and feel. Do them in the order shown as part of your warm-up or alone on off-days.

DRILL #1

Pendulum Arm Swing

The Goal: Turn your arms into fast-moving pendulums that swing on a vertical plane at your side. You'll run faster with fewer injuries.

Here's why: Arm and leg motion are oppositionally synchronized or "contralateral" (the right leg rises forward at the same time as the left arm), so fast arms = fast legs. According to Dr. Tom Miller, author of *Programmed to Run*, arm turnover rate dictates leg speed and arm movement precedes the leg by a couple milliseconds.

Forster stresses that the arm should swing pistonlike on a vertical plane in order to minimize the counterbalancing (twisting) of your trunk, and therefore direct more of your energy into forward motion and less into potential injury. Beware what he calls the "Tyrannosaurus Syndrome," the elbows-out/hands-up form that short-circuits the pendulum swing and promotes body rotation.

Since a short pendulum or lever takes less effort to swing than a long one, "shorten" your arms by keeping the elbows bent at less than 90 degrees. Don't let your arms get way out in front of you. "The longer the pendulum, the slower the swing," says Forster.

Initiate all arm movement from the shoulder joint; the elbow *should not move at all.* "If I put your elbow in a cast, you'd still be able to run with proper mechanics," says Forster.

Drive the backswing hard. "Reach back like you're going to put your hand in your pocket," he says. This isn't as simple as it sounds; while the forward swing is easy, our backswing is often limited by tight, rhythm-wrecking pectoral muscles, according to Forster. (See the stretching techniques in Chapter 12 to stretch pecs and arms.)

"It's incredible to me that some coaches don't talk about arm swing," he says. "They say, 'he's so fast already that I'm not going to mess with his form.' But I say if he's fast already, he'll be even faster with better biomechanics. Besides, recreational athletes need all the efficiency they can get; they don't have the motor of a Carl Lewis."

The Drill:

a. Elbow position: Bent at sub-90-degree angle.

b. Vertical arm swing: Don't let elbows flare out and hands cross over the chest. Tip: To maintain the vertical path, pretend you're scraping the ground with your elbows.

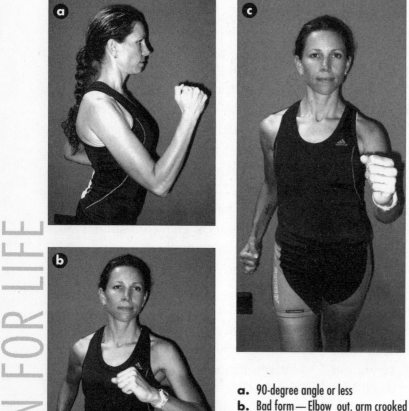

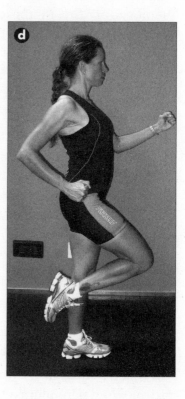

a. 90-degree angle or less
b. Bad form—Elbow out, arm crooked
c. Good form—Elbow vertical
d. Swing Elbow to the rear

c. Hand position: Relaxed, with thumb up and pinky finger down. Tip: Pretend you are pulling a horizontal rope attached to a distant bell tower. As you pull, it rings a bell. That also prevents shoulder shrugging.

d. Generous backswings from the shoulder joint.

e. Standing with legs unmoving in front of a mirror (for feedback) drive arms forward and backward at a faster-than-normal pace (180+ per minute) and bigger-than-normal amplitude. This burns in the neuromuscular pathway. Do sets of 30 seconds.

DRILL #2

High-Knee Prancing

The Goal: To give your foot/lower leg enough time in the air to be able to hit the ground moving backward, not forward, thus propelling you forward and reducing the braking effect of a heel strike. Think of an animal "pawing the ground." If you don't raise the knee, the foot would actually hit the ground on a forward arc, which breaks your forward momentum. A high knee allows you to hit the ground directly below your center of gravity, instead of in front.

Note: Lifting your knees high is not easy. "That's because our hip flexor, the iliopsoas muscle, is dormant in the general public," says Forster. "The iliopsoas is not active in modern life unless you walk stairs and hike steep hills. Otherwise, we

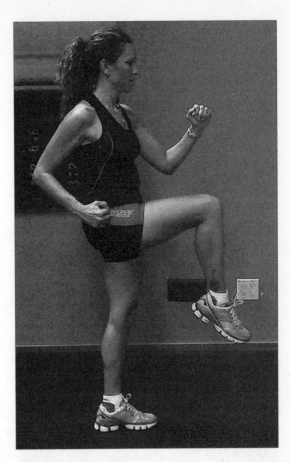

Clydesdale high knee drill.

don't use it. We use other muscles to lift our knee up and get out of our car. So we have to wake it up." High-knee prancing does that.

The Drill: Exaggerated running in place: Lift your knees abnormally high, like a Clydesdale horse. Do not kick out like a showgirl. Just high knees. Include vertical arm swing. Do 3 sets of 30 seconds. If you have space, move forward very slowly over 10 to 15 yards. After one set, jog a little bit, then do it

21

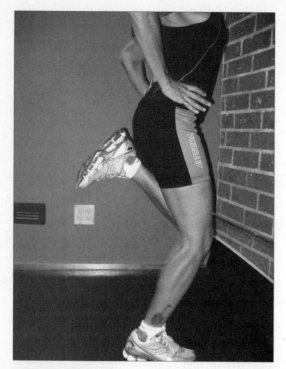

Butt kick/heel raise drill.

again. "Don't do too many at first—you could blow out a hip flexor," says Forster.

DRILL #3

Butt Kick

The Goal: Training the heel to get up to the butt while running has three functions: 1) Strengthens the hamstrings, which help pull the leg back underneath you when it's out in front of your body. 2) Shortens your leg pendulum, allowing it swing forward through the air into landing position with less force requirement. Again, physics dictates it's easier to

swing a shorter pendulum than a longer pendulum, even if it's the same weight, because more of the mass is closer to the axis of rotation. 3) Sets up a short-stride, forefoot/midfoot landing under your center of mass.

The Drill: Keeping knees in place (the opposite of Drill #2), kick yourself in the ass. Heel to glute. All the while, maintain vertical arm swing. You can do it in place or slowly move forward over 10 yards. Do 3 sets of 30 seconds.

DRILL #4

Russian Cossack Dance

The Goal: Train the glute to pull the foot back to a position below your center of gravity, not ahead of it, so that the foot can deliver forward propulsion.

The Drill: With arms folded across your chest like a genie, raise a straight leg up in front of you. Pull the straight leg down on an arc, so that the foot lands directly below your hips/your center of gravity, not ahead of it. You should look like you're doing a Russian Cossack dance. Do 3 sets of 30 seconds .

DRILL #5

Ultrafast Turnover

The Goal: The ideal cadence is 180 strides per minute—higher than most people are used to. To get comfortable with the pace, this drill pushes it even

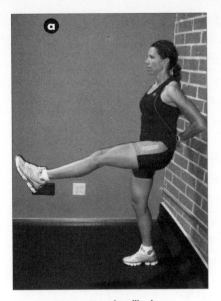 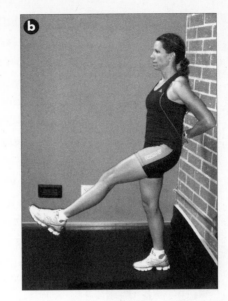 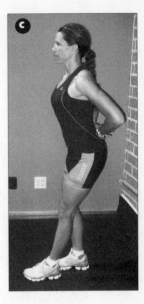

a. b. c. Cossack pullback.

more. The rapid turnover reduces your foot's time on the ground, meaning less time to pronate and get injured.

The Drill: Do the butt-kick drill, with proper vertical arm swing at 200+ strides per minute. Do 3 sets of 15 seconds, resting for 15 seconds in between while jogging in form.

With proper form now "burned in" to your muscle memory, proceed with your normal running workout. Of course, the hard part is sticking with it over time. Old habits are hard to unlearn. Changing your running form requires constant vigilance. They say it takes 3 weeks to change a habit and 6 months to lock it in for good.

Soft Running also requires some conditioning. Your body will not be used to the rapid turnover and high heel lift; initially your heart rate will rise as you reach for more oxygen. The higher leg lift puts more stress on your hip flexors, hamstrings, and butt. The forefoot/mid-foot landing puts extra stress on the calves and Achilles tendons.

Some of the conditioning for those muscles should come from the weight room, according to Forster. Find these exercises in Chapter 7. Otherwise, the conditioning will come over time. Tip: initially alternate 2 minutes with the new form, and 8 minutes your old way, then work up to 3 and 7, 4 and 6, and so on until you can run softly 100% of the time.

RUN FOR LIFE

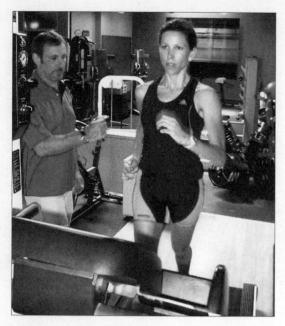

"Straighten your arm swing," says
Robert Forster to 40–45 age-group star Angela Lariva.

Pose Method runners told me that it took anywhere from two weeks to six months to accommodate to the new form. Of course, to instantly ramp up the learning and biomechanical curves, grab the Grips and take your shoes off.

There is a lot to digest in this chapter. Maybe you won't use it all. But try it little by little, drill by drill. From Day 1, you'll run more efficiently and limit the cumulative wear and tear. You'll get injured less and probably see less falloff in your times. And as the years roll on, the running won't stop.

THE KENYAN COUNTERPOINT

Learning how to run "soft" sounds easy, but is in fact a time-consuming process—a fact that causes many traditionalists to question whether a running technique that must be learned is worthwhile in the first place. Who better to ask than the Kenyans? Not only are they the world's most dominant distance runners, they're renowned for a "soft" gait and economical running style that is somewhat reminiscent of what is described in this section of *Run for Life*.

In January 2004, I traveled to Kenya, trekked through the Rift Valley, and met several past and present champions gathered in the town of Eldoret for the 11th annual Fila Discovery Races, Kenya's national championships for 5- to 18-year-olds. When I brought up the subject of form, they uniformly insisted that their form is as varied—and unlearned—as that of any runner anywhere.

Kip Keino shook his head when I showed him an article I had written about the Pose Method. "No, no, no. There is no correct running form—and you can't learn it," said the famed 1500-meter gold-medalist from the 1968 Olympics in Mexico City, now the head of Kenya's Olympic Committee. "Form is God-given. You're born that way. If you systematize it, you destroy it."

"Kenya's success is not dependent on form. No runner's is," said Paul Tergat, who set the marathon world record time of 2:04:55 in 2003 in Berlin (since broken by Haile Gebreselassie's 2:03:59 in Berlin in 2008). "Look at Emil Zátopek." Tergat was referring to the 1948 and '52 Czech Olympic gold medalist who had a form, said one pundit, that resembled running while "on the brink of an epileptic seizure."

Elijah Lagut, winner of the 2000 Boston Marathon, told me, "I do run soft, but nobody told me to do that. In fact, I run like the Pose method. Romanov copied me!"

Up and down the line—Sammy Korir, who ran a second behind Tergat (2:04:56) in Berlin '03, Joseph Chebet, 1999 Boston and New York winner; and Martin Lel, 2003 NYC winner and fourth fastest of all time (2:05:15)—they agreed: Kenyans do not learn or even discuss form.

That's the way their coach wants it. "It's crazy to try to alter form. Even an average guy shouldn't change. You can't run thinking of all this stuff—how to move your feet, your body, your hands, as you run—it's too distracting," said Dr. Gabriele Rosa, the Italian who in 1994 founded the training-camps program credited for much of Kenya's long-distance success. "It's all training, nothing else. Look at the form of [England's] Paula Radcliff; she got the world record (2:15:25, in London in 2003) with her head twitching all over the place."

Of course, just because the Kenyans are not taught a standardized running form, it doesn't necessarily mean that they don't have one. "Athletes often say one thing—but don't understand what they do. They all imitate the local hero—and in Kenya the local hero is a world record holder," says Richard Benyo, editor of *Marathon & Beyond* magazine. Fact: Three-fourths of Kenya's top runners have remarkably similar backgrounds. They come from one tribe—the 3-million-strong Kalengin. As kids, they walk and run everywhere barefooted; and as pros they live and train together in groups every day, all year long.

The only Kenyan who admitted considering form an issue was Margaret Okayo, winner of the 2003 and 2001 New York City marathons and 2002 Boston, but she may not have been serious. "Yes, I may change my form," she revealed with a smile. "I am thinking about bobbing my head [like Radcliff]."

The bottom line regarding a Kenyan form? "Everybody in Kenya runs different," said Lagut. "It's not like the Japanese. They all run alike."

CHAPTER 3

SECRET WEAPON IN THE ARMS RACE

If you can't keep your arms vertical, the e3 Grips do it for you

Rich Hanna was the 100k U.S. national champion in 1994 and 1995, but his competitive running career was nearly over by 2001 due to recurrent injuries, particularly a chronic tear of the soleus muscle of his left calf. "I felt like I lost a couple years in my prime," he said. "I tried everything—hardcore deep-tissue massage, magnetic insoles. Nothing worked. I was desperate. So I tried the Grips."

After two weeks of running while clutching a pair of purple e3 Fitness Grips, 2-ounce, plastic hand forms, Hanna's various ailments nearly disappeared. Several months later, Grips in hand, the 36-year-old placed second at both the U.S. 100k nationals and the World Championships, the highest finish at the latter by an American male ever.

"I think the Grips got me more in balance—they relax my shoulders and line them up with my hips," says the Sacramento coach and race organizer. Friends noticed he no longer listed to the left as he ran, which he now thinks was the cause of his torn calves.

"I will not run now without the Grips," says Hanna, who at 43 won the Masters division at the 2008 Way Too Cool 50k in 3:38, his 3rd-fastest time there, even beating one of his three overall winning times back in his prime. "Tons of local runners will say the same thing. I think Steve's a genius."

That would be Stephen Tamaribuchi, the Sacramento Shiatsu massage therapist who developed the Grips in 1997. He came to his epiphany—that the position of the thumbs

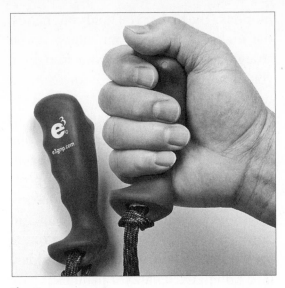
The grips.

helps control the stability of the entire body—literally by accident. A broken back in high school and torn neck muscles in college left him arthritic and unable to raise his hands over his head by age 29. While in therapy, observing how his body moved, he discovered that a bent-thumb position seemed to relieve the pain in his neck and back.

"It turns out that bending the thumb as if you're pressing a button tightens two ligaments that roll your elbow inward toward your ribs. That, in turn, controls shoulder stability," explains Tamaribuchi. (Try it; you can actually see your wrist and forearm tighten and feel an inward pull on the elbow.)

That discovery caused him to arrive at an unconventional top-down view of posture and motion, that, like the old song, can be summarized as "The arm bone's connected to the leg bone." In short, Tamaribuchi found that correctly positioning the hand stabilized everything down to the feet.

It works like this: A bent thumb on a knife-edge hand tucks the elbow into the ribs, which stabilizes and squares the shoulders. That centralizes the core and minimizes the side-to-side rocking of the hips, keeping a runner's legs striding in an ideal, "neutral" path. Tamaribuchi says the result is less stress on joints, on lateral structures like IT bands, and reduced pronation, translating to fewer injuries.

I couldn't disagree, given that the Grips had instantly cured my hip pain in 1999 and allowed me to finish the Boston Marathon. But what about all the runners

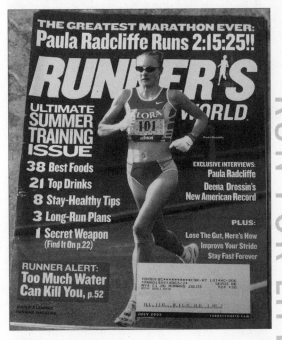
Radcliff: Example of bad arm swing.

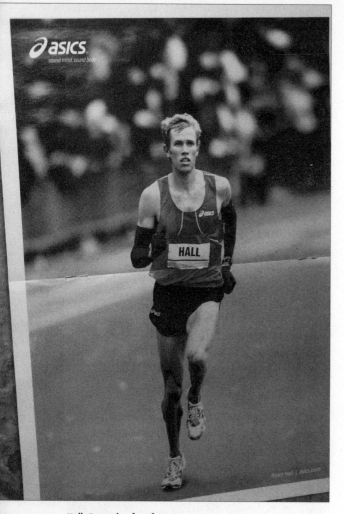

Hall: Example of perfect arm swing.

motions. The higher you hold your hands, the higher you raise your knees. If you straighten your arms out, you straighten your legs out. Hand speed correlates to turnover."

To the amusement of patrons of a Starbucks in Irvine, California, one late night in March 2008, Tamaribuchi demonstrated the effect of hand position on whole-body stability by having me stand up and turn my palm up and down; a down-facing palm would rotate the elbow outward and roll the shoulders in; a knife-edged hand or palm facing up would pull the elbow back in and square and stabilize the shoulders. When he tugged at me with my palms turned up and/or holding the Grips, I was more stable and less easily moved. When I walked up and down the store with the palms in the up position, I felt natural and balanced; with palms down, much less so.

The explanation, Tamaribuchi said, is that putting palms in the thumbs-up position forces everything to the center. Running with your elbows tucked in, you use more of your central core than your obliques, more of your vastus medialis (the interior section of your quadriceps) than your vastus lateralis (the outside section).

By contrast, running with elbows splayed out like chicken wings throws your form out of whack. "If you bring a hand over the midline of your body, it

and coaches, even soft-running gurus like Nicholas Romanov of the Pose Method, who believe that arm and hand position doesn't matter?

"To say that arm action has nothing to do with efficient running is crazy," said Tamaribuchi. "The arms control the leg rotates the humerus (upper arm) inward, which makes your body rotate," he says. "This wrecks your mechanical efficiency, which wants everything directed in a forward motion."

All this leads to three basic Tamaribuchi rules:

- Don't run with hands (or fists) facing palm-down. That turns the elbow outward, rolls the shoulders forward, forces the hands to cross the body's center line, and sets off a chain reaction of inefficiency.
- Do run with knife-edged hands with a bent thumb and elbows brushing against the ribs. That keeps the elbow in, and keeps you working efficiently through your central core.
- Don't ever let elbows roll out.

"Remember that the elbows-out position changes everything down the line," Tamaribuchi says. "Ideally, you should run with an erect back and knee lifts straight up through the midline of the thigh. But swinging your hands across the body, you give yourself kyphosis—shoulders and back are rounded; hips counter-rotate as they swing in and out; the femur externally rotates, instead of moving straight up. That makes the knee lift out to the side and the feet land funny, all pronated. You know what happens next? Injuries."

"The mechanical inefficiency tears up your body," says Tamaribuchi, who works with the U.S. Ski Team, advises athletes at the Olympic Training center, and per-

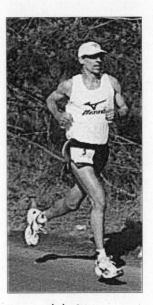

Hanna, with the Grips.

suaded Michael Stember, 1500-meter runner in the 2000 Olympics, and Dena Kastor, 2004 marathon silver medalist, to use the Grips. "You put unnatural stress on the IT bands and hip flexors as you shift the body in that direction. Instead of using the medial muscles of your body efficiently, you must use compensatory muscles to create stability.

"You need to work with your body, not against it," he says. "And it's not that difficult—just learn to control your arms. It's a lot easier than controlling your legs."

And if you can't control your arms, no problem. The Grips do it for you instantly.

RUN FOR LIFE

Of course, fewer injuries means more running longevity. "If you can stay injury-free, it keeps running fun," says Hanna. "You never want to stop doing something fun."

Part of the fun is going faster, and the Grips offer that, too. "I've done experiments on the track with some of my runners," he says. "I'll have them run a lap at 80% of perceived exertion with and without the Grips, and secretly time them. They always cut 1 to 1½ seconds off their lap time with the Grips."

There are two reasons for that, he thinks. "You run aligned, so your body wastes less energy. And since you reduce body sway and feet weaving back and forth, you go straight from point A to point B. So with the Grips, you actually run a shorter distance."

CHAPTER 4

THE BAREFOOT REVOLUTION

Olympic coaches and a barefoot guru agree: Going shoeless, for a minute or a marathon, strengthens feet and instantly confers Soft-Running form and injury reduction

"No shirt, no shoes, no entry," reads a sign in the window of the Secret Spot restaurant on Pacific Coast Highway in Huntington Beach, California, but the words "no shoes" are half-blacked out.

"They did that because I'm half their business," jokes Ken Saxton, who lives with his wife in a condo next door. Known as "The Barefoot Runner," the longhaired, long-bearded Saxton hasn't worn shoes (except on airlines) since 1987—not while ordering a tofu burrito, not while working his computer programmer job at Long Beach State University, and certainly not while running. He's averaged 10 shoeless marathons a year since 2002, including 14 in 2006 at age 51. His bare feet are fleet, too, as he qualified for Boston in 2004 and '05.

And there's one more amazing barefoot feat: Saxton says he's never been injured in over two decades of unshod running, even during a crazy 16-day period in '06 when he ran four marathons. "Okay, I was a little worn-out," he says, "but not hurt."

Saxton's sole-baring achievements have made him the pied piper of a tiny, but mushrooming barefoot running movement. Helped by the interest in "barefoot running shoes" like the Nike Free and the Vibram FiveFingers ("better than regular shoes, but they still deaden your feet," he says; see "Barefoot Shoes" sidebar, p.35) his Runningbarefoot.org website is up to 200 to 300 hits a day and his e-mail list to 1,500 members—5 times more than in 2002. Three barefooters ran the L.A. Marathon with him in 2003; 8 did in 2007. The Omaha Marathon even started a barefoot division.

Saxton's shoeless odyssey officially began when, as he puts it, "I just got tired of wearing out shoes, and shoes wearing out my feet." That occurred in 1987, when, after years of mostly running barefoot on the beach, he wore shoes at the Long Beach Marathon, his first-ever 26.2-miler, finishing in 5 hours, 5 minutes. "My feet were so beat up and blistered at the end that I had to walk the last two miles," he said. "After that, I gave up racing for ten years—and tried running barefoot on the streets out of desperation."

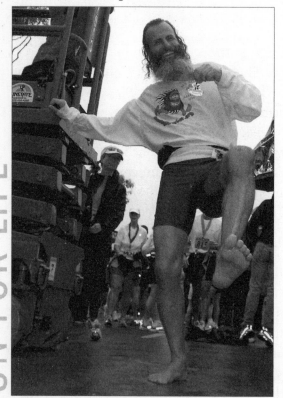

Ken Saxton at the 2004 OC Marathon.

He was hooked after one shoeless run on pavement. "Barefoot, I immediately felt great," he says. "I ran softer, lighter, landing on my forefoot and picking up my feet very quickly. But I actually wasn't thinking at all about my form. Taking on a more shock-absorbing form was automatic—like my body was getting instant biofeedback from the bottom of my feet, and simply knew what to do."

In 1997, after months of training with local off-road legend Bill McDermott (see Chapter 6), Saxton started racing again. He was surprised to finish the hilly, 10-mile Chino Hills Road Less Traveled in 1 hour, 11 minutes—good for 8th place in his 40–45 age-group. Even more surprising was the crowd reaction.

"I felt almost like a celebrity," he said. "Many of the runners 'interviewed' me after the event." So many asked if it hurt his feet to run barefoot that he began to answer their question with a question: "Doesn't it hurt to run with *those* on your feet?"

Saxton followed his first barefoot marathon, the 1998 Napa Valley Trail Marathon, with a barefoot 50k a month later. He set his PR of 3:18 at the Pacific Shoreline Marathon in Huntington Beach just before I visited him at his home in February 2004. Confident, self-effacing, and prone to funny quips, he floored me when he said he planned to (and ultimately did) run a marathon a month that year.

"Twelve marathons?" I said incredulously. "Don't they say that you can't run more than two or three marathons a year without hurting yourself?"

"That's with shoes on," he replied.

OLYMPIANS USE IT, TOO

Some might dismiss Saxton's barefooted devotion as the quirky karma of a kooky vegetarian hippie, but it's hard to ignore respected coaches who advocate the same thing.

A call to the Olympic Training Center in Chula Vista, California, led me to venerable middle- and short-distance coach Brooks Johnson, who had enthusiastically made use of barefoot running since the sixties.

"To counteract the negative effect of shoes, you should spend as much time running barefoot as possible," said Johnson, who gained fame for his work with Regina Jacobs, Patti Sue Plummer, and other future Olympians at Stanford University from 1979 to 1992. "Putting padding between your foot and the ground weakens foot muscles and dulls the proprioceptive sensors that tell them when to fire. Your toes, for instance, dig in when you lean forward while barefooted,

RUNNING CORRECTLY—NATURALLY

Just by taking your shoes off, you will naturally adopt the form of the guy at the right—which also happens to be the low-impact, highly efficient form used by elite runners. By running barefoot a few minutes a day, you, too, can teach yourself to run like this even when you put your shoes back on.

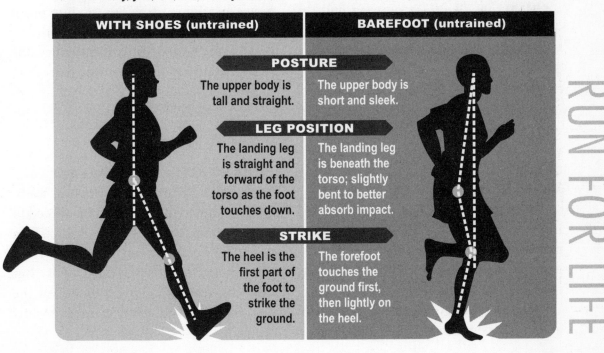

WITH SHOES (untrained)	BAREFOOT (untrained)
POSTURE	
The upper body is tall and straight.	The upper body is short and sleek.
LEG POSITION	
The landing leg is straight and forward of the torso as the foot touches down.	The landing leg is beneath the torso; slightly bent to better absorb impact.
STRIKE	
The heel is the first part of the foot to strike the ground.	The forefoot touches the ground first, then lightly on the heel.

RUN FOR LIFE

but don't with shoes on. And the rocking and rolling on top of that unstable padding causes all kinds of knee problems, like chondromalacia. Barefoot running gets the foot back to normal."

In other words, shoes do a nice job of protecting your feet from rocks, needles, and glass, but over time they desensitize the feet, make them lazy and weak, and trigger a chain reaction up the entire leg that can lead to shin splints, jogger's knee, and IT-Band strains. Big cushiony heels can just add to the problem, shortening calf muscles and the Achilles tendon.

The fix: Go au naturel. Barefooting stretches out the calves and gets foot muscles properly functioning again, like strength training for feet. "You see a lot of athletes with great engines but flat tires," said Johnson. "Barefoot running quickly pumps the tires back up."

Johnson said he had Plummer, 5th in the 5000-meter at the 1992 Olympics, running barefoot so much that her foot expanded one shoe size. At the OTC in 2004, he and coach Joe Vehill, in charge of distance runners like Deena Drossin Kastor, had all their athletes warm up and warm down with barefoot running every day.

"Remember that barefoot running isn't new," said Vehill. "We've been running on sand for a long time. But it's actually become more important as shoe technology has gotten better."

He and the iconoclastic Johnson don't agree on everything—Vehill encourages his runners to run "tall" (straight up), while Johnson, like the Pose Method's Nicholas Romanov, favors a forward lean. But strong feet are a must for all, which is why the OTC coaches to this day use barefoot running and a number of other foot-strengtheners: toe raises, plyometrics, stairstep calf raises, toe-in, toe-out exercises with surgical tubing, and scrunching up towels and picking up marbles with their toes.

The theory is that Western kids, wearing shoes by age two, weaken their feet. Contrast that with Kenyans, who often cavort shoeless into junior high. An exception Johnson noted was Mary Decker, who almost exclusively ran barefoot before age 16, just like her South African rival Zola Budd, the barefoot sensation of the '80s. As for proof that a barefooter can win in competition, that's easy: Ethiopia's Abebe Bikila, sans shoes, won the 1960 Olympic marathon in Rome.

WHAT IT FEELS LIKE

At the OTC, the athletes run barefoot on grass. But Saxton runs on trails, asphalt, and concrete. When he offered to take me on a 3-miler on the Bolsa Chica beach bike path down the street from his condo, I eagerly nodded okay. But inwardly, I was spooked. I looked at the blacktop. I looked at my toenails. And I cringed. . . .

BAREFOOT SHOES TOE THE LINE

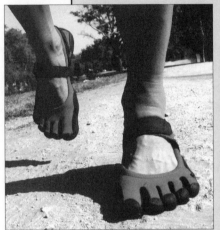

Whether you can replicate "barefoot running" once you lace up your shoes isn't easy. After a couple of weeks of barefoot drills, some runners will naturally make the switch to the balls of their feet during their regular runs, while some need months. For those who want to ease the transition into barefooting, Nike introduced its highly flexible, thin-soled Free in 2004. But those only went halfway. If you want to go nearly 100%, but are still leery of stepping on wayward rocks and twigs, there's only one game in town: FiveFingers.

The Vibram FiveFingers is a "foot glove" with individual toes and a formfitting quarter-inch-thick sole. Made by the world's most well-known maker of hiking shoe soles, they debuted in 2007 as a climbing shoe, but were quickly discovered by barefooters and barefoot wannabes. The perfect missing link between barefoot running and shoes, it can be used alone or in conjunction with Injinji five-toed socks. FiveFingers is the best of both worlds for those who want to make use of Soft Running but want to avoid the learning curve that comes with doing it in shoes.

But from the second we started, I was feeling no pain. In fact, I felt like I was running more smoothly and more stably than I ever had in my life. My forefoot landed lightly and mapped the contours of the blacktop like a blind man reading Braille. My air-cooled toes automatically spread wide and dug in, gripping the asphalt like Firestone 500s. Naturally and effortlessly, my body ran "soft"—slightly crouched, knees bent like springs to absorb shock, forefoot landing, rapid turnover, no possibility of a heel strike. Any momentary landing on a pebble was minimized by the light touch and the instant-reaction foot pickup.

As we finished, I was speechless. My feet didn't hurt a bit. And neither did my left knee, recovering slowly from a 6-month-old torn-meniscus surgery and normally a bit painful after a run. Undoubtedly, running barefoot seems softer on your joints than running in shoes.

The best part of it? I didn't have to do a thing. No tinkering with this and that, no self-monitoring. It was like regular Soft Running, but without all the thinking. Just take off your shoes and run!

Even if you're a lifelong heel-striker, running barefoot instinctively lands you on your forefeet and gives you the shorter, more rapid strides of an elite runner. And if you insist on heel striking, I guarantee that you will only do it once (unless you enjoy pain).

Videos that Ken and I shot of each other showed classic, shock-absorbing soft-running form. But there was none of the forward lean of the Pose Method, which cites barefoot running as an inspiration. Both of us ran squat-legged with vertical backs.

The only irritation came an hour later, as my soles were a bit raw after our run. Ken warned me that I had pushed the envelope for a first-timer. (It'd be smart to start with a few minutes of barefooting, and build up over a month, like the Pose Method.) But my feet normalized after two days as if nothing had happened, and looked no different.

That raises the question: What do Saxton's feet look like after years of running barefoot? The answer: Pretty normal. As we sat on his living room carpet, I grabbed his right foot and ran my fingers across the sole to check. No massive calluses, no noticeable scarring and cracking. The only sign there was something afoot was an enhanced muscularity, abnormally widespread toes, and a distinct lack of foot odor.

"That's *shoe* odor," he corrected.

CHAPTER 5

ROMANOV'S CONTROLLED FALLING

You become a "lean" machine with the groundbreaking Pose Method, a unique take on Soft Running that relies on gravity to pull you along

I wrote about the Pose Method, a groundbreaking version of Soft Running, for Runner's World *and* Men's Fitness *magazines after attending a seminar in 2003. The Pose is based on the unique concept of "controlled falling," which theoretically uses gravity to do the work, not your legs. Although it does not consider arm swing an important issue and makes no recommendations about it, I think the classic vertical swing described in the previous pages works perfectly with the Pose. The Pose Method is routinely picked apart, criticized, modified, and copied. The creation of Russian sports scientist Nicholas Romanov, it plays an influential role in any discussion of healthy longevity running.*

1979, Moscow, USSR—

Nicholas Romanov, 27, stands before a panel of stone-faced Ministry of Sports bureaucrats, awaiting a response to his presentation. His subject: a new running technique he has developed—one he claims will increase speed and reduce injuries for all runners, especially the elite Communist athletes who can use it to dominate the West at the next year's Olympics in Moscow. Romanov, a senior lecturer at Chuvash Pedagogical University, expects huge applause from his comrades for his great contribution to the Motherland, to Socialism, to sport. But their reaction startles him.

"Did our government give you permission to develop this method?" they say menacingly.

Romanov freezes. In the golden age of Brezhnev, that statement can be interpreted as a code phrase for "provocateur" or "traitor." His attempts to explain are cut short. "The gall. The insolence," they rant. "What in the hell do you think? That you—*you*?—know more about running than running coaches? And that *you* can teach people how to do what they already know how to do naturally?"

Good questions. Romanov, at that time getting his Ph.D. in sports culture and pedagogy, was not a runner. He'd been a university high jumper who regularly cleared 7 feet—running all of eight steps. Required to develop training schedules for runners as part of his degree, he panicked; he'd never liked running much and knew nothing about it. Since high jumping was all about technique, he first searched for books about proper running technique—and found none. Lots of information about training, but nothing about proper form? Romanov was intrigued. So he began looking at newsreel footage of the greatest modern sprinters and distance runners. He looked at ancient Greek Olympians as depicted on museum murals and pottery. He even analyzed the biomechanics of cheetahs, the fastest animals. He drew some conclusions:

A great runner leans his whole body forward. He runs "shorter" than his height by several inches, landing on his forefoot, with legs springy and slightly bent, like the hind legs of a dog. His foot touches the ground almost directly under the center of his body's mass and turns over rapidly, minimizing contact with the ground—like you do when you're barefoot. Ultimately, a great runner looks fluid, light on his feet, skimming the surface like a flat rock skipping across a pond. He's efficient, like he's getting more miles per gallon, his smooth footfalls blending into a seamless flow.

It's quite a contrast to the bobbing, jarring form of average runners, says Romanov, with their long, slow-moving strides, heel crash-landings, and quadriceps blast-offs—their blunt-force braking and strenuous propulsion, repeated over and over.

After months of observations came an "ah-ha" moment. "Efficient running doesn't involve propulsion at all—that's too much work," said Romanov. "In fact, exactly the opposite is happening: Efficient runners let gravity pull them forward. Efficient running is really falling—controlled falling."

Romanov was electrified. With "controlled falling," he felt he'd stumbled upon a universal theory of running—principles that applied to everyone, sprinter to marathoner, über-athlete to regular Ivan. If he could put it all into a learnable program, any runner could lower heart rates, raise speeds, and reduce joint and muscle injuries.

In 1981, Romanov named his running form "The Pose Technique," best visualized as an ideal position, or pose. Here's how gravity sets the Pose in motion, and theoretically saves energy and reduces fatigue:

Following a bent-knee, forefoot landing, the entire foot bottom makes brief ground contact before the heel is flicked butt-ward. Firing the hamstring to pick the heel up within an inch of the butt is not easy, but ultimately produces a net energy savings. That's because it puts the airborne foot in position to swing forward like a pendulum and simply falls to earth with little muscular effort—all due to the body's forward lean. "This is why the Pose is more 'efficient' than traditional running's push off the ground," says Romanov, "which requires a great expenditure of energy from the quads and calves."

In other words, pull is easier than push. The "cheap" heel pull-up of the Pose replaces the "expensive" toe push-off of traditional running. (Note: Firing the hamstring to flick the heel up is unnatural at first, and may require some hamstring strengthening. Some useful visualizations to accomplish this flicking motion include imagining that you are running barefoot on broken glass, stepping on hot coals, or running down steep stairs In each case, you don't push down—you pull up.)

To speed up with the Pose, the runner simply increases his body lean; in order to not fall over, turnover will naturally increase. Picture a unicyclist: The more he leans, the faster he has to spin the pedals to keep from falling over.

Not surprisingly, Romanov says that the Pose's reliance on gravity for forward motion effectively turns the legs into wheels. "The fastest runners can go 12 meters per second," he says, "but objects fall at 58 meters per second. That means you can fall five times as fast as you can run. Therefore, legs should not play a major role in propulsion. They are just carriers, like wheels."

Although intrigued by reports that Romanov's athletes stayed healthier ("Injuries just disappeared due to the softer landings and less ballistic shock to the knees and hips," he said), skeptical Soviet officials couldn't get past Romanov's basic premise: That running was not a natural skill for most, but had to be learned.

"We must learn how to shoot a basketball, to hit a golf ball, to play tennis," he cried. "Why shouldn't we learn how to run?"

Few listened. Romanov toiled in coaching obscurity for the next 13 years, his influence limited to a small, devoted group of juniors and second tier believers that eventually included a Soviet 15k champion. Then the Wall came down and Romanov did what millions of dreamers with crazy ideas had done before him: He came to America.

TRIATHLETES ADOPTED IT FIRST

In 1994, Romanov moved his family to Florida, where he hoped to reunite

PRINCIPLES OF THE POSE

The rules are similar to those of general Soft Running, outlined in Chapter 2, with a few critical additions and emphases:

Lean Machine: At all times, angle/tilt your body forward to the point where you feel like you will fall forward. Do not bend at the waist. To go faster, lean more.

Short Strides with Bent Leg: No long strides allowed; otherwise, soft-tissue strains and knee-rattling heel-striking will result.

Legs as Wheels: Think of legs as carries or "wheels," not directly responsible for propulsion. Pick feet up off ground instantly to keep momentum and cut injuries.

Flick it: Don't yank the foot up; flick it up just enough to get it off the ground an inch or so. It'll shoot up like a rubber band, going higher the faster you're running.

Free Fall: Once airborne, don't reach with your stride. You're in flight, carried by your mass. The foot travels in a natural arc, then drops like a plumb line with no muscle activity.

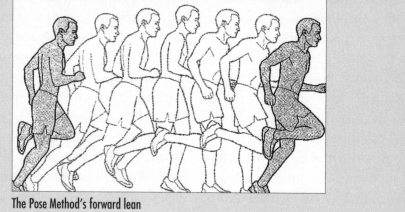

The Pose Method's forward lean

with his elder daughter, who'd married an American. He had trouble getting work as a university professor and running coach, his positions in the USSR, and was living in near poverty in a backwoods trailer on an ostrich farm in Loxahatchee, west of West Palm Beach. That ended when he was "discovered" by Kyle Sage, then a pro triathlete and assistant coach at a junior development camp, who'd heard a rumor "about a Russian with a bunch of far-out ideas."

Sage drove out to see Romanov, spent the afternoon "hopping around on one leg" (a Pose warm-up drill), and invited him to speak at a seminar. Within days, Romanov was quickly networked into the triathlon world, which has a reputation for being unusually open to discussions of form, given the importance of technique in swimming and cycling.

He worked with Sage as consultant to the U.S. Triathlon Junior team throughout the '90s, and was hired as a coach by the British triathlon team in 1999. Top British triathletes, including Andrew Johns and 2002 world champion Leanda Cave, use the Pose. So does top U.S. triathlete Hunter Kemper, who says, "When I get in trouble, I check my turnover and my lean, and I'm back on track."

As Romanov's seminars picked up speed, the testimonials from runners of all ages and abilities began piling up. Here's some I interviewed:

- Mel Wicks, Toledo, Ohio, a financial planner and 25-year runner who guessed he'd been injured one-third of the time pre-Pose: He'd been injury-free since starting the Pose Method at age 63 in 2003.
- Sean Hylton, a 36-year-old Ironman triathlete from Naples, Florida: He raised his weekly mileage from 35 to 50 per week, yet cut his recovery time from long runs from five to two days.
- Joel Andres, a Los Angeles lawyer-turned-personal-trainer who herniated two discs in his lower back in 2001 while lifting weights: "Two neurosurgeons told me I would never run again," he said. Since adopting the Pose in January 2003 at age 39, all his back

and IT-band problems disappeared, and 10k time dropped 9 minutes.

- Pat Manocchia, owner of the La Pallestra gym in Manhattan, who heard Romanov explain the Pose "through his thick Russian accent" in 1996: "My first reaction was, 'either this guy's out of his mind, or he's a genius,'" he said. Manocchia taught it to clients, including shock jock Howard Stern, and immediately saw injury rates and recovery times tumble. "You get faster due to injury reduction—not raw speed," he explained. "My clients' lower-leg, knee, and IT-band injuries went to nothing because you can train more and maintain race pace longer with less muscle damage. Take Howard—he's a serious runner—we run four or five days a week together—but he used to get injured all the time. No more."
- Kip Grossman, a banker from Laguna Beach, California, who ran a half marathon 20 minutes faster than normal at a 10% lower heart rate two days after a Pose seminar in late 2002, at age 41: "I felt so good the next day that I ran 10 miles just for fun," he said. "Normally, I'd have been laying in bed, totally wasted, my muscles screaming in pain. Instead, I felt like a million bucks." He was so impressed that he personally flew Romanov out to his home to conduct a private weekend seminar, where I met him.

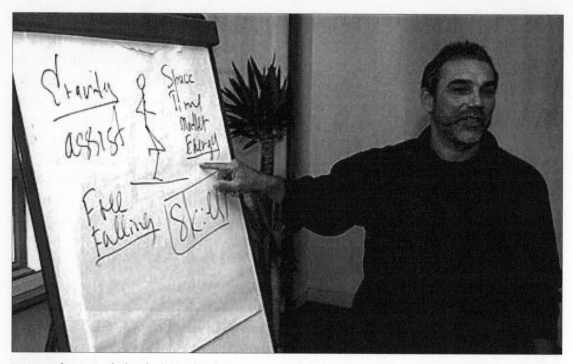

Romanov takes running back to the drawing board.

IMPACT REDUCTION:
THE HARD PROOF

Despite his successes, Romanov was still rankled that the Pose's "controlled falling" construct still drew sneers from the American running establishment—just as it did from Cold War–era Soviet athletic authorities.

So in August 2002, determined to have his method legitimized by the broader running community, Romanov contacted Dr. Timothy Noakes while accompanying the British triathlon team on a trip to South Africa. "'No one else will study this,'" he told me," says Noakes. "'They think it's a waste of time.' I listened to him, was intrigued that its running mechanics were quite different, and said, 'Let's do it.' It's my responsibility as a scientist to see if he has something." Noakes measured Romanov himself in his lab at the University of Cape Town and found reduced knee loading and impact. Two months later, Romanov returned and spent 5 days training 20 heel-to-toe runners to run the Pose Method.

The results: "We found a substantial decline in impact forces at the knee joint—I was quite surprised at the magnitude of the change," Noakes said, noting that the reduction for nearly all the runners was "than more 30%, some as high as 50%. We have seen nothing else that does this—not shoes, no matter how padded.

"My opinion: He really does have something," says Noakes. "I think the Pose and barefoot running (he sees the two as virtually the same thing) are advantageous in preventing injuries, which is quite important since we know that roughly 60% of runners get injured every year. It is highly probable that the Pose method would translate to less injuries."

Noakes did issue a warning that applies to the Pose and all Soft Running methods: "You have to absorb the shock somewhere, and you absorb it in the Achilles tendon and the calf. Some of the test subjects had calf pain."

Romanov wasn't surprised. "It isn't until the second week that the calf muscles start adapting to the new biomechanics of the Pose," he said. "These people had five days—not enough time to get used to the new load."

Some people, even Pose lovers, need more than two weeks to adapt. "After several months, I still needed to remind myself to pull my heel up quicker," says Grossman. "My biggest problem is tensing up on the balls of my feet. If you don't learn to relax as you land, your calves explode."

Rich Strauss, a triathlon coach in Pasadena, California, who says he's had no injuries since 2000 "due to Romanov," eases his clients into the Pose very much like Phase IV does with its soft-running program. "I call it Form Fartlek. I say, 'Do 8 minutes your old way, and two the Pose way, and repeat. Then after a few days, do 7 old and three Pose, and keep working down to all Pose." Romanov views such mixing as confusing, but Strauss says it allows people to maintain their fitness during the transition.

Many Posers suggest an adaptation phase of a month or two, as well as Romanov's hamstring and core-strengthening exercises. "By 3 months, you can master the Pose," says triathlon coach Joe Sparks, who taught the aforementioned Mel Wicks and claims the Pose helped him, at age 47 following a torn meniscus operation, to run his first sub-40-minute 10k. "But you have to start very slow, gradually developing the strength and flexibility in the calves. You have to treat this as a skill. And you don't learn a new skill overnight."

Or, as Romanov puts it: "Can you go play Wimbledon after two tennis lessons?"

Of course, some people don't get it at all. "Most of the others in my class stuck with the Pose, but it never really did click for me," says Jen Hood, a fitness trainer and runner from Perrysburg, Ohio. "It makes a lot of sense. I definitely take shorter strides now, especially on the downhills. I even implemented a lot of Pose drills with my own students. But I went from comfortable to uncomfortable and couldn't keep up without much harder breathing. After 5 months, I reverted to my old form."

While the Pose's emphasis on using gravity to pull you along may not work for everyone, one well-known biomechanist felt it had lessons that could benefit most runners. "The Pose is a very sound, practical concept," says Ray M. Fredericksen, who works in the biomechanics department at the University of Michigan and is an advisor for *Runner's World* magazine. "It's being termed a new method, but it has a lot of historical validity. The forefoot landing isn't far off. Most efficient runners are midfoot strikers, no doubt about that. And running is a matter of momentum, of picking your foot up off the ground and swinging your limb going forward. Naturally, you will lean."

Old habits and mind-sets don't die easily. After I attended the Pose seminar, I ran into Mark Allen, the retired 6-time Hawaii Ironman winner, at a trade show. When I told one of triathlon's greatest runners about the Pose's forefoot landing, his reaction was surprising, yet typical: "That's stupid!" he blurted. Having talked to Allen many times during my time as an editor at *Triathlete* magazine in the nineties, that seemed uncharacteristic, given that he was a known pioneer of innovative training methods.

A year later, however, after hearing positive comments about the Pose and attending a seminar, Allen had a new perspective. "The essence of the Pose makes sense," he said, "but its main benefit is that it gives you a checklist, a system of things you can think about to run better. And that's a good thing."

CHAPTER 6

HEAD FOR THE HILLS

Location, location, location. Trail running, the original "Soft Running," cuts the shock, strengthens feet and legs, and frees your mind. Here, top trail stars reveal their secrets for off-road success.

It's softer, so there's less impact. Its surface is varied, so your foot lands at different angles, strengthening feet, toes, and ankles and reducing repetitive-motion injuries. The scenery is undulating, natural, and car-free, so you feel like you get a challenging, pollution-free mini-vacation. And the constant ebb and flow of high-heartrate climbs and low-rate descents even tricks you into interval training, a key to fitness and longevity (See Section 4). No wonder 6.7 million runners hit the dirt in 2008, triple that of a decade before, according to the All-American Trail Running Association. Many, however, quickly find that doing it safely takes more than lacing up a pair of granola-colored trail shoes.

"You've got to run with a different technique, different clothes, and even have a different mind-set," says Ann Trason, the 14-time winner of the Western States 100 ultra-endurances race.

That's because trail running is to road running what mountain biking is to road cycling: way more technical. Although any dirt or grass trails deliver great shock reduction and leg-muscle strengthening, we're not talking about running on your local golf course here. Negotiating the challenging, remote, and steep outback requires special technique and special gear.

The best way to learn? "Just do what I did," says 5-time Western States winner Tim Tweitmeyer. "Buy a house on the route."

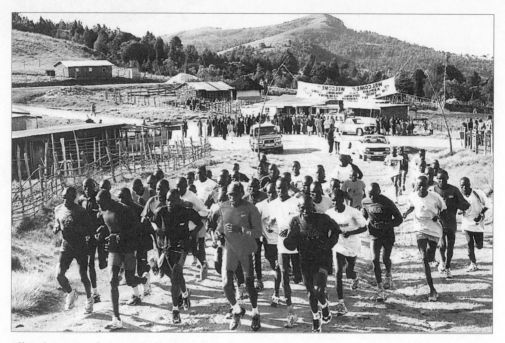

Off-road training in the Kenyan highlands.

If living on the American River in Auburn, California isn't in your plans, don't fret. Here Tweitmeyer, Trason, and other off-road experts offer some pointers to help you hit the ground running.

1. Pay Attention: While the most common "street" running injuries tend to be of the repetitive motion variety—knee pain, tendonitis, plantar fasciitis—dirt injuries are most likely to include broken ribs, twisted ankles, bee stings, and bruises caused by tripping and falling on your face, according to AATRA President Nancy Hobbs. Trails aren't perfectly groomed, like city streets, and often come booby-trapped with rocks, roots, and distracting scenery ready to turn you into a human avalanche. Mountain bikers and mogul skiers make good trail runners because of the way they watch the terrain. Basic rule: Look two steps ahead and down.

Especially pay attention on descents. I tripped slightly running down a steep 3,000-foot descent during the 2008 TransRockies Run and went flying about 20 feet. Good thing that I observed rule #8 (wear gloves).

2. Run Crouched: Keep legs slightly bent and elbows up. That lowers your center of gravity and provides balance, keeping you from falling on the uneven surface and poised to move side to side around obstacles. "I think of it like dancing," says Danelle Ballangee, one of America's best "sky" (high-altitude) racers. "You gotta be ready to move every which way."

3. Keep Your Head Up on Climbs: Don't look down too much on ascents, adds Bellangee. You need all the oxygen you can get on the upside, she says, so tilt your head up, open your windpipe, and breathe deep. This is critical at high elevation.

4. Walk the Steeps: Don't be embarrassed to walk the tough grades. It's hardly slower than running and is far easier on your heart and lungs. "On my first 50-miler, I was shocked to see somebody walk past me," admits Ann Trason. "If you're a beginner, walk a lot until your body gets used to it."

5. Smooth, Toes-First Descents: Fight the urge to cruise downhill on your heels. The forefoot provides far more control. "Running fast downhill is where you can make up a lot of time on the field," advised Bill McDermott, who did that so often during his record 13 wins and 31 straight finishes of California's legendary Catalina Island off-road marathon that he earned the nickname The Downhill Devil. "Concentrate on taking long, smooth steps, almost like you're riding a mountain bike. You won't trash your quads if you're smooth."

6. The "Four Times" Rule: My quads hurt for four days after my 3,000-foot TransRockies descent because I did not observe the Four Times rule. "Your quads will hurt after the first three times you run downhill. They're not used to the pounding," says Trason. The fourth time, when they've adapted to the stress of extreme eccentric contractions, is usually the charm.

7. Pack Water: With no fountains in the mountains and most streams polluted, even heading out for a quickie without a hydration backpack, fanny pack, or water bottle is dangerous.

"You get so caught up in it that you always stay out longer than planned," says Ben Hian, a former #1-ranked trail racer. "The steep terrain works you harder than you think, so dehydration can set in fast."

8. Wear Gloves and Pack a Jacket: Even the best trail runners fall sometimes, so wear full-finger gloves. And since mountain weather is unpredictable, stuff a wind- or waterproof jacket in your pack. Careful runners in the Rockies even carry a space blanket as protection in a bad storm.

9. Think Time, Not Mileage: Roadies are used to measuring their performances by miles, but trail runners should gauge theirs by time. "It's a change of mind-set," says Hian. "You go out for an hour—not for 10 miles." If basking in nature doesn't change your mileage mentality, the lack of markers in the woods will.

RUN FOR LIFE

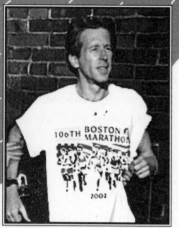

BILL RODGERS

The Babe Ruth of the Marathon

For five years, Bill Rodgers dominated the marathon like no one before or since: four wins each at the Boston and New York Marathons from 1975 to 1980; two American records at Boston (2:09:55 in 1975 and 2:09:27 in 1979); and a win at the 1977 Fukuoka Marathon, making him the only runner ever to hold the championship of all three major marathons at once. In 1978, he won 27 of the 30 races he entered, including the Pepsi 10,000-meter nationals (new world 10K mark of 28:36.3). All told, he ran 28 of his 58 marathons under 2:15, winning 21. He went on to make his career in the sport, opening a store, the Bill Rodgers Running Center in Boston, in 1977 with his brother Charlie and joining Frank Shorter in the fight for prize money for runners. Born in 1947 in Hartford, Connecticut, and graduating with a B.A. in sociology from Wesleyan University, he gave up marathons for good after finishing Boston in 1996, but has remained an active and successful age-group runner (in '03 he won every 55–59 division race he entered), and an approachable, gregarious spokesman for the sport who is in demand at events around the world. What you may not know, and what I discovered in our *Run for Life* interview on October 30, 2007, is the struggle that came before the success. After college, Rodgers had hit rock bottom, had an epiphany, then began his stunning rise to dominance. That's where we'll start.

It was 1972. I'd quit my running. I'd taken up smoking—I was a Winston smoker. It was kinda weird.

But the thing was—when a track meet came on TV, I wanted to watch it. And I was rooming with my high school buddy and longtime friend who was on the track team as well. We lived right around the corner from the Boston Marathon site, just a quarter mile away. So we would bike over there—we actually had motorcycles, we were doing the Easy Rider thing. I had long hair—wasn't a hippie so to speak, more of a political person. I saw the Boston Marathon for the first time and I was just totally stunned. I couldn't believe how incredibly huge and exciting it was. When my old roommate Amby Burfoot [long-time editor of Runner's World] won it in '68 back in college, it wasn't on TV. So I had no idea what it was like.

But when you're up there, right at the finish line, and there's thousands and thousands of people watching the race . . . wow. A 70-year-old race or something. In Massachusetts, in Boston, and in New England it was a big event, even then. People are off work that day. It's a huge celebration.

I watched the Boston Marathon for two years. I saw Amby, I saw Jeff Galloway finish in '72. He made the Olympic team. My old college roommates were making the Olympic team and doing this and that. And I was sort of like sitting there and smoking my cigarettes all Saturday night. It was stupid.

And then my motorcycle got stolen one day.

That motorcycle was all I had in the world. I had no money. I had a very low-paying job—take-home was like 75 bucks a week. It was just enough to cover the rent.

When I lost that motorcycle, a used Triumph 650 I had bought with $1,000 borrowed from my good buddy—it was the clincher. From there, two different thoughts came together: I wasn't married or had any kids, except for my brother's family. And I didn't have my running. I had nothing left.

I looked at Boston and said, "That's what I want to do. That's a lot more fun. That is something. This is a mind boggler." So I decided I would get back.

I joined the Boston YMCA, which was pretty cheap in those days. And I started running a little and using light weights and the rowing machine. I wanted to get back, get fit again.

I gradually cut back the cigarettes and started running outside, around the park near where I lived. And then started doing some races.

THE BEGINNING

We had a stable, active life as kids, and had a lot of fun. There are four kids in my family, Charlie, a year older,

and two younger sisters. We were all active kids, rode our bikes a lot. We'd walk five miles through the woods no problem. We'd go out every day—we played basketball, baseball, football, hockey, we did everything.

We hiked, we hunted with bows and arrows and BB guns for ducks. I was in Boy Scouts; we camped out a lot. My parents were not active; they were working hard to put us through college. My dad, Charles Rodgers, was the head of the mechanical-engineering department at Hartford State College. He was an intellectual type of guy, which he still is, but he always tried to stay fit by walking. My mom, Katherine, a nurses' aide for 20 years, actually became a runner in her mid-50s. She's a very high-energy person. They are now both 84 or so, and very healthy. My mom's still a walker, and my dad walks a bit, too. They're lucky.

I was a pretty active kid, and whenever I ran, in the schoolyard and neighborhood, I thought I was fast. And that translated into becoming a cross-country runner. Just before I joined the team there was the gym-class mile, everyone in the school runs it, and the coaches time it and look for talent. When I was a sophomore, I ran the fastest time in the school: 6:10.

So suddenly, I was the fastest kid in the school and next thing you know I was running cross-country and winning my first race. I guess I was pretty fit from all that biking and hiking as a kid.

My brother Charlie and a good friend and I all joined the team together. We had moved out of my hometown of Hartford to Newington, a suburb, and got a really superb coach, Frank O'Roark. He was the guy who, probably more than anyone else, really believed in me.

Running clicked for me immediately. I liked it, I had fun with it, I liked the competition. Sophomore year I was the fastest kid in the mile and 2-mile. I wasn't thinking of a 4-minute mile. I was thinking of a 5-minute mile! I had some ability, but I wasn't any Craig Virgin or Alberto Salazar. There was quite a bit of American success at the time; we all knew about Jim Ryun; we saw Billy Mills take his gold medal (at the 1964 Olympics). But I couldn't relate to them—people were just too far

RUN FOR LIFE

away. I didn't have any big, grand goal. I never even thought of the Olympics. I watched it on TV. I'd read the results in the paper and see my name there and that was great.

We didn't train so hard that, like some athletes, you'd want to quit. I trained moderately compared to the athletes of today. The friendship and the camaraderie was the big thing. I don't think that's understood too much; people always talk baseball-football when the subject is "team" events. But cross-country and track—the team thing is very powerful.

No question it [my success] was a boost socially. People at school knew I was a top runner and put me in the yearbook. At a state level, I was at a higher level than most of the kids in my school in the team sports. People understood that, even though it wasn't like the stadium was filled with people when we ran.

I was undefeated my senior year in cross-country. I won the Class A state championships. But when I went to what they call the State Open, which is all three Division schools, I got beat, took 2nd. Then on the track, I ran the 2-mile in 9:36, and took 3rd. So I was one of the top kids in New England, but I wasn't that fast. I ran the New England cross-country and track championships, and I would come in like 8th. I would run 9:55 or something.

Thinking about college, my parents said, "Well, are you going to keep running?" And I said, "Yeah!"

I got a lot of letters from people. But I wanted to stay at a nearby local college. I checked out the University of Connecticut, Providence College, Colby College in Maine, Trinity in Hartford, and Wesleyan. And I liked Wesleyan. It was a terrific academic school and nearby in Middletown. The buildings are beautiful, stunningly beautiful. Very high academic level, Division 3 school. I said, "This place is fantastic."

And Amby Burfoot, the state 2-mile state champion, was in college there. I had gotten to know him a bit because I raced his younger brother Gary. And Jeff Galloway was there, too.

Academics was a priority at Wesleyan, and I only did fair in high school—B- or B average. But Wesleyan looked

at you in a more rounded way. They don't give athletic scholarships. Sports were considered in the gentleman's way of the amateur era. You know, "Sports are a part of life, but they are not the be-all, end-all." And I liked that.

Turns out my roommate in my freshman year was Amby, a junior. That year, he placed 6th at the NCAA cross-country nationals championships. Pretty good for a little Division 3 school. So, with him and Galloway, a senior, I had a chance to run with some of the top guys in the country. Amby won the 1968 Boston as a senior. Amby beat everybody. He was undefeated for four years.

I did okay as a runner there. After Amby and Jeff, I was the top distance runner on the team. Academically, things were hard. But Wesleyan was very good for me in that it was a low-key athletic environment. I could live a normal life as a college kid. Visit friends. It wasn't like I was aiming for the Olympic team.

I didn't have a big dream at that point. Not at all. I wanted to do well, and win my cross-country meets, of course, and I trained hard.

Amby's the guy who got me out on the road. He'd do a hilly 25-miler when he was training for Boston. He was doing 140 miles a week as a college senior.

He took me out on my first 15-miler, as a freshman. As a sophomore, I did a 25-mile run with him, 10 miles over my longest run, and it was quite an experience. I actually did pretty well with it, but then with about 2 miles to go, he turned to me and said, "Bill, I gotta go"—and he took off. I guess we had just been jogging, and I thought we were just flying or something.

Although I had just practically run a marathon, I had no interest in running one. I had no idea what it was about.

The marathon was almost cultlike back then. It was such a small group of participants. Yet they had the exact same passion as the top runners in the world today—I don't think that's ever changed. Amby had this drive to win that I was amazed by. I think ultimately it lit a spark in me, too. His high school coach was Johnny Kelly, who won the Boston Marathon in 1957, so that motivated him. Amby was kind of like a surrealistic character. He was like the white Abebe Bikila (the Ethiopian); he was skinny, above six feet tall. I saw Bikila run at the Olympic Games on TV. And here I could run with the guy who could run the marathon like Bikila! And I could try to stay with him. It was fantastic.

We became friends. We see each other now at least once a year at various races. And he's still running—and he's still beating me here and there. He's very fit. Sixty-one. Did the Comrades 56-miler this past year, so he's doing really well.

I was a good runner, a solid runner, a racer. And I liked that. But I never thought about cranking it up. My best achievement in college, my senior year indoors, I broke 9 minutes for 2 miles. When I graduated from college in June of 1970, that was it. I quit running entirely for three years. And I became a smoker.

VIETNAM AND THE LOST YEARS

It was during the Vietnam War, which I was very much against. A lot of things were happening: Kent State, student strike, 700 colleges in the U.S. shut down, we didn't have classes for a time—the whole country was going through tough, tough times. It was the end of my senior year, and suddenly, I had big things on my mind.

I didn't support the war. I didn't think it was good for our country. So I applied for Conscientious Objector status.

The Supreme Court said if you had a religious basis for being a Conscientious Objector, they would look at that. You had to get a bunch of people speaking up on your behalf, and sometimes people wouldn't do that for me, because they supported the war effort. And that was really hard—they would label me unpatriotic. However, it was starting to change in America. More and more people were starting to say, "what exactly do we want to achieve"? And I did, my brother did it, another friend on the track team. We all felt the same war about the war, politically and in every way.

I've always been fairly religious. I'm a lapsed Catholic, you could say. But I've always been religious on a personal level. So it was part religious, part political. I grew up with Martin Luther King, the Kennedys, when the country was undergoing a lot of changes, which I thought were for

the better. Maybe the hardest thing that the country went though was the Vietnam War, particularly the people who went over there, it was tough on them, brutal. Sometimes, they didn't come back the same people.

I really admired Muhammad Ali for his stand on the war. He took a beating on it personally. Our society, our governmental leadership—he was vilified. But that's the way politics are.

I sort of held my beliefs more inside, but I was also very strong in my beliefs. I thought I was going to have to leave the country. I was actually thinking about hopping on a freighter and going to New Zealand. I never really thought of Canada. All I knew is that I was going to go over there and kill people. If I had to go to jail, I'd rather go to jail. It was a big tragedy for our country.

There was no reason to keep running. When you leave a team environment, like a track team, you think it's over. That's how it was. They quit their sport. Even running, much easier to keep doing than other sports, was still tiny then. There was no reason to keep it up.

Anyway, I quit running, and I didn't know what I was going to do. Finally, they said yes to my Conscientious Objector application. I passed my physical in the army, and they said, "Now you owe 2 years to the U.S. government."

My brother (who also got the Objector status) did two years as a drug-and-alcohol counselor in Connecticut. And I worked at a Boston hospital as an escort messenger; that is, I pushed people around on stretchers, and I took patients down to the operating room or hematology, dead people down to the morgue, took blood samples out. It was a fascinating experience, and I learned a lot. It had to be very low pay, as if you were a private in the army.

So I did that for a couple years. I was smoking. Then my motorcycle got stolen …

THE RUNNING BOOM

The bike got stolen in early '72. I got married, then built up my mileage real quick. I was on a mission. It took a year to do a marathon, and me three years to become a world-class runner.

RUN FOR LIFE

I was already running 100 miles a week by the time I saw Frank Shorter win the gold medal at the 1972 Olympics on TV. I said, "Wow, this is mind-boggling. Who is this guy?" Then it turned out that we ran against Yale, which is just down the road from Wesleyan. In fact, Amby Burfoot beat Frank when we were in college. Frank was a year up on me class-wise.

I started running twice a day, which I remember Amby doing at Wesleyan—eight miles in the morning and seven or 12 miles at night. Put in the miles. Heavy mileage. Started doing some New England road races. Sometimes I'd start winning 'em. Everything: 15k, 10k, 20k. Then ran my first marathon—a disastrous experience. I hit the wall.

It was the 1973 Boston. You could qualify in those days with a 30k race, and I had placed 3rd in a Massachusetts 30k. The winner that day, in fact, was none other than Amby. So we both ran Boston that year. I know where he finished, but I dropped out. I made it to the top of Heartbreak, and that was it. I was just so dehydrated. It was a warm day, maybe 75.

I was living in a section of Boston that was pretty close to Heartbreak Hill, which was at the 21-and-a-half mile mark. By 13 or 15 miles, I was already whipped too hard, dehydrated, I didn't drink enough. I made all the beginner mistakes.

I quit running for 3 months.

It was a big learning experience to fail and really take a beating in my first marathon. But I didn't want to let go of it, so a few months later I started up again, 120 miles a week. And then, I ran a tiny little marathon in Massachusetts, a 5-loop YMCA race. I won that in 2 hours, 28 minutes.

For a while, I was actually out of job. In '74, I started working at a school for mentally handicapped people—challenged, as they say today—who are, the term was "retarded," years ago. That was another learning experience. I was there for a year and something. I really enjoyed that work. And I could run there.

I had a relative when I was a kid who had cerebral palsy, and he was mentally challenged. So I knew about it, it really struck me to go to school and see, "woo, some people really got a bad deal in life." I studied sociology.

I was interested in history and economics, English. Later I became a special ed. teacher, maybe influenced by my dad in a subtle way.

I joined the Greater Boston Track Club, which had a terrific coach, Billy Squires, who coached Dick Beardsley and Greg Meyer. We had a powerhouse distance team. We won the national cross-country championships, lotta road titles. One of my teammates worked at Boston College. He gave me some information, I applied to grad school, went there and got a degree in special ed. I got my degree the year I won the '75 Boston—the big breakthrough for me—and started teaching in the fall. I taught for two years.

In '74, I did my second Boston Marathon and placed 14th. But I was in 4th place for most of it, through 21 miles. But I was still learning the marathon, how to pace myself, how to take drinks, and how to train.

I was doing okay in the shorter races. In '74, I won the 7-mile Falmouth Road Race on Cape Cod, and I beat Marty Liquori, a top track man. He raced Ryun in the mile. He was the big gun there; no one knew who I was, and I beat him.

That was a huge boost to beat Marty. And I really whipped him—he wasn't near me. I wasn't going to let a miler beat me over seven miles.

I have to admit, I was cocky. But you have to be. It's part of all top runners. You have to have this attitude, because if you don't, how can you win? You are trained to build this within yourself. That's the competitive nature. And if you don't have it, well, you're not going to win a race like that. And that's okay. But I had it and I enjoyed it.

The club was a big part of it. We all pushed and helped each other. It was that old team thing again. You can't do it on your own. You need the group. You can never push yourself as hard as someone is pushing you. And I wasn't the only one who did well. Greg Meyer, Bobby Hodge, Mike Roach. We took every team title we raced. We'd travel around the country and win events. We had a lot of psychological, emotional momentum that gave us a lot of strength. It's kind of the way I see the Kenyans today come in groups of four, five, or six.

RUN FOR LIFE

We ran together all the time. Long runs on the weekend. Road runs of 9, 12, 15 miles during the week. We would run like the Kenyans: we'd start easy, then we'd start picking up the pace. Sometimes, we'd really push in the end. Same way the Kenyans train.

So, we had a terrific team, and it was great fun. Many of us on the team became marathoners. Alberto Salazar was a local high schooler, and he was running with us on weekends. Greg Meyer came over from Michigan. We had 30 to 40 guys, and women, too, like Patty Catelano. It was very exciting. Craig Virgin came on the scene a bit later. We saw Prefontaine out there in '72, made that brilliant move as a young kid. It was an exciting time.

And it was seeing the first running boom as you ran down the street. You started seeing a lot of people out there. It was kind of an era of innocence; you waved to everybody you saw. It was kind of a bond, like "yup, you're doing it too—let's go for it." It was very unique. I don't see that today—I see it somewhat, the bond's still there, but it just different. I think the runners who waved had the abstract dream about the Olympic Games, something like that, something special. The bond of going for the Olympic Games and representing your country, that's truly different, totally underappreciated in the U.S., where it's all big commercial stadium team sports.

ME AND FRANK

Frank Shorter and I went head-to-head quite a lot over the years. He beat me in our first races. The first time we ever raced was to make the world cross-country championships team in '75, and he won. But I defeated him a month later at the 1975 world cross- country championships in Rabat, Morocco; I took a bronze medal there and he was 20th. That was actually my first world-class breakthrough race. The next month, I won Boston, and the Olympics was suddenly a possibility.

I said, wow, I was the fastest marathoner in the world that year. I had beaten Frank, the defending Olympic marathon gold medalist, so I was one of the top guys running distances in those days. Or I thought I was. (laughs)

So I went to the Olympic Trials, in May of '76, and raced Frank. It was virtually a two-man race; we ran away from the rest of the field. But he edged me. Frank's a terrific strategic runner, a very smart runner. He won in 2 hours, 11 minutes, 50 seconds. I was 2:11:58. It was just to make the team. But he was the defending gold medalist. Maybe he just wanted to make the point that he was still going for the gold.

Frank had a brilliant day in the Olympics and took silver. I had a terrible day and took 40th. I think Frank was better than I at peaking, and also better running in the heat and humidity. I never really liked that. I could run seven miles, like the Falmouth Road Race, in the heat, but in the marathon, I think I have a lot of trouble with not taking adequate fluids. It was really depressing to bottom out in the Olympic Games. I finished the race, but I was stopping and walking, I had a lot of cramps, my hamstrings, my calves. I ran 2:25. It was a big comedown. But that's sport. That's marathoning.

Then I got a lucky break. Fred Lebow, the New York Road Runners Club president, came to the Falmouth Road race two weeks after the Olympic games. Frank and I were racing each other. And he invited both of us to the first Five Borough New York City Marathon. And we both said, "Yeah, we'll come." That was my Olympic race. It was just a few months late, though. Ha!

I was in good shape. I'd increased my mileage. Got back to doing more speed work. Before the Olympic Games, I didn't do enough speed work, and it cost me a lot. I learned from that.

The day of the New York City Marathon was a beautiful day to run. Low humidity. Sunny. Frank was there, I think he took 2nd or 3rd. I won the race. But you know, he'd gotten another Olympic medal. And I think to try to come back from that and try to win, after you've made your mark, against someone really out to.... I was highly motivated. Nothing to lose, everything to gain.

I think it takes about three years for your body to become accustomed to it, maybe at any level—beginner level or world-class as a professional runner. Certainly it took me three years; so that I could handle the training and still race the marathon. So by the time New York rolled around, my body had reached a certain level of strength, cardiovascularly and muscularly, to where I could handle the training and the race.

Certainly, by the time I won Boston in '75, the running boom was already on, kicked off by Frank in '72. By '76, Frank and I were spearheading the boom together, he with his Olympics win and me winning the two biggest marathons in the world at that time. We were very lucky in that regard. We became competitors, rivals, and later, friends. So I think that helped, too, in that there were two guys duking it out, and we were both Americans. We were lucky from that perspective. It was kind of the early days in professional marathoning as a sport. Without the Kenyans, Mexicans, Brazilians, Tanzanians, Ethiopians of today, it was easier to put together a big string of wins. I hit it just right, I guess. So both of us helped the boom. The media could see it and take notice

He ran Boston in '78, 2:16, I believe. I think he would have run Boston earlier, when he was the best in the world—because he was ranked best in the world three times, the same as I was. We had similar careers in some ways, and very different in others. But they wouldn't bring him in. Boston was almost absurdly amateur. The amateur rules were held to very strongly. They weren't always elsewhere in the world in track and other sports, but it was in Boston. So Frank would run another race—he ran Fukuoka four times instead and won that. I think if he had run in Boston, honestly, in the years when he was best in the world—'71 through '76—he'd have won Boston, too. But they didn't bring him in, didn't make any effort. The sport was sort of undeveloped in that sense. Today, if you're an Olympic medalist, the race directors are looking for you.

GETTING PAID

After I won Boston in '75, I got invited to other marathons around the world. I got invited to a marathon in Holland, a marathon in Fukuoka in southern Japan, which was kind of the world championships of marathoning. It is to Japan as the Boston Marathon is to the U.S. Frank won it four times. I won it in '77. Took third my first year. But it

was so exciting to go to Japan, where marathoning was like king of sports. It was just striking to see the way that marathoning is so understood there. Going back the last 100 years, Japan would have to be considered the world's number-one marathon country. Definitely. They've had Olympic medalists, world record holders, Boston winners going way back.

It was exciting to take part in international events— you'd meet runners from New Zealand, Poland, Finland. There weren't many Africans in those days. In the '70s, the Kenyans were more aiming for the track at that time. With Frank's gold medal in '72, the boom went worldwide, country to country. U.S. to Europe to Brazil.

Kenya had the great talent from the days of Kip Keino. But it was more middle distance, maybe 10000-meter and steeplechase.

I was a teacher in '75 and '76, full-time. It was very tricky. The whole amateur thing was strictly enforced. Track officials, writers, the publisher of Runner's World yelled at me that he was going to write a big story that we were paid to take part in races. Instead of support, we got negativity. We were Olympians, and we were treated like dirt half the time, because people didn't understand how hard it was to train well for track and field. They were looking at baseball, thinking they were terrific athletes. They were clueless. There was a certain cluelessness about that. And we were all trying to be a "professional"—Frank, myself, all of us out there at the time, all trying to be professional, high-level athletes. I think status was changing—we were training more than people ever did.

Change was happening in the sports world. We had to train, but had no money. You can do that for a while, some sports more than others, but marathoning is a twice-a-day training thing. Also, we saw others profiting from the sport, so why were the athletes treated poorly? You know you have this skill, and you're working tremendously hard to be as good as you can, but nonetheless, "we don't think you deserve to be paid for it." I saw that sort of thing happen over a period of time. U.S. athletes had to work to make expense money. We were given a plane ticket, hotel, and per diem—that was within the rules. You got a Team USA uniform and it was an honor to compete for your country. But then I'd meet athletes from other countries and begin to notice. "Hey, this guy from Russia, he doesn't really have another job. He's supported by the government of Russia." And same thing with this guy from Finland. Or Great Britain. Amateurism is a little bit fraudulent.

This all came to a head in 1980 with the Olympic boycott, when the U.S. boycotted Moscow. The marathoners, distance racers, the road racers, we formed an association to fight for allowing distance runners to be paid. The Association of Road Racing Athletes was formed. And that group put on the first prize money road race in the U.S. in a long time—since the turn of the century: The Cascade Runoff in Portland, Oregon.

We had talked to USA Track and Field. They said, "No, you can't do this. We are going to suspend you. You have to abide by international rules, amateur rules. You are not going to be able to compete in the Olympic Games." Not only that, each country's track-and-field leadership works with each other. New Zealand, let's say, would work with the U.S., and they'd say, "We'll make sure our athletes can't go to races in the U.S. if you make sure your athletes can't come here." So they'd work together to kind of keep us down.

After the Olympic boycott, we had enough unity to forge our own destiny. We had nothing to lose. We put on the Cascade race, it was successful, American Greg Meyer won the men's, won $10,000. And suddenly the whole sport, particularly road racing here in the U.S., started to have to change. It became an issue. And other races started saying, what do we do? A lot of them waffled. The Boston Marathon was one of the last of the big American races to change. They didn't change until '86. New York changed earlier, but even then it had to be forced. It's the way things happen, I guess. You have to fight for it to change.

In '77 my brother and I opened a shoe store. I put my name on it, The Bill Rodger Running Center, rather than paying a franchise fee—I didn't have the money to do that. A little store in Boston. That allowed me to travel to races and train as a professional, much better than when I was

a teacher. I was training twice a day and trying to teach. It was hard, in the sense of coming back, then you'd have to have a substitute teacher there and the kids would lose focus. You really couldn't do it. It was a full-time job to be a high-level athlete.

Everyone was telling me, "Bill, you ought to open a running store." Other people like Jeff Galloway had already done that. Frank Shorter did it. A lot of runners were teachers in previous decades because it allowed them to train and compete during the summer. The next step was to open your running store as the running boom evolved and there was a market for shoes and gear. And right after that we opened up a running clothing line. I put my name on that, same as Frank Shorter did. That went really well for a number of years. So we were allowed, finally, to start making a living doing that—just like everyone else in America. (laughs)

And other countries started to change, too. Today, it's quite different, and it's great to see the professional athletes well-paid.

We still sell a T-shirt with the words THE MARATHON CAN HUMBLE YOU on it. I said that in '75, because I'd won Boston that year in the fastest time in the world, then I went to that marathon in Holland a few months later and I ended up dropping out.

So I ended up writing an article for Runner's World, and that was definitely my feeling: The marathon can humble anyone. Even if you have a gold medal, everyone is a bit vulnerable in this sport. Your training doesn't go just right, you have a little bit of a weakness, catch a bit of a flu, someone's a little bit hungrier, trains a little better, a little smarter … whatever. Just competition, you know.

But I had a lot of fun all those years. I was able to travel all over the world. I actually won a marathon on five continents. It was pure fun to meet runners all over. Even when I didn't race—I remember one time when I went to the first Moscow International Marathon, their first prize money race. Fred Lebow and the New York Road Runners Club was there. I went with a group of American runners, and we met the Russian runners. This is about—I think—the early '90s. I saw Gorbachev at Lenin Stadium and all that.

Ran the Beijing marathon, ran in Australia. The athletes are all the same. In South America, I won the Rio marathon in '81, I won the Amsterdam in '77, and Stockholm in '81. I won the Melbourne Marathon—is Australia a continent?—in '82. The fifth continent was Asia: I won Fukuoka and Kyoto in Japan, both in '77. So it's a global sport. That's one of the unique things about it—it's global, like soccer. Even more global now, because the Africans are out there. Nairobi, Addis Abbaba. India is going big now. Beijing—I dropped out there.

I stopped winning races in the early eighties. I won Miami in January '83. I ran Boston a couple months later in 2:11:58—not a bad time—but I took 10th. With a pretty good time like that, the level of the sport was rising up. A lot of young Americans were coming up, getting serious.

Yeah, it was a bit of shock to be back that far. Greg Myer won it in 2:09 flat. I was starting to lose my focus. My first win was in '75—eight years earlier.

The lifespan of a competitive marathoner is usually five years, something like that. Let's see: I was at 2:09 in '75 and 2:11 in '83. In '84 I ran the trails, but I was 36.

And I ran a lot of marathons by then. I was a heavy racer, and that affected me. If you only run one a year, maybe you can do more. Also, I got married again in '83 and had my daughter Elise in '85. In the first marriage [ended in '81], there were no children. So I could be just a runner. I didn't have a house, just lived in an apartment, train full-time. Yes, I had a job for a while, and opened a business, but it was still me, me, me just running. But when you have kids, things shift, big-time. And I was getting older. And I had victories already. You can't do it forever. No one does.

Well, I think today the top marathoners don't race quite as much. But the top marathons are more competitive than ever. So the standards of training and recovery are more scientific. The runners are truly full-time professionals. Of course, people like Frank, and myself, and Greg Myer, we were trying to be professionals in a system we had to fight. On the other hand, I think it was a little more relaxed than today when it's so competitive.

Our times are comparable to most of the best of today, except for the high-altitude-born runners. But there are some breakthrough athletes, like Steve Jones of Wales, who ran 2:07. But the Kenyans and Ethiopians have kind of redefined the sport at the very top level—and the Japanese, too. Their national record is 2:06. When I was racing them, it was 2:08—and only one runner had done that. Now there are half a dozen. So there's a little more depth at the top—particularly from the altitude-born Africans. Huge difference. Then another issue, I think, is that there is drug use in the sport, as there is in all sports. That wasn't prevalent when I was a marathoner. It may have been there, but it was very low-key—probably more on the track.

STAYING AGE-GROUP FIT: TRICKY AS HELL

In '88 I turned 40, and I tried to win Boston Masters, Age 40 Division. I came in 2nd. It was close. Being an age-group runner is like a quest—you still want to stay with it. I quit once and I don't want to quit again. I still love the sport. But I'm certainly not going to win the Boston Marathon again. That was clear even many years earlier. But that was okay. I was happy with my life, my two daughters, born in '85 and '90. So my life's changed. But I love the low-key side of it, the camaraderie, the fitness side. And I still race a lot—as much as I ever used to. But I was just slower and back farther. But I still tried to win my age-group.

I love the old 78-year-olds who say they can't wait to come back at 80. The epitome of the human spirit. Sports kind of represent that indomitable side that everyone has in them that whether it is supported or uncorked or something, a lot of people don't know, or they miss, or didn't have someone who believed in them, for some reason they never got out there. Never found their sport. Which is sad, because I think everyone is an athlete,

Staying fit as you get older is tricky as hell. I had 58 marathon starts and finished 50 in a 20-some-year career. But I never had problems with my knees or cartilage. I never had a back injury in my life. I did have aches and pains, and got Achilles tendonitis and plantar fasciitis when

I was 40. But I never had surgery. I had the best of health and fitness, didn't see the doctor much.

Some of that is just running. If you're a walker, runner, a cyclist, a rower, or a swimmer you can say good-bye to the doctor for a long, long period of time.

The injuries come because runners are so into their sport. It's this quest where they changed their life for the better so much—reversed heart disease, lost weight. So they can't stand to take off a day. They overdo it. Do 100 marathons and never stretch or rest enough. I think the biggest weakness most of us have—myself included—is not resting enough. And learning how to stay fit as you get older is a big mystery. I don't think there's been too much research done on the best way to train. Should you train four days a week, and swim three days a week? When I was younger, it was "more is better."

You still need to recover and cross-train. At 60, I absolutely rest more now. When I was training for the marathon, I used to do 130 miles a week. Now I do like 50—and that's hard. I'm as tired if not more. I'm still trying to find the best way to train. Do you know Owen Anderson? I'm doing a clinic with him in February. He knows so much about training. I was asking him how much rest you need. Should you take off like a month off every year? Just don't do your sport. Let your body take a vacation....

I've never done that. From '72, I never took time off until I broke my right leg four years ago—my tibia. An interesting experience. I think I had a stress fracture. Maybe my body was telling me (laughs) "Bill, you have to do something different."

It's a fluke thing. It happens because you overdid it. Didn't rest enough. You trained hard, hard, hard, hard. And your body said, "Wait a second. You need to rest more. And if you're not going to rest, I'm going to make you rest."

My mom has osteoporosis. They said I was low normal—osteopenia. I take that medication Boniva.

It may have been a result of overtraining and not resting enough. I was 55 years old. I was doing 50 miles a week and training harder. I was a bit faster then.

I eat better now than when I was winning marathons. I probably had too much sugar and fat, because I had to have a lot of calories back then. You can get away with it as a young person.

I still don't have an ideal diet, but I've learned a lot. I eat a lot of complex carbohydrates. In the morning, I'll have toast with peanut butter and jelly on it, coffee, orange juice, then I'll run and come back and have some cereal, some fruit. At night I'll have chicken, tuna fish, something like that, some bread, vegetables. But I still like my sugar—always been a sugar addict. Chocolate chip cookies, another great Massachusetts invention. Toll House cookies were invented in Wakefield, Massachusetts. All endurance athletes love their cookies. I've never been a PowerBar eater. I gotta really be hungry to eat that kind of stuff.

I don't do much crosstraining. When I first broke my leg on my comeback, I bought an exercise bike. But as soon as I could just run, I've hardly used the bike since, because I'm already tired from the running. Cycling seems to tighten up my quads; I'm a little leery about going out on the road, getting hit by a car. We are a car culture. You've gotta watch your butt.

But I try to go the gym—I just went today. I haven't done it for a long time. I've always used weights on my own more. When I was 40 years old, if I ran a long one I'd go to the pool afterward to swim 10, 15, 20 minutes. Good way to lower your temperature, stretch out your legs. The gym—a little gym near where I live—easy to use. Of course, back in '73, I joined the Y. When I broke my leg, I used the pool there for water running. For rehab— that was how I came back. After that, gradually I'd start walking, then I'd run. I'd use the floatation belt, where the feet aren't touching the ground.

I tried AQx (water resistance shoes)—interesting technology. I know other runners who have done similar training. Like Priscilla Welch, the top woman over 40 in the marathon. She got injured, went to the pool for aqua jogging, and kept her fitness at a pretty high level. I think she won New York at the age of 40, about 20 years ago.

Today, I did 10 minutes in the pool, crawl, backstroke. The water running is a huge part of recovery. That's what rest is, right? It's physical but also mental.

On form, I think Pose running, Chi running, and those soft running methods are great—really just going back to our roots. After all, our ancestors ran over the plains, and fields, through the forest. We are made to run on grass or dirt. Asphalt is for cars and bikes, right? I was very lucky because Amby got me doing that in college. He was a big trail runner. His coach, Johnny Kelly, taught him. Abebe Bikila ran barefooted.

Run naturally, don't worry too much about form. Be relaxed. Gradually extend your distance. Not overdoing it too, too much on any particular day. Try to be steady. Consistency is everything. That's how you get stronger. That's what Amby tried to teach me.

The rest part, too. All these things are key.

The drop-off in the numbers of older runners is demographic and cultural. The baby boomers start at age 60, and the generation just ahead wasn't as active. They didn't have doctors telling them not to smoke. I think there are more 50-, 60-, 70-year-old runners than there have ever been, by far. Before it was just Johnny Kelly and a few others. Now, there are thousands.

I can still crack a 7-minute mile at some of my races for ten miles—and I'll get beaten! Lot of 'em started late—in their 30s, 40s, or 50s, or later. I see that a lot. And these people are so determined. They've found something that changed their life. They feel so much better physically. Health-wise, energy-wise. They feel better, they look better.

Some runners do get injured—the guys who really push it. Guys who are competitive runners. Like me. I broke my leg. Shorter has had some surgeries. I had other friends who didn't stretch enough, rest enough. They just raced, raced, raced. Now we know that there is more to it than just that—gotta stretch, use weights, eat better. We are starting to learn all these things.

You've gotta run less as you get older. If you want to be really good, you still have to work hard, but you have to be smart about it. You may be fit enough to go faster, but you're so tired because you didn't rest enough and you're running too far.

Interval training is better than going out and running a lot of empty miles. I do intervals once a week, a long run once a week, weights once a week, swim once a week, stretch three–four days a week. I always did something in the gym. But I didn't do much for my legs, actually. I did curls and presses with a 20-pound weight throughout most of my career. No push-ups, and I never used machines. I think today, most people benefit from crosstraining and weight work, and I was no exception to that. It's key for beginners and older folks, but I have also seen some runners who don't look like they had a muscle in their arms, and they are superb distance runners. So it's primarily a cardiovascular sport where you develop terrific muscle strength in your legs and back.

When I was doing the marathon, for 20 years from '73 to '92, I guess (I ran the 100th Boston in '96), for strength training I did hill repeats. That's quadriceps-strength training. I didn't need to hit the gym—that was always my theory. I think you may need the weights if you have an injury develop or have a certain weak spot. I didn't seem to have that really when I was younger, because I always did stretching, too. I didn't do a lot, but did something after almost each run.

I run almost every day. I think that's been a mistake, though. I've been thinking about taking a day or two off, though.

The number one thing is to get more rest. Once you hit 50, I don't know if running every day is smart anymore. Now I win my age-group sometimes, but get beat by people who run less. I don't feel strong. They are resting, doing more quality.

I'll be 60 in December. My goal: I want to see if I can beat one of the top 60-year-olds in the country. I want to win my age-group in a 10k and a half marathon. A lot of people can whip my butt.

As for running to 100, that's so far away. I can't even guess. When I was 15 or 16, I didn't think I'd be running at 60. My goal is to be fit. Beyond that, I only know one thing: I don't want to be a couch potato or go back to smoking.

RUN FOR LIFE

RUN STRONG

At a recent gathering of marathon runners, one observer looked around the room and said in disbelief, "Some of you people look like chickens that are only fit to make soup out of." He was right. Dr. Alan Clark told me that after six months on a running program, friends would approach my wife in private and speak with a concerned air about my gaunt appearance and ask how long I had been ill. Her explanation—that I was a long-distance runner—would leave them scratching their heads.

—The Complete Book of Running, *p. 75, by Jim Fixx*

Fact: If you don't strength-train, you won't be running at 100.

Runners may not want to hear that. Most seem to hate going to the gym, regarding it as the antithesis of what they love about the sport. Instead of leaves crackling underfoot, birds chirping, and daffodils perfuming the air, you get a treadmill or a leg press next to a grunting, sweaty fellow named Larry exuding a decidedly less-blissful aroma.

On top of that, most runners could care less about looking "buffed." But if you want to blast through the century mark in full stride, you need to aim for serious buffitude starting at age 35 or 40. That's when your muscle mass begins a natural decline that can only be stemmed by vigorous resistance training. The workouts should be all-body. You need strong upper-body muscles to remain functional in everyday life activities like putting books in a bookcase, lifting heavy grocery bags, and rotating the steering wheel of a car. You need strong butt, quad, hamstring, and calf muscles not only to run or walk but also to armor your joints against osteoarthritis by keeping them aligned and cushioned. You need a strong core to hold it all together. You need a fast reaction time to keep you safe when unexpected obstacles—cars and dogs and coffee tables—crop up and try their best to break your collarbone or hip.

Quick-reaction speed-strength, also known as power, is an absolute necessity for meeting the challenges of longevity running and the challenges of real life. It requires lifting heavy weights fast, which is taxing but gets you finished quicker. If you're going to go to the gym anyway, you may as well make the best use of your time. It's called "power training."

This section presents two ways to do power training; the first is a traditional gym-based program with some body-weight, freeweight, and machine exercises, but done at double- or triple-speed. The second, found in the sidebar, is CrossFit, a radical, unconventional, super-high-intensity program that gives you a different workout every day for a month. Sweeping military and law enforcement agencies and rapidly spreading into the mainstream, CrossFit takes "double-time" to a dizzying new level. The best part of it: Both regimens can be mixed and matched. Any way you do it, power training will make you stronger, faster, and better equipped to run into a superfit future.

CHAPTER 7

THE FOUNTAIN-OF-YOUTH POWER WORKOUT

Rapid-contraction weight lifting ramps up human growth hormone release and armors you against aging

You may think your muscles are strong now, but they're really not—unless you're 25 or 30. Any muscles older than that have already started to go downhill, and normal steady-state running won't bring them back. Only strength training and serious interval training (which is covered in the next chapter) can do that.

At age 30 or 35, your muscle mass starts to deteriorate anywhere from .5% to 1% a year, depending on what expert you talk to. Then it gets worse. After 50, the deterioration speeds up. Every decade, the atrophy doubles. By 80, muscles almost seem to evaporate—including the muscles in your legs. If you don't believe it, just look around: old runners start to look shriveled—because they are. So while it's true that steady-state aerobic exercise like running, cycling, and swimming can help slow the rate of decline, don't be fooled. It's not enough.

Shrinking muscle hurts you in ways you haven't thought of. It is linked to bone loss, a weakened immune system, degraded posture, and increased incidence of diseases like cancer and diabetes. Insidiously, it is replaced by fat. For every 10 pounds of lean muscle mass we carry, 500 calories per day is consumed to maintain it. So ever-smaller muscles leave us fatter.

Result: You may weigh the same at 48 as you did at 18, but your body composition is more fat, less muscle.

Then there's power loss. In 2002, researchers at Johns Hopkins and Boston Universities discovered that, with age, muscular power falls off much faster than muscular strength and size. And, just as with strength, power loss accelerates with age.

Lack of power is a big deal. It can cost you your life.

Defined as the ability to use your strength quickly in response to changing situations, power is essential for human function. It gives you instant reaction time, the explosive, microsecond adjustments that give you the balance and agility that can be the difference between success and failure. Examples: a 45-year-old racquetball player might still be able to bench-press 200 pounds like he did at 35, but because his power is down 5% he can't retrieve that shot in the dead corner anymore; a 60-year-old mountain biker may still be able to climb the same hills almost as fast as he did at 40, but wipes out on the descents because his muscles can't react to roots and drop-offs as quickly; a 75-year-old might still give you an iron-grip handshake, since his strength is still 80% of what it was decades earlier. But with his power down 50%, he might lose his balance as he gets up from a table, fall, and break his hip.

Power will give an 85-year-old the instant acceleration he needs to get across the street when the crosswalk light turns red, or duck out of the way when a car makes a sudden right-hand turn in front of him. Power is a key to athletics—and to survival.

Technically, power reflects ability to generate muscular work per unit of time; more simply, Power = Force x Velocity. In a 2003 article in the *Journal Of Gerontology*, researchers found that power was two to three times more important than strength in helping older people maintain mobility and physical performance.

"Older" is relative, by the way. It can apply to 37-year-olds trying to stay as mobile as 24-year-olds, like Michael Jordan in the nineties. He observed a rigorous "power training" program after age 30, as do many of this era's older pro athletes. Trainers have known for years that weight training that focuses on maintaining power is necessary to keep aging pros at the top of their game. Power training is weight lifting with the intensity dial turned to "all-out." No leisurely set of 20 biceps curls with 3-pound weights here. You must push fairly heavy weights *fast*, because you move fast in life.

What we didn't know until recently is that this power training is vital for average folks too, especially as they age. In other words, *there is a very good argument for everyone to be weight training like professional athletes after age 30 or 35*. If you're not doing it after 50, you're hurting yourself. It's so important that if you have to choose between a run and a weight session, many experts say lift weights.

Endorphins make you feel good for a couple hours, but 40 minutes of building big, powerful muscles will make you feel younger for a week.

So, get over your gym-phobia and get ready to work. Getting younger and faster won't be easy. Power training means hitting *heavy* weights *fast* and *frequently*. Done right, it's a physical and psychological challenge, taking more effort than regular weight training, but thankfully over quicker. Power-focused weight training is the most effective antidote to aging, bar none. Avoid it at your own risk.

Below, a little more background to drive in the point, followed by a sample 40-minute strength workout that hits your whole body hard and strengthens running-specific danger zones.

A. YOUR GOAL

Build Fast-Twitch Fibers With Fast Contractions

You may have heard of "superslow" weight lifting, whose proponents touted amazing health benefits from short sessions of agonizingly slow lifts; hundreds of copycat magazine articles promoted it in the early 2000s. Well, forget it. To restore size and power, do exactly the opposite: Go "superfast."

A 2002 Boston University study led by Roger A. Fielding, Ph.D., found that rapid contractile movements, such as a speedy upstroke on a leg extension,

can quickly bring back your thick, powerful "fast-twitch" muscle fibers—even in 73-year-old grandmothers who never worked out a day in their lives. Short, bulky, and white-tinted, fast-twitch fibers (known as Type 2) contract two to three times faster than the smoother, longer, aerobic-oriented, red-colored "slow-twitch" fibers (known as Type 1)—30 to 70 twitches per second versus 10 to 30 twitches per second. Type 1 muscle fibers pace themselves because they are "on" all the time, responsible for much of our day-to-day muscular activity, including steady-state aerobics. They don't start to waste away much until age 60 or 70.

The fast-twitch Type 2s, on the other hand, lie dormant until called to action. Until then, they atrophy, withering substantially by age 50 and virtually disappearing in old age without stimulation. Regular aerobic activity is not enough to stimulate them.

On the bright side, fading fast-twitch fibers don't hurt you as much in pure endurance activities, which is why many marathon runners and cyclists have done well into their late 30s and even 40s. On the dark side, the rapid falloff in fast-twitch fibers severely impacts reaction time in more skill-oriented tasks and wrecks balance in old age. It'll diminish a runner's finish-line kick, or a football player's first step. At 45, tennis players are several steps slower on the court. At 70, you might fall and crack your ribs on the same tricky trail you've run on for years, because now you can't react quick enough to avoid tripping on a root.

Researcher Fielding split his Boston University test group of 73-year-old women into two groups: super-fast leg extensions and regular-speed contractions. He found that the super-fast group had similar strength gains as the regular group, but got far greater gains in fast-twitch fiber volume and peak power output.

"But why wait until 73?" he asked me. "In younger people, they'll come back even faster." In fact, it's much harder for oldies to regain power, and worsens with age. A 2008 University of New Hampshire comparison of inactive older women (age 65 to 84) and younger females (18 to 33), all of whom engaged in an 8-week knee-extension program, found identical 12% gains in both groups' quadriceps strength, but a huge disparity in power increases— 9% to 35%. The reason? Due to age-related withering and lack of stimulation from what UNH study director Dain LaRoche calls "the low-intensity activities older people tend to do—walking, gardening," there are simply fewer Type 2 fibers to grow back.

The take-home: Wait too long, and it could be too late. "I would advise people to actively engage in resistance training once they hit their 60s," said Scott Trappe, director of Ball State University's Human Performance Lab, which published a 2008 study similar to that of UNH. "Once you hit the threshold of 80, [growth] may not be possible." Noting that lifting light weights may not be intense enough to stress Type 2s, UNH's LaRoche offers advice you'll hear again and again: "Use resistance heavy enough to fatigue muscles in 8 to 12 repetitions."

Again, runners should not make the mistake of assuming that their legs don't need heavy, rapid-contraction strength training. Aging puts every muscle in the body at risk. Masters sprinters manage to keep greater muscle mass because their high-intensity anaerobic intervals are a lot like lifting weights (see Section 3). But normal runners tend to shrivel. So you have to hit *all* the muscles of the legs, with extra attention to the calves (see section E., below) and the VMO, the inner portion of the quads (see section F).

B. THE HGH WORKOUT

Do No-Rest Circuit Training with 3 sets of 8-to-12 reps to "failure"

The gym is an effective one-stop shop, usually filled with enough equipment to blast every part of your body. Using a mix of freeweights, body-weight exercises, and weight machines, the program below cycles through 3 sets in 40 minutes, doable if you use rapid contractions, cut the socializing, and are willing to get uncomfortable.

If you're uncomfortable with the word "uncomfortable," keep your eyes on the prize: You have to push hard enough to wake up and stress those sleeping, shrinking fast-twitch fibers. How hard? "At least 70% of maximum perceived one-rep effort, in order to produce cellular and metabolic changes that yield stronger muscles," says well-known muscle guru Dr. William Kraemer, Ph.D., a kinesiology, physiology, neurobiology, and Human Performance Lab professor at the University of Connecticut, and former president of the National Strength and Conditioning Association. That translates to maxing out at the aforementioned 8 to 12 repetitions, known as going to "failure."

Failure is the point of overload, at which you can no longer move the weight at all, or do so without breaking form. It leaves you straining, breathing hard, and the particular muscle exhausted. Have you ever seen the young woman talking on her cell phone while doing 5 minutes on the leg-extension machine with a 10-pound weight? She is wasting her time—and yours. Politely explain to her that she is not getting any human growth hormone that way. (I'll explain in a minute.)

What this high-intensity effort leaves in its wake are microtears in the proteins that control the contraction of muscle cells. Naturally, this tearing is traumatic to the muscle being worked out. If it could talk, it would be screaming, "I am being stressed to the breaking point. I am falling apart. I need to get stronger immediately, so send reinforcements fast!"

The reinforcements are protein, and they are called to the battlefront by hormones, including the glamour boy of bodily chemicals, human growth hormone. Lactic acid, which flooded the muscle in response to the anaerobic overload, cues the pituitary gland to secrete HGH, the body's fountain of youth. It promotes lean muscle mass, body fat reduction, youthful skin, thick bones, strong connective tissue, and deeper sleep. It will make your muscles grow at any age.

When HGH arrives on the scene, it directs satellite protein cells to swarm torn areas, like the way blood plasma coagulates at a cut. Protein is the glue a muscle uses to put itself back together. Thus, the healing/strengthening process begins. (This is why you should eat more protein when you lift weights; it'll be used to rebuild your muscles.)

Working out hard is the key. "Just cut out the talking and work out to failure to maximize the spurt," says Kraemer.

The adult body reacts quickly and positively to this sudden jolt of HGH, almost as if it's pleasantly surprised. And it is, in a way, considering that your body's production of HGH tumbles after your mid-20s, some say by as much as 24% per decade. It's no mystery why; you're done growing—it's not needed anymore. So, whereas your body produces about 500 micrograms of HGH a day at age 20, it drops to 200 milligrams at forty, and 25 milligrams at 80. You know the result: muscle-mass shrinkage and body fat increases.

Fortunately, the HGH factory doesn't ever completely shut down, and will respond instantly when you put demands on it.

Can you strength-train enough to negate the relentless muscle deterioration that comes with aging? That is unknown. But clearly, you can slow the slide and do some rebuilding—it all depends how often you send the right orders to the factory. And that's dependent on how hard and how often you are willing to take yourself to the gym, how many muscles you work, and whether you can summon the effort to push them to failure.

While I don't love lifting weights, I'm afraid not to. Strong, fast muscles are what make everything else possible, and

THE CROSSFIT FUTURE

Strength, aerobics, and superfitness in 20 minutes of fury

I'm hyperventilating. Twelve minutes into what I thought was a simple, 20-minute workout of pull-ups, kettlebell swings, and 1-minute runs, I'm bent over with my hands on my knees, mouth wide open, head spinning, shoulders numb, and torso heaving with giant belly breaths. I'm spent, I feel nauseated.

"Hurry up!" urges my trainer. "You're on the verge of being beaten by a 38-year-old housewife who is 4 months pregnant!" As a lifelong runner, cyclist, and gym rat, I thought I was fit—until my first day of CrossFit.

Probably the world's hottest workout program right now, CrossFit combines the ultra-intensity strength-training philosophy of Chapter 7 with the ultra-intensity intervals of Chapter 10.

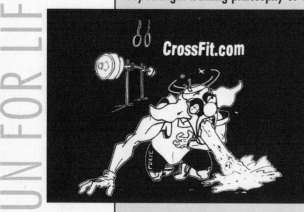

CrossFit mascot Pukey the Clown

But instead of conventional weights, it uses a random mix of common calisthenics, gymnastics, and gym exercises like squats, push-ups, pull-ups, dips, deadlifts, medicine-ball throws, handstands, and just about any physical thing you can think of. The workouts—different every day, posted on the www.CrossFit.com website, and often named after women ("because they reminded me of hurricanes," says Greg Glassman, the gymnast–turned-personal trainer–turned fitness guru who created them)—are timed and compared against others over the Internet. That assures a manic,

66

are essential to keeping running to 100 a realistic goal. The rapid-contractions/no-rest paradigm at least gets the workout over as fast as possible.

Of course, increasing numbers of people would rather just skip the workout and get an injection of synthetic HGH. They lose weight and get more muscular, too. Manufactured for clinical use since the 1980s and approved by the FDA in 1996, artificial HGH is used by an estimated 100,000 Americans today. But it's expensive ($500 to $1,000 a month) and controversial due to questions over its effectiveness and potential side effects. While your own exercise-induced spurts of HGH target only the muscles that ask for it, injected HGH may make other things grow, the theory goes, such as tumors. The FDA only approves its use to treat severe

head-spinning pace that, done right, ought to leave you quite uncomfortable. In fact, the CrossFit mascot, imprinted on a popular T-shirt, is Pukey the Clown, a muscle-bound bozo spewing green bile, a rare involuntary reaction to the lactic acid that floods into the bloodstream with anaerobic workouts.

The shirt, and the superb all-round functional fitness, are hot properties among thousands of CrossFitting police departments, SWAT teams, Navy Seals, and units of the Canadian, U.S., British and Australian armed forces. But that's just the tip of the CrossFit iceberg. Authorized trainers in the U.S. multiplied by 20-fold from 2005 to 2008 — from 50 to over 1,000. In research I conducted for articles in *Men's Journal* and *the Los Angeles Times*, I found

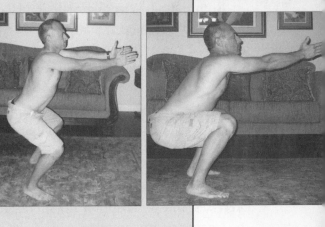

Air Squats typify CrossFit's emphasis on functional movements.

athletes of all types and ages — professional mixed martial artists, triathletes, housewives — using CrossFit to build what they all seemed to claim was the best shape of their lives — and doing it all in 20 minutes a day or less.

Is there something here for runners who would like to do a 10k at age 100?

I think so. CrossFit, largely underground until it exploded out of Glassman's Santa Cruz garage gym in 2005, may be the best example of what I call the "Unified Theory of Fitness" — that strength *and* cardio, both done in all-out bursts, ward off aging by cueing the body to flood itself with HGH and other hormones that keep you strong and young. The brutal, mixed-up, amped-up, double-espresso workouts blast your entire body while providing adequate recovery time for growth.

"It's natural because it's the way we worked out as kids—lotta different stuff all the time, done all-out," said Glassman. "It became clear that a single, blended workout of gymnastics, lifting, and aerobics, done at an all-out pace, generated better all-round fitness than training each discipline separately on alternate days. 'Segmented' trainers can't keep up with us on our workouts."

Glassman got a pat on the back in 2005 when the Canadian Infantry School in Gagetown, New Brunswick, conducted a 7-week trial of CrossFit versus its own rigorous Canadian Fitness Manual training plan. The results: CrossFit scored higher in every fitness category and was ranked more enjoyable by most of the 110 officer candidates tested.

Test organizer Captain J. T. Williams admitted, however, that a minority did not enjoy CrossFit's intensity or find its competitive aspects motivating. That was no surprise to Glassman, who says that 80% of the people who try it don't stick with it.

hormone deficiencies in children and adults. There are risks if taken by healthy aging adults, according to a study on aging in the *Journal of the American Medical Association*, including signs of diabetes or glucose intolerance, fluid retention, joint pain, and carpal tunnel syndrome.

Bottom line: Why take artificial HGH if you can produce it naturally? In the gym, you can precisely target it to your muscles with no worries of side effects.

C. THE IMPORTANCE OF SEQUENCE

Packing in three sets of 8 to 12 reps to "failure" over a dozen or more strength exercises, the prescription for increasing the frequency and amplitude of the HGH spurts that grow muscle, could take you all night, But it can be completed in 40 minutes by organizing the workout in groups of non-overlapping exercises, such as push-pull or upper-lower. An example of push-pull: Follow a chest exercise (push-ups, bench or seated press), paired with a complementary, oppositional movement like a seated row, which works the back. The chest rests as the back is worked, eliminating downtime. You can pair up leg extension (quads) with leg curls (hamstrings.) Based on the proximity of the machines, you can sequence three or four exercises (i.e., dips/leg press/pull-ups/leg extension), keeping the pressure on by blasting one station and move on to the next. (For body-weight exercises like pull-ups, squats, and dips, go to "failure" by doing as many reps as you can). If a machine is occupied, skip it and move to

I understand why. On my first day of CrossFit, after I finished three rounds of "Helen" — 21 kettle bell swings, 12 pull-ups, and a quarter-mile run — I was so exhausted that I had to lie down in my car for half an hour. And that was with a time of 17 minutes, 35 seconds — a minute behind the pregnant woman and more than double the Helen world record of 7:35, set by a Santa Cruz police officer.

Fortunately, your body gets stronger fast. Over the next two months of doing CrossFit three days a week, I cut three minutes off my Helen, saw gains in nearly all strength categories, and could run uphill noticeably faster than ever before.

And although I've never soiled my tank top, I wear my Pukey T-shirt with pride. After you make it through a couple CrossFit workouts — tossing your cookies or not — you feel like you've earned it.

the next to keep the momentum going. This way, you can hit your whole body hard, head to toe, in 40 minutes, and don't need to do it again for three or four days.

D. BUILD-IN REST AND RECOVERY

Ironically, while you need more intensity with age (to maintain the fast-twitch fibers), safety requires you to take it easier, too: Use lighter weights on your first set to warm up, take more recovery time (rest and sleep) between workouts, and gradually build up to heavier workouts over time. Since muscle fibers need at least 48 hours to recover from a hard workout, never lift two days in a row. I've found that a hard workout keeps me strong for a full week. Some advocate alternating heavy

and light workouts. "If you're 35 or older, make every second workout a 'recovery workout' (below 80% of max), and every fifth week an easy week," says Dan Wirth, president of Sierra Fitness Health Clubs of America and a former University of Arizona strength coach.

E. TO KEEP MUSCLES FRESH, MIX IT UP

To prevent gradual decline, Wirth and many other coaches promote cross-training and "Periodization"—working muscles with different weights, reps, and exercises every couple of months.

Ironically, while the Periodization program described in Chapter 26 is applied to running/aerobic training, Romanian coaching guru Tudor Bompa actually developed its principles for strength training. He noticed that muscles "learn." As you get stronger, a movement that initially took 10 muscle fibers to move soon takes 9 fibers, then 8. To keep firing all the fibers, you need to change your routine— the exercises you do, the sequence you do them in, the loads, the number of reps. Do heavy weight and low reps one month, then light weight and higher reps the next. Change technique; on pullups change your grip from underhand to overhand. Instead of an overhead barbell press do handstand push-ups against a wall. Change brands of machines; a Universal incline-press has different biomechanics from an Icarian. Dump the machines for body-weight exercises like squats, dips, and pull-ups that work many muscles at once.

The ultimate mixed-up workout plan is CrossFit (see page 66), which hits you with a new group of functional, compound-joint exercises and anaerobic intervals over the Internet (CrossFit.com) every day. Done for time, the full-speed workouts yield something unheard of until now: simultaneous gains in strength, power, endurance, and speed. CrossFit is sweeping through law enforcement and military circles because it's so effective so fast—as little as 20 minutes per day.

F. WORKOUT RULES

Muscles can be rebuilt, but joints aren't so lucky. Microthin synovial membrane, already a tissue-thin lining that covers bone ends with lubrication slicker than wet ice, thins and wears with age. Knees' meniscus cushions rip. The femur dangles precariously from the cavity of the shoulder blades, making the shoulder prone to impingement and rotator cuff injuries. Blood, barely able to penetrate joints due to lack of capillaries in tendons and ligaments, delivers fewer healing nutrients with age. What to do?

Four things: warm up, do full-range-of-motion exercises safely by using good form and natural exercises, emphasize pulls, and cool down.

1. Extensive warm-up

No matter if you're young or old— but especially if you're old—don't do any serious strength training or running without getting your body prepared for action: pre-lubricating knees, elbows, and shoulders with synovial fluid, raising your heart rate, and working up a light sweat. A good start is stretching and yoga (see Section 5), Symmetry posture exercises (Section 3), and various exercises, such as neck rolls, shoulder shrugs, alternating arm circles, hip circles, trunk rotations (hands on hips, rotating in circles), knee circles, and leg swings (side to side like windshield wipers, and forward and back, like kicking a soccer ball). If you're short on time, ease into all-body movements like jumping jacks, the elliptical machine, and squats.

2. Aim for safe, full range-of-motion exercises by using good form, body-weight exercises, and cable machines

Many trainers and therapists nowadays warn against extreme ranges of motion for all strength exercises, regardless of age, due to potential joint injuries. But for running to 100, you need full range of motion to keep your muscles strong and flexible with age. What to do?

Good form is key. To keep the kneecap in its track in the base of the femur, do machine squats by pressing through your heels and avoid the first half of leg extensions. During body-weight squats, a superb exercise you can do anywhere: Start with feet positioned wider than shoulders, toes pointed outwards at 30 degrees, head up, back arched, and weight entirely on your heels. Then push your hips backward, raise arms overhead, and lower your butt to within a foot of the floor (as if you are taking aim at an old-fashioned Asian pit toilet). Then push up through your heels to a standing position. On first try, 5 or 6 of these will rocket your heartrate. Do 25 and you are a machine.

As for the shoulder, some call for dumping the military press and the apple pie of the weight room, the bench press. The latter can pin the scapula between bar and bench, causing the humerus (upper arm bone) to grind into and overload the glenohumeral joint which is supported only by tendons and ligaments. The solution: Replace the military with more natural exercises like handstand pushups and overhead barbell presses; replace the bench with a standing cable machine press, which frees the scapula and requires hip, stomach, and lower back to stabilize the body. In fact, use cable weight machines as much as possible; they are better for you than fixed-path machines because they combine some of the instability and real-world body bracing of free weights with the convenience of selectorized machines. Do as many exercises as possible on them, observing the 8-to-12 reps to failure rule.

3. Do more pulling exercises

"It's easy to push and harder to pull—so we get lazy on pulls," says James T. Bell, Ph.D., president and founder of the International Fitness Professionals Association. The imbalance is exacerbated by sitting at a computer all day and by falling in love with yourself in the mirror, causing you to overemphasize frontal muscles. Solution? "Do more backside exercises to balance it—upper and lower body," he says. More lat pulldowns, pull-ups, and rows than presses. More hamstrings than quads—three times as much, some say.

4. Cool down with a recovery spin and stretching

After lifting, your capillaries are dilated and pooling with lactic acid. An

RUN FOR LIFE

easy cardio workout, such as a bike or full-body elliptical, is a good way to pump it out. Then, before you shower, stretch. Stretching becomes more important with age. Elasticity of tissues drops with age; instead of bending and stretching, they break, says Bob Forster. "So stretch more and avoid injuries that are hard on these tissues," he says.

G. MUSCLES THAT NEED SPECIAL ATTENTION

You need to strengthen neglected and weak muscles and build up others that will protect knees and lower back. The first group includes the hip flexors and backside muscles such as the calves, butt, and hamstrings.

a. Calf Muscles play a key role in superfit aging and absolutely must be hammered with weights regularly for four reasons:

1. Load: They bear more of the load with Soft Running's forefoot landing, as well as hill running. Strength training helps them stave off fatigue.

2. Withering: Calves will have a higher propensity than other muscles to get weak as you age. They and the forearms are "distal" muscles, which tend to wither faster because they're routinely stressed less than muscles nearer the body's core, according to Michael Bemben, Ph.D., director of the Neuromuscular Research Lab at the University of Oklahoma. (Also

work the triceps, the backside upper arm muscle, as it is predominantly—90%—composed of fast-twitch fibers.)

3. Injury prevention: Strong, flexible calves help ward off plantar fasciitis, one of running's most common foot ailments. PF is often linked to a tight soleus/tibialis posterior area in the lower leg. The tibialis posterior is a muscle located just underneath the soleus and gastrocnemius and connects from the arch of the foot all the way to the back of the knee. Work the calf and you also work it.

4. Pump: Calves play a little-known, but important role as a "second heart pump" that assists the return flow of blood to the heart.

Calf exercises: Standard weighted calf raises, either via standing or seated weight machine or pushing up on your toes while holding weights in each hand, are great. However, I think the most thorough, convenient, and practical way to work the calf any time, anywhere, with body weight only is the Deep Calf Raise, courtesy of Dr. Michael Yessis, the inventor of Active-Isolated Stretching and the author of *Explosive Running*. Standing on the ball of one foot on the edge of a curb or step, lower your heel as far as it'll stretch, then explode upward onto your toes. Do as many as fast as you can, going to failure (I do about twenty-five). You get a maximum strength and stretching workout all at once. It's also great as a warm-up exercise for a workout or a race.

b. *Butt:* Strong glutes are essential for posture and proper running form, but they are surprisingly underdeveloped in most runners. Cable kickbacks are a good way to strengthen the butt. Other machines at the gym that build booty include the leg press (push through your heels), the standing hip-rotation machine (be sure to keep a straight leg as you push the pad back), and the old favorite a man would not normally be caught dead on, the "Butt Blaster." Hey, get over it. It works. Push them all heavy and fast.

c. *Hip Flexors:* The higher knee lift will stress the hip flexors. Strengthen them with cable knee lifts, attaching the cable to your ankle.

d. *Hamstrings:* Already neglected vis-à-vis the mirror-centric quads, the hams will need to be built up to handle the heel flick of the soft-running technique.

H. STRENGTHEN "DANGER ZONE" MUSCLES

Keeping the muscles that surround and stabilize the knees and low back strong is essential for running longevity because they will stabilize those joints and reduce long-term injuries.

a. *Lower back:* Lumbar spine deterioration is one of the hidden tragedies of running. A lifetime of sitting tightens the spinae erector muscles that flank the spine and weakens the transverse abdominus, the deep ab muscles that draw the belly button to the spine. The relentless pounding of running can turn the discs between the vertebrae into jelly, not only causing osteoarthritis and back pain, but risking impinging the nerves of the spinal cord. Do these exercises to armor the lower back:

1. *Back extension:* Lying belly down, raise your head and upper back to work the spiny erectors. Caution: Don't hyperextend.

2. *Dying bug:* Lying faceup with your arms at your sides, press the small of your back to the mat and tighten your core by making a "pssst" sound. Then raise and lower opposite legs and arms at once without moving the spine. Reverse.

3. *Transverse abdominus (TA):* Standing with light dumbbells at chest level, twist side to side as you draw a sideways figure eight.

4. *Cross crunches:* Fold left leg over right knee and cross over with elbows to hit TA, intercostals, and obliques.

b. *The Knee:* Running longevity demands that you take steps to protect the knee—running's most valuable and vulnerable joint. The biggie: Avoid what some call "Runner's Knee," which represents two different conditions: patellar tendonitis, a strain of the tendon that connects the kneecap to the quadriceps,

RUN FOR LIFE

and chondromalacia, a flaking-off and wearing-away of the cartilage inside the knee joint that leaves you with a painful clicking and scraping. Chrondro is the much worse of the two; while tendonitis heals with rest, cartilage does not regrow.

To protect what cartilage you have, you must take active steps to prevent "lateral tracking," in which the kneecap is pulled to the outside by a tight IT band and a too-strong vastus lateralis (VL—the outside section of the quadriceps), which tends to get overdeveloped in relation to the vastus lateralis oblique (VMO), the muscle on the inside of the quadriceps, just above the kneecap. The vast majority of knee problems are related to this lateral tracking.

Normally, the V-shaped underside of the kneecap smoothly rides in a groove in the bottom of the femur. But when it is pulled to the lateral side, it scrapes the side of the groove, scraping off cartilage and wearing out your meniscus. Bone-on-bone, chrondromalacia—and osteoarthritis—has now begun.

The lateral tracking issue is even more critical for women. Wider hips and the bigger Q angle (angle between hip and the knee) also mean that there may be more "pull" on the kneecap, which can cause pain when running uphill. Kneecap cartilage also seems to wear down more in women than in men. And women's kneecaps slide around more from side to side, in part because women have more estrogen, which can make women's ligaments more flexible than men's.

Best bet for stopping lateral tracking in its tracks: Stretch the IT band and vastus lateralis (VL) and strengthen the weak VMO. Also strengthen the hamstrings; it has been known for two decades that "antagonist muscles exerts nearly constant opposing torque throughout joint range of motion." (*American Journal of Sports Medicine*, 1988.)

Studies have routinely shown that strong quadriceps have less cartilage loss behind the kneecap. But there's a problem: Those with a tendency to overdevelop the lateral side can't just hop on the leg-extension machine and pump away. It is not easy to find a good "isolation" exercise for the VMO (inside of the quad) that won't also strengthen the VL (the outside of the quad).

Phase IV's Bob Forster is against using the leg-extension machine, as he believes it creates shearing force on the kneecap. He says the VMO can be targeted with the leg press, pushing through the forefoot.

But James T. Bell, the IFPA president, says a leg-extension machine works safely and effectively if used correctly. The key: Point the toes out and roll the entire leg like a log to the outside. That way, the knee tracks with the toes. Don't just flap the ankles outward; that puts stress on the knee capsule.

Bell says that deep squats can also strengthen the VMO. But in direct

RUN FOR LIFE

contradiction to a high-intensity program like CrossFit, which relies heavily on large quantities of rapid-fire squats, he believes that the squat is the rare strength exercise that you *should not* do rapidly. His reason? The VMO doesn't become activated until you squat below the knee-hip line—a deep squat. "The knee needs a slight dislocation to go that far," says Bell. "So do the squat, slow, controlled, no ballistic motion whatever. The knee will accommodate the deep squat if you don't exceed the knee/toe line, which puts stress on the knee capsule. Also, don't twist the tibia in relation to the femur."

Given the agreement about the benefit of the squat, but the conflicting views on its safety, be sensible: If you are doing them at a rapid pace and feel pain, check your form, slow the pace, or stop.

Finally, as you strengthen any of your body's muscles, be sure to stretch them. Important for the VMO: the Side Lying Quad Stretch found in Chapter 12.

SUMMARY

With the exception of ultra-intense intervals (see Chapter 10), running doesn't build muscle and power. *All muscles of the body decline with neglect; in the weight room, hit as many of them as possible.* In 40 minutes, racing from exercise to exercise, blasting 8-to-12 reps to failure, you can do a 3-set, head-to-toe circuit-training workout that ignites a powerful, fast-twitch-building, fat-stripping spurt of HGH. Start with the following exercises pictured on the next page (grouped in 3 segments to allow for efficient circuit training); mix them up and add others over time to stay fresh. Order doesn't matter, but to save time and keep motivated, pair alternating front/back and upper/lower exercises such as push-ups and rows, and pull-ups and dips. Warm-up with a light set and warm-down with easy aerobics to regain flexibility. In between, push it like your athletic life depends on it. *Because it does.*

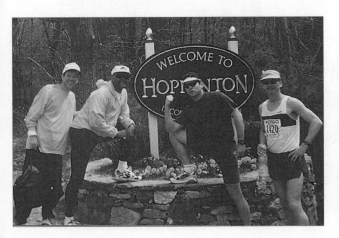

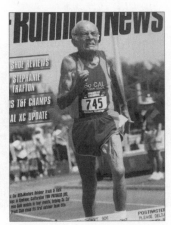

Remember: You may stay naturally robust into your early 40s, but runners won't retain muscle mass without strength training after age 50.

40-MINUTE ALL-BODY WEIGHT WORKOUT

Warm-up:
Squat Thrust with Medicine Ball (or weight plate)

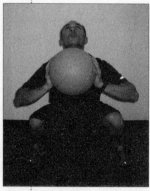
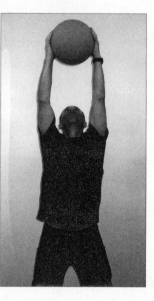
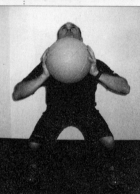

Group 1 sample exercises:
Deep Calf Raises, bottom and top positions

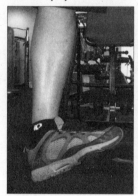
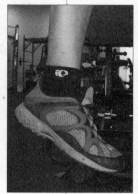

Dips

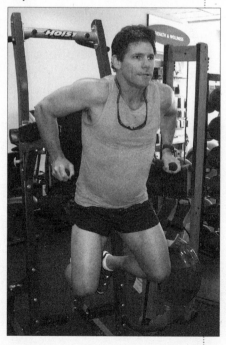

Abdominal Twist with Medicine Ball (or weight plate)

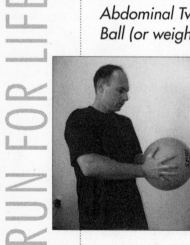
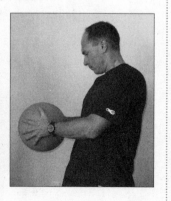

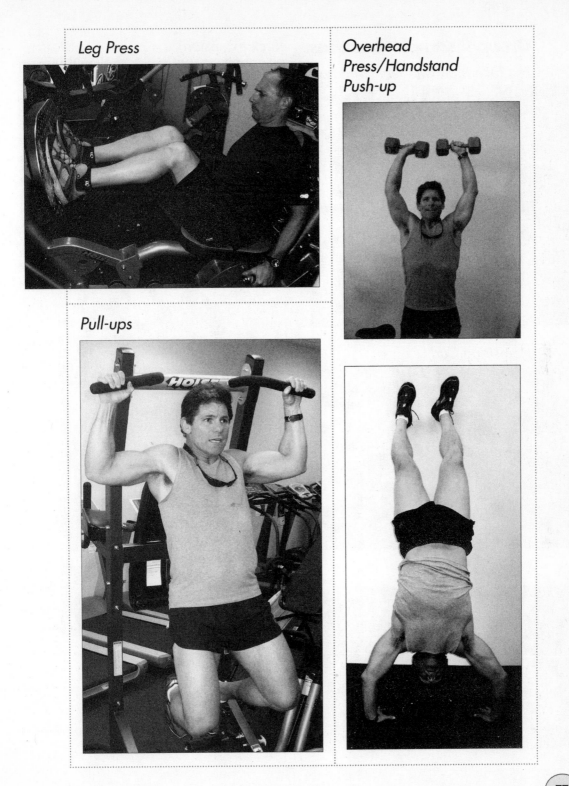

Leg Press

Overhead Press/Handstand Push-up

Pull-ups

Group 2 sample exercises:

Leg Extension with feet turned out

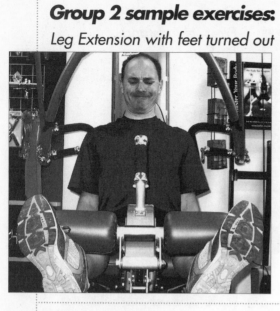

Back Extension

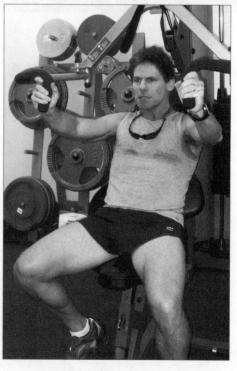

Chest Press, Push-up, Bench Press

Hamstring Curl

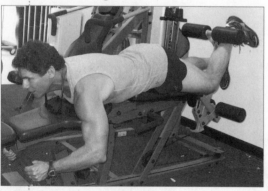

Phase IV Sit-ups

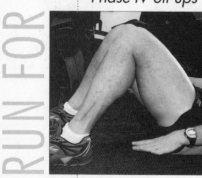

Seated Row

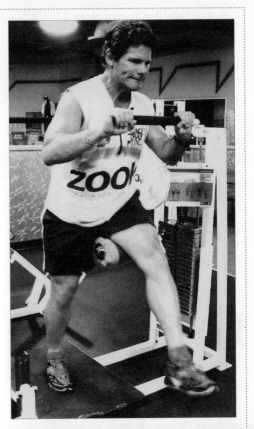

Group 3
sample exercises:

Various butt exercises:
Cable Kickback/Hip Rotation
Machine/Butt Blaster

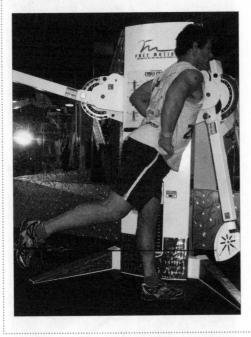

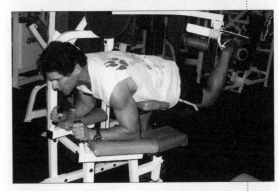

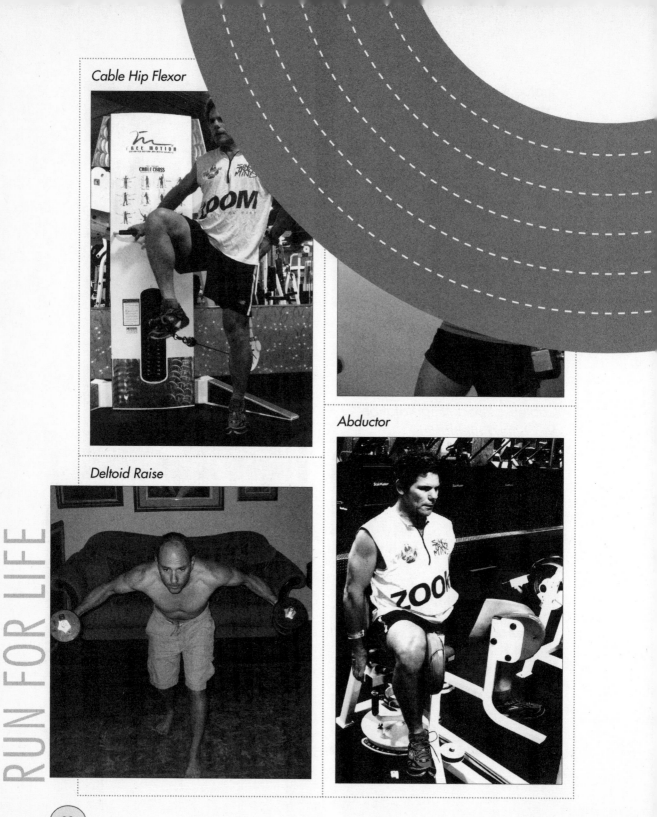

Cable Hip Flexor

Deltoid Raise

Abductor

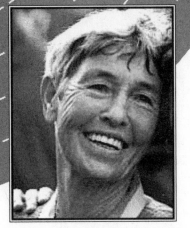

HELEN KLEIN

The Role Model of the Ages

Seven days into the 1995 Eco-Challenge—a 10-day, round-the-clock, 400-mile hiking, mountain climbing, kayaking, river rafting, rope-climbing adventure race in Utah—a number of middle-of-the-pack teams were camped overnight at a riverside checkpoint. That's where I got a lecture on how I should be wearing running shoes, not hiking boots, by a tough, skinny little grandmother named Helen Klein. (She was right; my feet were all blistered; hers weren't.) She was 72 at the time, making her a good three decades older than everyone else, including her own teammates. That provided great publicity for her team Operation Smile, which was raising money for third-world oral surgeries. "*Dateline NBC* would not have covered us if I weren't on it," she told me. "They were also watching a team of New York City cops. On the third day, the female cop had to drop out, so the whole team was out. So if I didn't finish, *Dateline* wouldn't have had a story. So that prompted me to finish."

It takes a lot more than icy rivers, the world's longest rope course, and a race billed at the time as the hardest endurance event in history to stop the unstoppable Klein. As of November 9, 2007, when the following interview was conducted, this retired nurse and mother of four had completed 86 marathons, 143 Ultras, and 28 100-mile races, along the way setting 75 world or age-group records, including the 80+ mark of 4:31. They all came after age 55, when she first started running.

Arguably the most famous female ultrarunner, role model, and race organizer in the world, the formerly non-athletic Klein always led a disciplined life that dovetailed perfectly with the challenges of long-distance running. Dedicating their lives to the sport, she and husband Norman tossed aside a thriving Kentucky dental practice to start a new life next to the route of the Western States 100. Running "within herself" and sticking to a dedicated weight training, healthy-diet, and don't-push-it philosophy, she does up to 10 races a year now and is a poster girl for superfit aging who's been studied by researchers like Dr. Ken Cooper (who sends a limo to pick her up).

"She's genetically lucky, but it doesn't matter what kind of genes you have—you can always trash 'em," says Norman, the Western States director for many years. "She does everything right. She wants to live and be reliant on herself. Our bedroom looks like a gymnasium. Over time, she's gotten more stringent. She cut out all snacks. Very disciplined, strict. It carries over to the events. That's what attracted me to her. She's tough."

Example: The 50k Shadow of the Giants race in 2002 when Helen was 80.

"Pacing her at the 18-mile mark, I let her go ahead," Norman said. "Her vision isn't the best. 'Watch out for that root,' I tell her. She did, but slammed her head on a branch. It was as if Mike Tyson hit her. Big gash in her forehead. Blood all over the place."

The former maxillofacial and oral surgeon took off his T-shirt, wrapped it around Helen's head, and tied it in a tourniquet. "She ran the last 18 miles faster than the first 13," he said. "After it was over, she had a hell of a gash. We stopped, ate, home after 10 P.M. I sat her down and put nine stitches in her head."

I was not athletic and didn't do anything athletic. Eighty-five years ago, when I was born on November 27, 1922, in Fairchance, Pennsylvania, girls did not do anything that made them sweat. My mother thought animals were dirty and didn't allow me to touch any. I was an only child. My mother was a strict disciplinarian. I was taught to knit, crochet, cook, and do everything that would make me a good housewife and a good mother. I did my own housecleaning—nothing particular about that. I was a great baker and a good student. I studied hard; things didn't come easy to me. I always worked hard to do my very best at everything

I did. I was told at home to finish everything I started. My mother's rule was: I wasn't allowed to quit, even if I didn't want to do it or didn't like it. If I started anything like piano lessons or dancing lessons, I had to do it for a year. That way, I could really make up my mind if I liked it or not. When we sat down at the table, I had to eat everything put on my plate, whether I wanted it or not. I had to make my bed before I left to go to school. So it was a strict upbringing.

Both my parents were fifth-generation Americans, non-religious Protestant Baptists. Dad was in construction.

I went to nurses' training at a hospital school. Girls were encouraged in those years for further education to become nurses or teachers or secretaries. Those were the things that were offered to us. So I chose nursing.

I got married the first time when I was 19. I had four children; they are now all between the ages of 51 and 63. I tried to pass on the "must finish" rule; they are all fairly accomplished people. All were born in New York City. I lived there for 25 years. All are now on the East Coast.

I didn't start work until the last one was in school. Became a full-time nurse. After 25 years, the marriage was not working. At 44, I married my second husband, Norman, an oral surgeon, age 30. I guess I started the older-woman/younger man trend, because it's very popular now. Everyone I talk to now, their husband's a little younger.

I was always young-looking for my age. Always healthy, never heavy. Kind of small, always looked 10, 15 years younger than what I was. Even today, no one believes that I'm 85 when I say it.

When Norman went into practice, I worked with him as his assistant. I did that for 8½ years, until I got tired of spending 24 hours together a day. So I left him—I didn't leave him, just the office.

We did scuba diving and spent a lot of time on beaches. Scuba was the only thing I did athletic. We took a college course together and became certified. We did that for seven years. We completely

RUN FOR LIFE

forgot about scuba diving when, 11 years after we got married, we took up running.

THE CHALLENGE

After Norman did his residency, he had to give two years to the army. He was put in the hospital at Fort Campbell, Kentucky. After he was done, I had worked in the hospital in Hopkinsville, the town next to the fort, and the doctor there convinced us to stay and open a practice. We did. And we practiced there until 1983.

A friend, who was an orthopedic surgeon at the hospital we worked at, tried to get Norman to run. He'd run every morning past our home in Hopkinsville, Kentucky. One day, he challenged Norman to run by putting up a flyer for a 10-mile race in our mailbox, and telling us that we had 10 weeks to get ready. Norman is not one to pass up a challenge, even though he was just a sports spectator—he knew more sports than anyone I've ever met. He used to watch games all the time; on weekends he would travel to football games and baseball games. And so he took the challenge. But I also took it with him.

We trained 10 weeks, did the 10-mile race, and have never stopped.

I was embarrassed to go out in, uh, shorts. Runner's shorts. Because there weren't any women running yet. There were only three or four men who ran in the town. But the race drew people from everywhere. There ended up to be 50 in the race—46 were men, and four were females. The other three females were cross-country high school girls and I was 55.

I won the 30-and-over trophy.

At the time of the race, I was no longer working. I was retired from nursing. And I wanted to stay healthy, so I'd been walking every day prior to running. After the race, I figured I'd just run three miles a day to stay healthy, because you do need exercise.

But Norman had greater ideas than me; he was going to train for a marathon. When he was young he said that he thought he might like to run Boston someday.

So he started running 6 miles a day. And I would run my three and even go a little further. But that's all.

Then he went to do his first marathon, and I went along just to watch. The Chicago Marathon was really hot that day, and he did not run as fast as I thought he should. I worried about him—I went to the finish line a couple of times to wait. I was a nervous wreck. I figured he's gonna do about 3:30; he didn't think that. It took him 4:15 or 4:20. About 200 yards from the finish line, he was barely moving. Not breathing at all, just little short puffs, and bent over. He didn't want to walk—wanted to run the whole thing. He'd lost his upper body form.

At the finish line, he lay down for two hours. And I was a nervous wreck. And I said "Never again. Never again am I going to stand and wait for you."

"If you are going to continue this, then I am going to train and do the races also. And you can wait for me." So that's what he's been doing.

He said, "That's great." And I went home and started training.

RUN WITHIN YOURSELF

From then on we did all the races together. However … Norman has gotten injured numerous times, simply because he is a type-A personality and he always wants to do better each time. Improve, improve. If a little is good, more is better. So he has sustained so many injuries. He's done 50 marathons, 50 ultras, and 2 Hawaii Ironmans, but for the last few years has been unable to run. And so …

They never learn.

There is a lesson here: Run relaxed and don't try to do every race a little bit faster. I never try for speed, to go better this year than I did last year. What I do is, there is a certain allotted time to finish to be official, the race closes at a certain time and has cutoffs along the way, I just make sure I make the cutoffs, so I'll be official.

This is the key to staying healthy.

I run within myself. I listen to my body. I know how to take care of myself. I know when I'm going to be in trouble, and I back off. If my pulse rate goes too fast, if I have any feelings that are bad feelings, I do something to take care of it.

I keep mantras running through my head. "Relax and move, relax and move," I keep telling myself. When you get a downer, when you get a monkey on your back and you want to quit, I overrule it with my mental toughness. I back off a little bit; I tell myself not to quit now. I take raisins or nuts or something that I carry with me to get some energy back. And a few minutes later, you feel better.

If I'm at a marathon, and getting tired, I tell myself, "I'll rest this afternoon." If I'm running 50 miles, I'll say, "I'll rest tonight." If I'm running 100 miles, I'll say, "I'll rest tomorrow—don't rest now."

I have missed the cutoff. The first time I tried the Western States 100 in 1983 we lived in Kentucky, where it was nice and warm. When I flew to California, they had 18 feet of snow banked up on the roadside and we had to run over 26 miles over snow at a couple thousand feet altitude up the mountain—the first 4½ miles in deep snow. At the midway point, I missed the cutoff by seven minutes. And I laid down on the trail and said, "Never again [will I do this]."

And then I went to the hotel and slept and got up in the morning to see Norman finish. While I was there, the clock had been turned off, the race was over, but all of the sudden there was this one woman coming to the finish line. The finish was on a track, a school track—you get off the mountain and turn to this school. The lady is coming around the track, covered in mud from head to toe. Everyone was applauding for her because she was going to finish even though she was 15 minutes over the cutoff. Everyone's applauding. The lady standing next to me said, "Is that Helen Klein?"

And I said, "Oh, I wish." Then I explained what happened.

I struck that "Never again," from my vocabulary. And I said, "Well, maybe." And so I never said "Never" again. Then, I said to Norman, "The only way I could really finish a race like that would be if I lived there and could train on that kind of terrain." Because I'm living in tobacco country farmland, flatland and I'm training to run a 100-mile mountain race.

Soon thereafter, we gave up everything in Kentucky and moved to California.

Then I trained on the trails, and the next year I finished the race.

I guess Norman is a positive, upbeat guy. Not as positive as me. He has a lot of negatives. (laughs) Yeah, he was happy to do that (move) so that I could finish that race. And I've been running ever since.

As for my husband's surgery career, when we left Kentucky, he gave it up. He came to California and tried to decide what he would like to do, because he was tired of people complaining—you know, people don't want to go to an oral surgeon, they don't want to have pain, and surgery is not fun, so he was tired of hearing it. He wanted to do something that would make people happy.

So he decided to take a real estate course and sell real estate. He did that for a year, but he wasn't too happy with that, either. Because he is very meticulous and organized, and most people's homes are not in that condition when they are selling. If the house wasn't spotless, he had a hard time pushing it.

After a year, the Western States 100 was advertising for a race director. So he and I applied for that. Six others applied as well. We got it. We directed it for 14 years.

When you direct it, you can't run it. He ran it twice before, but that was it. I started nine times and finished four—and the reason was always the snow. Because I'm lightweight, I land lightly—that's another reason I don't get injured: I don't pound. I'm supposed to weigh 109. Dr. Cooper did a physical on me at his clinic in Dallas, and told me that was my ideal weight. Right now I'm at 105.

HIGHLIGHTS OF 29 YEARS OF RUNNING

All of the hundreds are great. The multiday races, too. I've run in every continent except Antarctica. I love third-world countries. So I love running in China, in Japan, Thailand—they are all highlights. I must say that I'm not competitive, but if someone tries to psyche me out at the beginning of a race, I'm going to beat them or die trying.

One of my highlights was a race across the Sahara Desert, the 1995 Marathon des Sable. One hundred forty-three miles; the longest day was 50 miles. I have no sense of direction; a map means nothing to me. I took a map course and I cannot read a map. Because they don't use a trail, and you do it by compass and map, I wouldn't do it unless I had someone to do it with me. So Norman said he would do it with me.

We got invited, and all our expenses paid up. Four miles into the race, Norman twisted his ankle and got two stress fractures. The doctor thought it was a sprain and taped it up, but after another mile, he couldn't go on. So he told me to go on. Well, I figured if he's not going to finish, one of us had to finish since we were invited. So even with my fear of getting lost—there is very little to see there—I figured if I could just keep someone in sight, I would be okay if they were going on the right course.

I walked the 10 miles to the next place you had to report. All you got was a liter of water at each stop.

You had to carry everything on your back, including all your food for the six days, and the map, everything in your back. It weighed 25 to 30 pounds.

The day Norman got injured, one man gained two hours on me. Over the next two days, he followed me, stayed right on my back, not close enough to talk to me, just a few feet. That annoyed me, because he had two hours on me. So all he had to do was follow me, and he wins.

On the 50-miler, when it was dark, I got away from him. I sort of stopped, and let him go on. I sort of backed away, moved over a few yards, got to the side and far enough ahead of him so he couldn't see the glow stick on my backpack. So I got ahead of him and made up quite a bit of time that day on him. Each day I made up a little more. So I beat him.

If he had been friendly, I wouldn't have thought of passing him. So don't ever psyche me out if you're in a race with me.

That was 2 weeks before the Eco-Challenge. I was 72 and he was 70. So I was on the stand with my award with four other men. I have that picture. And it was a great award, made from an old, old rock.

In Morocco, I did get blisters on my feet from that hot rocks and sand and dunes. It healed before the Eco-Challenge. But I did get problems with the bottom of my feet there, too, but not as bad.

WEIGHTS' DUAL BENEFITS: STRONGER BONES, BETTER FORM

We didn't have a plan. We wanted to do races in various places, and so we'd just train for those. We'd just run every day. Then in 1983, when I came to Western States, I met an older runner who had belonged to a study of a Masters running group at Barnes Hospital at Washington University in St. Louis. He said they had no woman in the study and would love to have me. When I went home, I called them, and they said "yes."

So every two years I would go to Barnes Hospital and stay overnight. They would do two days of studies on me. Put me on a treadmill and run, run, run and they would draw blood and test it. They found out that my body was kind of a lot younger than my years.

They said I had the bones of a 30-year-old. Actually, the last time I had an EKG, my doctor told me that I had the heart of a 20-year-old. I got good results every year I went except for 1988. They did a bone scan on me. My legs and my spine were thicker, like a 30-year-old, but my arms did not come up to that. It had to be the lack of weight-bearing exercise. So they asked me to start weight lifting.

RUN FOR LIFE

I came home, joined a club, and started weight lifting. Prior to that when I would run up the mountain, I'd run the flats and power-walk fast up; when I'd try to run up, I couldn't get enough oxygen. I thought it was because I had small lungs, but actually it was because I'd lose my form. I'd get tired and bent; I slumped a little. That would press in on my diaphragm. I would lie down when I could breathe well on the trail for a moment, oh maybe 30 seconds or a minute, breathe deeply, then get up and go again. Well, I started weight lifting. And 2 years when I went back for the next study, my arm-bone density was the same as my spine and legs. And I didn't have to stop when I'd be going up the mountain because I kept my form better.

Because my muscles were now also stronger in the back from that, I didn't lose my form. Interesting, when I'm running I always tell myself "keep your shoulders back and down" so that I have good form. I haven't had any injuries because of the way I run. I have good biomechanics.

I never had a coach. I read about ChiRunning—it's a lot like I run. It's natural. I try to land lightly, and not pound, pound, pound. I land on my forefoot, but I bring my heels down on every step. Because if you don't, you get plantar fasciitis—that's the plantar connects your toes to your heel, that curls up when you run uphill or downhill. And you don't bring your heel down, it causes plantar fasciitis.

A lot of runners don't do weights of any kind, but they should. Actually, you don't put on weight [when you do it], like many seem to fear; you build muscle and lose fat. You tone your muscles; they look better.

I do it three times a week. Freeweights. One 12-pounder in each hand. All the normal things, curls, lay down and do presses, et cetera. Machines for pull downs—50 pounds.

But no leg exercises. I just do running for that. My legs aren't shriveling. They were always strong because I did lift a lot of patients in the ER. When the ambulance comes in, you run over and lift that patient. You get a good strong body. I know how to lift with my legs so I never hurt my back. Directing races, we have to lift cases of Coke and all kinds of things. So although my legs are a bit loose when I run—not as tight as they used to be—they look the same as they always did. Everybody knows me from the back, anyway, because of my legs.

I do some yoga and Pilates to keep my core strength. I'm not a sitter, I go, go, go.

RIGOROUS DAILY ROUTINE + CLASSIC HEALTHY DIET

I get up at 4 A.M. every day. Long races start at 5, 6 in the morning. If you're not accustomed to getting up then, you don't start well. I have a hot tub on my patio. I get under the jets for 15 minutes and stretch. I keep it at 102 degrees and I get myself all warmed up. Then I come in and eat my breakfast, clean up my kitchen, and make my bed.

I eat a very healthy diet. I make my own almond butter. Out of raw almonds, toasted in the oven with no oil or salt for 15 minutes, then grind them in a Vita-Mix machine. I make my own bread—not white bread, but whole wheat, pumpernickel, or rye. I have an orange juice before the hot tub, then I come in for an almond butter and banana sandwich on my homemade bread, have a cup of coffee. No soft drinks, although I'll have an occasional Coke in long races, along with my usual Gatorade and sports drinks, to stay awake. I then do work around the house for about an hour and a half maybe. Then I go run.

I used to run 10 miles every day. But now I don't feel safe out there alone. So women I run with generally don't want to run that far, so I run maybe 6 miles, and Norman runs with me sometimes. On the weekends it's safer and I run longer.

Every day there are murders and rapes. I live along the American River—there is a bike and equestrian trail right along it where I train. There are a lot of wooded areas with wild animals, and there are many,

many times people get accosted on it. Women are not safe alone, really.

Norman goes on short runs with me. He works a lot of races. We have our own races—a 100- and a 53-miler that we direct. And we have the Helen Klein 50-mile, 50k, and 30k races in September and November. I run the 30k—18.6 miles. It's a good training run for the marathon.

After the 6-mile run, I have my second breakfast. Cereal, banana, fruit. Generally oatmeal or polenta with fruit, and another cup of coffee.

I really would like to be a vegetarian, because I like all the happy foods—the lentils, the peas, the grains, all those things that are healthy. But Norman doesn't like all those things and needs to have some meat. So I eat four ounces of lean meat—beef, fish, or chicken.

After the second breakfast, it's 10 A.M. I do laundry—we have lots of laundry due to all the activities we do. Then it's lunchtime. I like soup, healthy soup. An apple with some cheese. I don't like processed food or fast foods. I have to eat at restaurants when I travel, and I travel a lot, so I like to eat healthy back at home. I eat lots of vegetables, healthy salad with very little dressing, lot of squash, cauliflower. Lots of colored vegetables. Not much butter—I always use olive oil in my cooking. I eat lots of fruit—4 or 5 a day, and a lots of grain, and small portions of turkey or meat. I take an antioxidant multivitamin every day.

I'm a healthy person. I don't have a lot of problems or use medication. I don't get colds or get sick.

After lunch, I work around my house or sit down to read. I've been reading more lately. I don't watch television. I walk around—just keep moving. I have friends come over and run with me. One gal comes and runs with me twice a week early in the morning. I coached her and she likes to run with me. She drives an hour and 15 minutes each way. We do 10, 15 miles together.

You have to push it—but not for speed. I never have any pain in my muscles or joints. Just the pain of exhaustion. On rare occasions, I do interval training. When I was doing 24-hour track runs for records, I would go on our bike path, marked every mile, running ¾ of a mile and walking a quarter. I would eat on the walk. When I got to the track, I'd run 3 laps and walk one, continuing that for 24 hours. The first time I did that, when I was about 65, I got the world record. 102 miles. I had gone 100, and the official said, "If you go 8 more laps, you'll get the world record."

A French lady then ran 102½ a couple of months later. So I went back and ran 103½. The next time I ran 105½. When I was 70, I ran 109½. The way I did it was—and I didn't get any faster—was that I would run four and walk one, instead of run three and walk one. So the only time I did speed training was for that.

No regular intervals. But on the bike path, there is a final straightaway at the end that I try to do all-out. Then I walk through the park home.

SLOWING DOWN

Yes, I have slowed down. When I was 80, I wanted to do a 4:45 at the California International Marathon because it would break the world record by about 20 minutes. So I trained my regular 10 miles a day, took one day off, ran 1½ miles to the gym, worked out, and ran home. On race day, I had a perfect day. It was cool, the way I run best, and I ran 4:31, and I broke the 80–84 world record by almost 39 minutes.

Well, it's five years later, and … I'm slower now. In my last five marathons, I've been running 5:15, 5:10. Fargo, North Dakota in 5:13; an all-woman's race in Spearfish, South Dakota in 5:17; the Portland Marathon—had a tough day in 5:40; the California International in 5:16; and the Napa Valley Marathon in March '07 in 5:15. In the last year, I've gotten even slower. I did 18.6 miles last Saturday. It took me 3:53.

I'm training for the California International again. I have to, because it's here; it runs from Folsom to the state capitol. At mile 10, I'm very near my home. I could turn down a hill and be home in 5 minutes. The race closes in 6 hours, so that's what I'm shooting for.

The record is 6:53 for an 85-year old. Everyone says that's a piece of cake—but it's not! 26.2 miles is not a piece of cake when you're 85. I could not understand why, when I was running better, how the time could get that much worse in five years. The lady who set the record of 6:53 took almost ten hours—9:53—when she did it at 90. I didn't understand the falloff, but now I know.

It's not that the deterioration accelerates, it's just the aging alone. If you're 85 … They say you lose 3% of your ability to use oxygen every decade. Your body is older and functions slower. But I'm happy it functions!

I won't lift weights with my legs because my legs aren't the problem. It's the whole body that's the problem. I'm not going to fight it—that would require going out and training really hard, and that's not the way I do things.

Can I run to 100? you ask. It's not impossible that I run at 100. I read a story about a guy running on the track at 100. But do I want to?

HIKING TO 100?

Actually, I'm getting bored with running. Because I've been doing it for so long, and I'm not accustomed to staying with anything that long and not having changed. It's become our whole life—we direct our own races, and, to pay back the people who volunteer at our races, we work their races. Maybe it's time for something else.

I don't have good balance on the bike. You saw me at the Eco-Challenge and you know that I fell. I put the bike away. I don't row or anything else. I don't have the time.

I like to hike and see where I've been. Because when you're running, you don't see it—you have to watch your footing. So we did start hiking; we've done several good hikes.

When I moved to California, I met a woman who was 68 and she was hiking the trails that we would be

running. I said to Norman then, "Boy, when I'm 68, I hope I'm able to do that." And here I am, 85 and still running, and we'd like to be hiking.

When we started running, we went to Nepal. And we hiked to the base camp of Mount Everest. We spent the whole month of March in Nepal, and did all the trails up to 18,000 feet. It was really great. I would really like to do that again. When I do quit running, I will hike. I don't think I'll ever get up Mt. Everest. But I have climbed a big mountain in China, and I climbed Mt. Fuji and slept up there.

Hiking and walking are different things. I only walk through the aid station to get a drink, then walk to the waste basket to toss the cup in. And now, I definitely can't afford to walk more because I can't run fast enough to walk and make the cutoffs.

On the 100-milers and 50-milers on trails (on the other hand) I always power-walk the uphills. Some of 'em are like 2- or 3-mile climbs. And you can't run that steep mountain. You can power-walk it just a few seconds slower than if you ran it, because you can't have a big stride when it's steep.

I've been trying to stop Norman from race-directing, and let's just go hike and see the world. Even if a marathon at 85 was my last one, it wouldn't bother me. But I wouldn't sit. I'd probably walk 5 miles every morning. And go hiking on the weekends or my off days. I want to be mobile as long as I'm on the earth. I don't want to be a bother to my children or my husband. I don't want anyone to have to take care of me. I'm very independent.

If I replace the running with walking and hiking, I'll eat less. I have to eat so much food—it's terrible. I'm eating every two hours now all day long—and I still lose weight when I race.

READY TO PASS THE TORCH

When I do my talks to groups, the most common question I get from non-runners is "Am I too old to start running?" I get a lot of 50-year-olds. I tell them I started at 55. I speak at a lot of nursing home facilities, so I talk to a lot of doctors and nurses. The 50-year-olds say, "Oooh, it's not too late for me."

People ask about diet. They all want to know what to eat. Any magazine or newspaper you pick up—it's all there. They say the things I've been saying all along. Been preaching that for years.

But I won't write a book. Here's a story that explains why: I'm left handed. I went to school later than my friends for first grade because of my November birthday, so my mother taught me to read and write so that I could keep up. On the first day of school, the teacher said, "If you can print your name now, pick up your pencil." Everybody had a pencil and a sheet of paper on their desk. I was so excited because I'm not only going to print my name, but I'm going to write it cursive. As I'm printing my name, the teacher comes down the aisle from the back and has a ruler in her hand—and she whacks my hand, knocks the pencil to the floor, and yells at me, "Pick up that pencil in your right hand." The girls were not allowed to use [their] left hands in school. Now, I don't know what the reasoning was behind it was, but they thought it was wrong.

So until the seventh grade, I had to use my right hand. I could write beautifully with my left, but I could not write with my right. So I struggled. When I got home, I would do my homework with my left hand, but try to make it look like my right hand's writing, so my teacher wouldn't think that my mother did my homework. So, now—that was the most traumatic thing that ever happened to me. And even now, when I pick up a pen or pencil to write, that's in my head. It's a terrible, terrible thing. So I'm not writing a book.

I actually had a book out, but I didn't write it. It's no longer in print. It came about when I did a testimonial for a running book. If I had seen that from the beginning when I started running, I wouldn't have learned by trial and error. Anyhow, the author came over to our house,

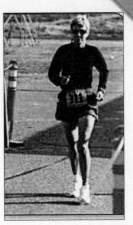

looked at 2 large boxes full of magazines and newspaper articles about me, and put together a book of quotes of mine he thought would be good for runners. I had a thousand printed and sold it. The name of it was, No Limits Living. I called it that due to my age and my sex. Because all these years, I've been trying to find what the limit is. And eventually I will come to it.

When I finished a couple of Western States, the oldest female and male finisher always got a clock from Dr. Wally Bortz, an octogenarian geriatrician who teaches at Stanford and is active in Palo Alto. He wrote a book, We Live Too Short and Die Too Long. He has patients who are 107, 105. He says you should be able to live to 125, with a good lifestyle and some good genes. When he gave me that book, I came home and read it in two nights. And I decided I wanted to live to 125. Then, a few years later, he wrote another book which he presented to me with the clock. It was called Dare to Be 100. I told Ruth Ann, his wife, that I wasn't going to let him take that extra 25 years away from me. But that may change.

With the world the way it is right now, with everything that's going on, I don't want to live to 125. Global warming. All the cheating in sports—in every form of sports, it's so bad. It's just not a good world right now. So I'll be happy with 100.

They all say, "Helen, you can't quit, you can't quit—you're our inspiration." But I think it's time for someone else to take over and be that inspiration. And I tell them, my answer is always, "Everyone that toes the start-line inspires me."

RUN FOR LIFE

HELEN KLEIN

RUN BALANCED

In early 2000, when I was 43, I went to a clinic and had my picture taken twice. First a profile shot of my body, then a head-on shot. After being printed out, the photos were overlaid with a grid of horizontal and vertical lines.

I was shocked.

My body was visibly, obviously out of balance. My right shoulder tilted up 2 inches higher than my left. My left hip was higher than the right. I was twisted to the right. I leaned forward on my toes with my butt sucked in, shoulders slumped, and my hands hanging on the front of my thighs, not on the side.

"It's no surprise—you're the typical aging athlete," I was told. "Your posture is corroding."

Typical? Aging? I thought I looked pretty good for my age, but there it was on the grid: clearly out of balance. And it dawned on me: Could this have anything to do with all these years of nagging injuries?

"You don't want to build a Ferrari on a bent frame," says the picture-taker, postural therapist Patrick Mummy, whose Sacramento- and San Diego–based Symmetry—The Pain Relief Clinics (SymmetryforHealth.com) have a unique track record of straightening people out. Symmetry uses a little-known treatment method called Postural Therapy, which is based on the theory that chronic pain is caused by muscular imbalances—simply, that some muscles are overused while corresponding muscles are underused. As the imbalances solidify, the body's symmetrical harmony is lost and the overworked muscles eventually begin to hurt. The pain can be stopped when we learn how to regain symmetry by shifting some of the load back to the underutilized muscles.

"You want to run to 100? By definition, Step One must be posture," Mummy says. "Otherwise, everything you do to build yourself up—the running, the weights, the cross-training—is reinforcing the problem."

Poor posture, which starts the minute that we stop running around as kids and start sitting at a desk, says Mummy, doesn't just look bad. And it doesn't only cause back pain, although that malady is so widespread that it is the number-one cause of missed work time in America. A drooping neck, a hunched back, rounded-forward shoulders—conditions increasingly seen even in computer-addicted 10-year-olds—restrict breathing and digestion, hurt athletic and fitness performance, and are the basis of a multitude of injuries and joint conditions. Think about it: Why did Scott Tinley and the other endurance athletes described in "Bionic Body Parts" (Chapter 23) each wear out just *one* side of their hips? Because they are imbalanced. Maybe if they'd gotten straightened out two decades ago, they wouldn't have had to spend $30,000 each to have a cobalt-chrome ball and cup installed in their hip sockets.

This section of *Run for Life* offers a way to solidify and permanent-ize the posture-correction issues that were first addressed in the Soft Running section by a vertical arm swing. It gives you a general 8-step posture-alignment plan that Mummy designed for runners, and starts with a striking case study that highlights the benefits of improving your posture.

CHAPTER 8

WHEN McCASKILL WENT STRAIGHT

Superrunner Dan McCaskill was desperate to stop his agonizing pain. Could postural therapy save his career?

It was painful to watch. Awkwardly, agonizingly, a man, apparently a cripple, shuffled along, one shoulder tilted at a weird angle relative to the other, his left leg dragging behind him as if it were broken. It seemed to take him forever to move 20 yards. The crowd began to notice and murmur comments of sympathy. Poor old guy.

Then 58-year-old Dan McCaskill shocked everyone. He finally limped his way to the podium, then leaned forward. It was 1999. For the fourth year in a row, he was handed the first-place medal for winning his age-group at the Torrey Pines 5k run.

Maybe the finest masters road racer in the San Diego area over the previous 20 years, McCaskill, then of Carlsbad, made a career of proving that you don't need to be able to walk to run. A retired Federal Agent with the U.S. Border Patrol and a former 82nd Airborne army paratrooper, McCaskill began running for fitness in the early seventies and soon was untouchable at races ranging from the 1,500 meters to the marathon. At age 39, he ran a 1:10 half marathon. At 40, he ran the fastest Masters 15k, 49:12, and a sub-32 10k. Training 75 to 100 miles a week, he became the national age-group 3000-meter steeplechase champion at 45. At 50, he won the national age-group 25k championship. At 55, he could still run a 34-minute 10k.

McCaskill's competed in so many races—over 1,000, he thinks—and won so many of them, that he can't remember times, dates, and even names of the events. But he has all of them—plus every daily workout in between—meticulously labeled, dated, and commented on in logbooks. Running and racing are his life.

"I've probably won my age-group at every race in San Diego," he guesses. "Nobody could touch me. In my 40s, I could win races outright."

He retired from work at 50 just so that he could concentrate on racing. As he neared 60, he could still finish in the overall top 25 of a 5k.

But while McCaskill thought he'd spend the rest of his days running happily into the sunset, his body stopped cooperating.

"Throughout my career, I'd always be crippled the day after the race, but I'd just take a pill and stretch," he says. "Then, in the nineties, the pain got so bad that I thought I'd have to give up running for good." In 1999, for the first time ever, he had to stop and drop out of two races because he was in so much pain.

A laundry list of injuries a kilometer long, starting in his youth, finally caught up with him. In high school, a broken femur kept McCaskill in traction for a month and a body cast for a year, leaving his left leg an inch longer than the right. He had two separated shoulders, skull fractures, and several cracked ribs from bike crashes in the eighties. Since 1981, he's been plagued by chronic sciatica, which tightens his left leg during races, causes a limp when he walks, and often forces him to drive his car while sitting on one cheek

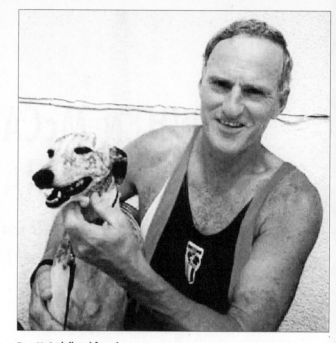

Dan McCaskill and friend.

of his ass. In 1984, his left Achilles tendon swelled to three times its normal size; on doctor's orders, he didn't run or bike for a year. The next year, when he got back up to 60 training miles a week, the Achilles flared again. He ran on it until he could stand no more, undergoing the first of five Achilles operations in 1994.

In short, McCaskill was a mess. He tried everything: massage therapy, physical therapy, yoga 5 days a week, anti-inflammatories, vegetarianism, chiropractic treatment.

By January 2000, with his right Achilles now as bad as his left one ever was, and his shoulders so misaligned that a tailor had to make him a suit with one

94

side of the collar sewn higher than the other, McCaskill knew he had to try something radical. His pain wasn't just ruining his running, it was distorting his body, wrecking his life. On the recommendation of a friend, he went to Symmetry.

TRUING A BATTERED WHEEL

On January 27, McCaskill drove to Rancho Bernardo and hobbled into Patrick Mummy's office.

"The second he walked in the door, it was obvious that Dan was the most inflexible man I'd ever seen," said Symmetry's cofounder and owner. "He was tighter than tight, no fluidity, total bilateral dysfunction and deviation."

A gait and postural analysis proved it. Mummy measured McCaskill like a cabinetmaker measuring kitchen wall dimensions. Using a pelvation meter (basically a fancy level), Mummy found that the left side of McCaskill's pelvis was angled 14 degrees, while the right side was angled 5 degrees—a whopping 9-degree disparity. His left shoulder blade was elevated 3 degrees. The hips and head tilted forward 4 degrees more than they should. The upper torso rotated right to left. The pelvis rotated left to right. The upper torso was offset to the left. McCaskill stood with too much weight on the right leg, both heels and on the inside of each foot.

McCaskill was like a bicycle rim way out of true; some spokes bore a heavy load while others did nothing at all. "His posture showed so many compensations and imbalances that it impacted his running, walking, and all his movements," said Mummy.

When it was time for the diagnosis, he didn't pull punches.

"To tell you the truth, I don't understand how you can walk," said Mummy. "To undo all your imbalances, it's going to take lots of work over the next ten weeks."

Mummy then made McCaskill an individualized, 10-position routine of stretching/strengthening exercises chosen to deemphasize his over-contracted muscles, particularly the unnatural left-hip elevation and the pelvic angle's huge left-right disparity. The positions involved laying on his back with legs twisted, pressing against walls, and bending over chairs.

McCaskill was to do the hourlong routine at home twice a day, holding each position for several minutes. Once he showed progress with these exercises, Mummy would give him progressively more strenuous exercises. Symmetry has a bank of 350 exercises, about 30% of them straight from yoga, all pictured in the book and CD-ROM *Symmetry: Relieve Pain, Optimize Physical Motion* that McCaskill took with him.

Asked how the exercises felt on Day 1, McCaskill replied succinctly: "It hurt like hell."

95

THE 10-WEEK PLAN

Like the old song, however, *it hurt so good.*

"Afterwards, my body was much more in alignment, looser, less painful. I had more range of motion in my movements. I walking much more fluid and balanced," says McCaskill. "It was a rarity for me." Technically, he was suddenly using his left side more equally with his right.

Through Week 1, McCaskill grew looser and his stride more fluid. He called some of the Symmetry positions "tortuous," and was plenty sore in the worked areas, but the payoff was clear. On the morning of Day 4, he noticed he could walk down the stairs with far less effort than normal, not holding on to the banisters for the first time in years.

On February 1, after 6 days of exercises, McCaskill returned to Symmetry. The results: his hip angle disparity improved from 9 degrees to 4 degrees, with significant improvement in his shoulders, standing posture, and walking gait. He went home with a new set of exercises that targeted his unnatural rotation.

"Some of them were even more painful than the first ones," said McCaskill. "My tendons, muscles, and bones were in complete rebellion."

Technically, he was right. He was experiencing what Mummy calls "transitional pain," where muscles resist as they are being reeducated to perform differently.

By Day 13, McCaskill was still sore, but felt a more balanced, longer stride with each run. His hip angle disparity dropped to 1 degree. Four days later, he did his first sustained high-intensity workout in years.

On Day 20 came a major breakthrough. For the first time in 25 years of running, McCaskill felt as if his left leg was "doing its job."

On Day 27, McCaskill noticed he hadn't taken a pain pill for a few days. He had much-improved range of motion in his shoulders and wasn't limping as much while walking. Four days later, he finished the Torrey Pines 5k race in 20:23, taking first in the 55–59s, his fifth win in a row. He still looked like hell at the awards ceremony, but felt surprisingly good. A few days later, he was astounded to find that he had no sciatica pain.

March 15 (Day 48) was a landmark day with a twist: Despite a perfect 10-degree/10-degree hip angle, and increasing range of motion on his right side and shoulders, nearly all of McCaskill's other measurements were worse. He had a great deal of muscular pain, and complained of a sudden decrease in left leg function.

The explanation, explains Mummy, is a final "transition phase," where the body tries one last time to fight the changes. "It's like the 'detox' phase in an alcoholic's recovery program, where the body is ridding itself of its last toxins," he says.

96

April 19 (Day 83) was Graduation Day, McCaskill's last appointment with Mummy. And it was beautiful. The "detox" theory was correct. Perfectly matching pelvic tilts. Shoulders level. No trunk rotations. Left hip elevated just ½ degree. Side view and frontal plane flawless.

McCaskill took a final set of exercises from Mummy to do on his own, then did a hard Fartlek workout. He felt smooth and balanced. His sciatica didn't act up. His limp was gone. He ran fluidly, with an even gait, and had no recovery pain later.

A string of wins followed. A 20:19 at the Clif Bar 5k. 21:58 at the Calloway 5k. A red-hot 19:48 at the Bonita Bunny Run 5k. 26:31 at the Temecula 4-miler. 42:18 at the Citrus 10k. 19:48 at Cal State San Marcos 5k. 26:47 at the Terry Fox 4-miler. A smokin' 19:53 3rd place at the Turf to Surf 5k. All pain-free.

Was McCaskill cured? Technically, no: He'd have to do postural exercises the rest of his life, or risk regression, warned Mummy. But in terms of lifestyle, he truly felt like a new man.

"I am no longer the walking dead," he said.

THE FOLLOW UP: REALITY STRIKES

I first interviewed McCaskill for *Competitor* magazine in mid-2000, then followed up in June 2008. He had moved inland to Fallbrook, in rural northern San Diego County, where he bought a big piece of property and was running an hour a day on dirt trails with his greyhounds. But life hadn't been as idyllic as it sounds.

In November 2000, after completing his 83-day Symmetry regimen and winning a slew of races, McCaskill had his fifth Achilles surgery. After a slow, painful recovery, he raced again the next March and began a 2-year winning streak that included a 22:28 at the Lake Elsinore 5k on November 22, 2003.

It was his last race.

"The pain was too great," he said. "My sciatica." After his Achilles operation, it came back worse than ever. Having moved an hour away from San Diego, he didn't care to make the drive back to see Symmetry in San Diego. The next year, Mummy moved to Sacramento. So McCaskill switched to yoga seven days a week and worked out with weights and exercise balls. He took lots of pain-killers. All the while, he kept running an hour a day with his dogs—but only slow, "junk" miles.

"I hurt too much to run hard, and had to take too many days off," he said. "I was getting slower. And I won't race if I can't be competitive—it'd be too embarrassing."

In 2005, an MRI told McCaskill what he had long feared: degeneration in his lumbar spine that was affecting the nerves of his spinal cord. It looked so bad that the doctor told him, "you ought to be paralyzed." Years of running 75- to 100-mile weeks while misaligned had given him severe stenosis and spondylosis in his

L-1 through L-5 vertebrae. Stenosis narrows the vertebrae tunnel and clogs it with bone spurs. Spondylosis narrows the space between adjacent vertebrae and causes them to loosen and shift around, like bricks after an earthquake. Both rub and pinch the spinal cord, leading to muscular weakness and severe pain in the neck, shoulder, arm, back, and/or leg.

"I needed it Roto-Rootered out," said McCaskill. No operation does that perfectly yet, but 9½ hours of arthroscopic surgery on December 31, 2007, scraped some of the bone spurs off. Now the sciatica pain in his right glute is gone—but replaced by constant pain in his right calf. Another operation doesn't excite him.

McCaskill's not into self-pity. He doesn't ponder the "what-ifs"—wondering what might have happened had something like Symmetry been around to straighten him out a couple decades earlier, before the damage was done. "Lots of people are a hell of a lot worse than me," he says. "I did pet-assisted therapy with my greyhounds at old folks' homes, and seeing them made me thankful for all I've been able to do. And I'm still healthy enough to run an hour a day—just not fast."

Besides the running, McCaskill gets an all-body workout during three or four hours a day of pruning, digging, and raking on his property. All the searching on the Internet for solutions to his pain over the years has made him something of a walking, talking medical encyclopedia. And an optimist.

"I keep thinking the 'immaculate solution' is right around the corner," he says. "They'll soon be able to inject stem cells into my spine and fix the nerve damage. They've already done it with rats, you know. If all goes as it should, give me a call in 2011."

That's when McCaskill turns 70—and starts staging his comeback.

CHAPTER 9

STAND TALL LIKE A KINDERGARTENER

Feel young again with the Symmetry 8-step runners' posture plan

Shoulders back. Chest forward. Back arched. Butt back and prominent. Stomach rounded, not sucked in. Belly button angled slightly downward. Ankle, knee, hip, shoulder, and ear vertically lined up. Shoulders and hips horizontally lined up. Body balanced, 50/50, side-to-side, front-to-back, ready for endless hours of nonstop motion. Posture perfect as nature intended it. It's a 5-year-old boy. If you want to run to 100, it would benefit you to try to look like him.

"Everyone blames running for breaking down the joints," says Patrick Mummy, who has a picture of the above boy in his office. "But running itself as a fitness activity is not the culprit. It's really due to the body not being in optimal balance, not being in symmetry. If you're properly aligned and balanced, there is no such thing as overuse injuries. You can run as much as you want—if you keep yourself balanced."

Well, what would you expect him to say? Posture is Mummy's business; not coincidentally, he named it Symmetry. But he makes a good point: Why do you wear out the right knee before the left? Why did the four people profiled in Chapter 23 get just one hip resurfaced, not two? For that matter, why do all kinds of body parts constantly go out of whack on runners? We all know what happens when one wheel of your car is out of alignment: the car pulls to one side and that tire wears out quicker. Well, the human body is many times more complex than a car.

Some of those imbalances come from compensations from injuries. But Mummy thinks many factors contribute, including a culture of sitting, lack of pulling exercises, and—surprise!—running.

"I can spot a runner who only runs a mile away," he says. "They aren't balanced; Their hips are forward of the knees, ankles, shoulders, and head. In a balanced body, all these are aligned on a vertical line."

Wait a second. Didn't he just say that running was *not* the problem?

The problem, Mummy says, is that runners usually only run and do nothing else. So, athletically, they only move in a linear fashion. They don't move side to side, or twist. They don't even move backward in the linear plane—only forward. This is not good given that the human body was designed to operate in these three planes of motion.

"When runners focus on the linear plane to the exclusion of the others, the muscles involved in forward movement get overdeveloped," he says. "This pulls your posture out of balance. Hips being forward of the knees puts tremendous pressure on the knees. Injuries are almost inevitable."

But we can't blame all posture problems on running. Your posture started corroding a lot earlier. "In fact, we know almost exactly when," says Mummy: "The day we ran off the playground and started sitting at a desk. At the ripe old age of 5, we begin to break down."

To fully understand why, let's go back to the 5-year-old boy with the perfect posture mentioned earlier, the one you see in the photo. His name is Conner.

It took Mummy many years to find Conner, but when he did, it was an "ah-ha" moment that changed everything. It started at San Diego State University in the early nineties, where Mummy was a top baseball player who suffered from chronic injuries. With no answers forthcoming from doctors, he began thinking his problems were posture-related. Armed with a degree in exercise physiology, he began borrowing from a grab bag of Eastern therapies, including martial arts, yoga,

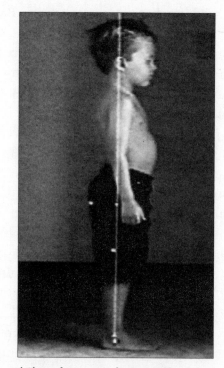

Your goal: The perfect posture of a 5-year-old.

and tai chi to "realign" out-of-balance bodies with stretching and strengthening exercises. But what actually was correct balance? Was it different for everyone, or was there an ideal form? Every adult that Mummy measured was different.

Then he measured kids.

"It was uncanny," he says. "Every 2- to 5-year-old I measured had the same three posture and balance characteristics: Number one, half the body's weight is in front of a vertical line that can be drawn from ear to shoulder to hip to knee to ankle, and half is behind. Two: The right and left sides of the shoulders and hips are level. And three: To facilitate rotation, the pelvis is canted at a 10-degree slope from the iliac crest, a posterior-to-anterior tilt that angles the belly button downward, not parallel to the floor."

To Mummy, it was clear that this uncorrupted position, technically where the sagittal (linear), transverse (sideways), and coronal (rotational) planes of motion all meet, is the true ideal posture—and that the idea that everyone has their own individual posture is hogwash.

"This is the perfect posture for motion, which we were designed to be in 80% of the day," says Mummy. He explains that the 10-degree tilt of the pelvis is the most effective angle to help the hip flexor do its job of pulling up the leg, a key to motion. The level hips give you a perfect ability to rotate side to side. The lined-up ankle, hip, and ear assure right-to-left balance.

When these three lines, or planes, are in alignment, the body is in "Dynamic Tension"—a postural state, Mummy claims, in which every muscle of the body is at the same tension, where breathing is optimized, where the core body is ready for action.

Unfortunately, this perfect state of Dynamic Tension is fleeting. Early in modern life, children begin to do something unnatural: They sit for long periods of time. They don't want to—they are forced to. And the posture breakdown begins.

As we sit, the less we move the pelvis, which Mummy calls the "fulcrum" of all of our movement and the "center of our energy." The hip flexor muscles begin to shorten, pulling up the pelvis, drawing your butt in under you, and making the lower-back muscles work harder. Shoulders crouch forward to write or type, hips cant to one side or the other (elevating one shoulder higher than the other), and repetitive motion creates right- or left-hand dominance. Add an accumulation of injuries and an overemphasis on chest presses instead of pulls, and you develop what Mummy calls the "suck and tuck": butt drawn in, belly pushed up, shoulders stooped, diaphragm collapsed and lower back flattened—an ache-ridden, constricted position that squeezes lungs and intestines.

Ironically, being athletic exacerbates the problem. "Athletes are actually worse off than sedentary people regarding posture," says Mummy. "They are not only out of balance, but they actively reinforce it. They are exercising on a misaligned posture."

Take runners, who are always in the sagittal plane.

"In the sagittal plane, you are always working your hip flexors, quads, and hamstrings," says Mummy. "While they get overused, the adductors and abductors (the lateral movers) and transverse abdominals (the twisters) get underused. Sitting at a desk all day long further atrophies the lateral stabilizers.

"The result: The butt pulls forward. IT bands tighten up because they are trying to keep you from falling over. The knees and hips start to wear out quicker—not from running too many miles, but from being out of place. After all, they have to overcompensate to make up for the imbalanced body position. They are no longer positioned correctly to take on the forces of gravity."

The perfected balanced human body, standing at rest, should have virtually no muscular tension, according to Mummy. It was designed to balance bone on bone in gravity, with subtle "intrinsic" muscles holding everything in place. The bigger "dynamic" muscles, the ones that move you, should be completely at rest.

Here's a way he says you can test this yourself: Standing on your heels with butt back, back arched, and shoulders back (so that ear, shoulder, hips, knees, and ankles are in a vertical line), push an index finger into your butt muscle. It's a big, dynamic muscle, intended for motion. It should be soft. If it's not, readjust until it is. Now you are in balance. But if you slouch your hips forward so that your naval retilts upward, the butt suddenly tightens up. Since you are no longer naturally in balance, the butt has to go to work to hold you upright.

Exacerbating the imbalances of running and sitting is aging, which deteriorates the function and strength of all the muscles, intrinsic and dynamic. Some wear out quicker than others, wreaking more havoc with posture and forcing more muscles to work overtime to compensate.

SOLUTIONS

Maintaining a natural posture in an unnatural environment is a challenge. "In

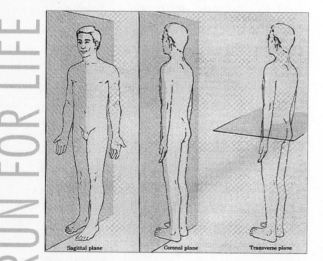

Sagittal plane   Coronal plane   Transverse plane

The 3 planes of perfect posture.

an ideal world, athletes would do multi-planal training—which is different than cross-training," Mummy says. "Traditional crosstraining sports like cycling and rowing are even more linear (in the sagittal plane) than running. Swimming has twisting, but since it's done in an anti-gravity environment, it doesn't work the coronal plane so much." According to Mummy, functional, multi-plane sports like tennis, basketball, boxing, soccer, and even Frisbee throwing, which involves twisting, backpedaling, and moving in all directions, would be good complements to running.

But a couple days a week of hitting backhands probably won't be enough to undo years of poor posture. This is where the Symmetry exercises come in. As he did with me and Dan McCaskill, Mummy measures the difference in height between pairs of hips and shoulders, checks the pelvic tilt, looks at side-to-side and front-to-back symmetry, feeds the data into a database of 300 stretching-strengthening exercises, and gets an 8-exercise printout of a body-straightening plan. As the athlete's posture changes and progresses, as you saw with McCaskill, so does the plan.

Many therapists prescribe orthotics and heel lifts, but Mummy is against that. He believes that the majority of leg-length discrepancies are not real, but caused by the body's imbalances. "We are so conditioned to go after pain sites, and not try to figure out the source of the pain," he says. "What are you going to do—resurface every joint in your body?"

That may be possible someday, given advances in medical science. But Mummy's general posture plan for runners who have a common case of the old "suck-and-tuck" is here now at a pretty good price: free.

SYMMETRY'S 8-STEP POSTURE ROUTINE FOR RUNNERS

The 8-exercise set below will take 10 to 12 minutes to complete. It'll help stretch hip flexors to restore correct pelvic tilt, reposition shoulders back, and equalize hips. Perform in the order given often, especially as part of a warm-up for weight lifting or aerobics.

EXERCISE #1

Static Floor

Purpose: Relaxes and evens spine muscles to prepare for exercise.
Time: 5 minutes

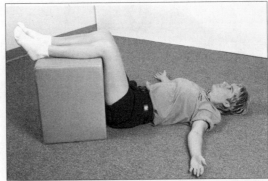

How to: Lie on your back with both legs on an 18-to-20-inch block or seat of a chair, knees bent to 90 degrees. Keep your arms out to your side with your palms up. Relax your back into the floor and breathe through your diaphragm.

EXERCISE #2

Piriformis Stretch (a.k.a. Crossover)

Purpose: Removes pelvic elevations, untwists the hips, and indirectly repositions shoulders.

Time: 1 minute per side

How to: Lie on your back with your knees bent, with your feet on the floor and hip-width. Cross your right ankle to left knee, pivot off the outside of your left foot, and rotate your right foot and left

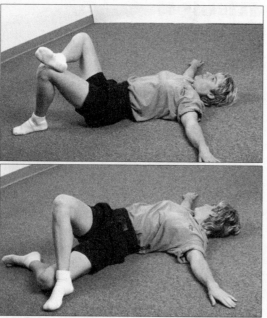

knee to the floor as one unit. Make sure to not let your left foot slide in as your rotate on its side. Keeping your right foot flat on the floor, press your right knee slightly away, feeling a stretch on the outside of the right hip. Place arms out to the side, relax your shoulders and stomach, and look the opposite direction.

Exercises #3, #4, and #5 all are designed to lessen pressure on the knees by repositioning the hips back and retilting them to their natural 10-degree downward tilt, ultimately reducing injuries. The problem: Because runners only move forward in the sagittal plane and don't move sideways, their abductors are neglected and weakened vis-à-vis the overdeveloped hip flexors, shifting the hips forward and tilting them up toward a zero-degree angle. With runners' hips almost always shifted forward of the ear-shoulder-knee-ankle line, the knees have to compensate, resulting in extra flexion and pressure.

EXERCISE #3

Hip Abduction/Adduction

Purpose: To even out the angle of the pelvis left to right at a uniform 10-degree tilt.

Quantity: 2 sets x 20 reps

How to: Lying on your back with your knees and hips bent at 90 degrees, place your feet hip-width and straight on a wall. Keep your feet straight (almost pigeon-toed), slowly spread your knees

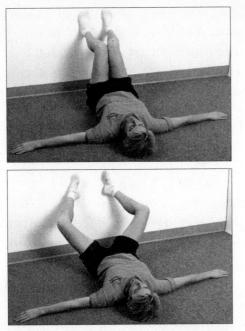

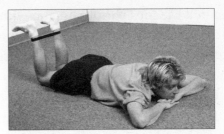

Using a strap can be an effective way to strengthen abductors.

apart while pivoting on the outside of your feet while keeping your heels on the wall, then bring your knees together, and then repeat. After each set, reposition your feet correctly on the wall if necessary. Relax your stomach and shoulders.

hips back and lower the belly button to the proper 10-degree tilt.

Quantity: 3 sets x 20 reps per leg

How to: Lie on your side with your head resting on your arm and extend your body as straight as possible. Bend the leg closest to the floor 90 degrees, tighten the other leg, and pull your toes back. Rotate straightened leg by pointing your knee to the floor and heel pointing to the ceiling, then raise your leg to the ceiling and back down again without rotating your hips. Keep your upper body rested. Alternate sides.

EXERCISE #4

Outer Thigh Lifts

Purpose: Stabilize and strengthen the outer muscles (abductors) to help pull the

EXERCISE #5

Triangle

Purpose: Another way—by using isometrics—to strengthen the abductors

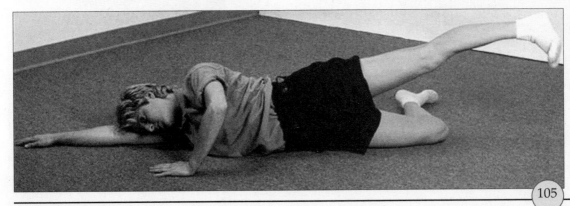

and pull the hips back to line up with the knees, ankles, and shoulders. As you bend laterally, the wall provides a reference point to align all the load-bearing joints from a profile view.

Time: 1 minute per side

How to: Standing with right foot perpendicular to wall (heel on wall), rotate left foot so that it is perpendicular to the right foot and 3 inches off the wall. Take a healthy step out with the left foot, keeping it 3 inches off the wall. Place arms out to your side with palms facing out. Tighten quads, and, keeping both glutes and shoulders on the wall, rotate the upper body from the waist toward the left foot.

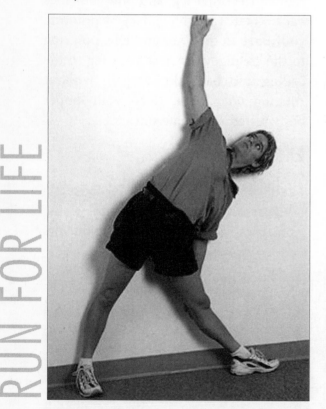

Slide down until the right glute starts to come off the wall, then hold position and take your right arm and stretch it over the top. Look up at right hand. *Breathe.* Try to hold one minute in that position.

EXERCISE #6

Joggers' Stretch (Assisted)

Purpose: Simply stretches out your hamstring. More importantly, it realigns your knees to be over the feet. Helps to track the knees better to get rid of knee pain.

Time: 1 minute per side.

How to: With your right foot flat on the floor, kneel down, placing your left knee directly behind the right foot. Curl your left toes under, making sure that your feet are straight and directly in line with each other. Place your hands on a chair in front of you and stand up, keeping your quads tight and your back flat, placing your feet flat on the floor without changing your foot position. Keep your hips square by

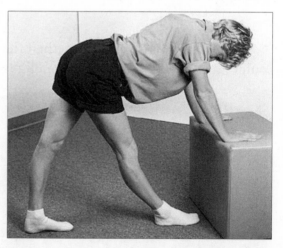

not allowing them to rotate. Shoulders and stomach should remain relaxed. Hold for 1 minute per position and return to the kneeling position when finished.

EXERCISE #7

Standing Overhead Reach

Purpose: Lengthens and decompresses your spine, making you taller and relieving pressure on discs squeezed by gravity and the pounding of running.

Time: 1 minute

How to: Place your forearms on a waist-high counter with your feet hip-width apart and your feet pointing straight ahead. Walk your feet back until your hips are directly over your ankles as you bend at your waist. With your quads tight, arch your lower back, allowing your head and stomach to drop toward the floor. Keep your stomach relaxed and maintain the weight on the balls of your feet. Feel it in your hamstrings and back.

EXERCISE #8

Wall Sit

Purpose: This is the glue that holds the previous exercises together, lowering your center of gravity by strengthening pelvic muscles and quads and unbowing your posture.

Time: 1 to 2 minutes

How to: With your lower back against a wall, slowly walk your feet away from the wall. Keeping your feet hip-width apart and straight ahead, slide down until your knees are at a 90-degree angle or just above. Press your lower back into the wall by placing the weight on your heels and not your toes. Keep stomach and shoulders relaxed. Feel it in your thighs.

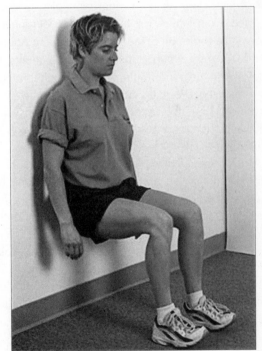

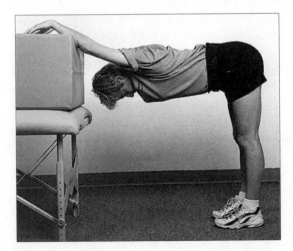

RUN FOR LIFE

FRANK SHORTER

The Leader of the Pack

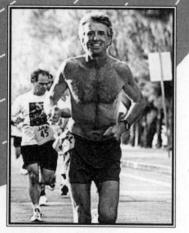

Honolulu marathon

He kicked off the running boom, historians say, with his win in the marathon at the 1972 Olympics. He invented a widely emulated business model that let runners make a living when it was rigged against them. He led the fight to let runners win prize money, like other world-class athletes. He served as chairman of the U.S. Anti-Doping Agency. Every step of the way, anywhere from 140,000 to 180,000 miles worth of them by various counts, it seems that Yale grad Frank Shorter put himself in a position to have maximum positive impact on the sport of running.

Running five miles a day by age 11 in his hometown of Middletown, New York, Shorter first achieved fame in his senior year of college by winning the NCAA 10,000-meter title in 1969, the first of five U.S. national 10k championships through 1977. He won his first marathon, Japan's prestigious Fukuoka, in 1971, then won three more in a row there. Clearly America's best distance runner and the Olympic favorite at the time of his '72 gold medal, it is widely accepted that he had a second Olympic gold medal stolen from him by a drug-taking East German in the 1976 Games. When Shorter's competitive running career ended at the beginning of the eighties, 30 million Americans were jogging for fitness (up from 2 million decade earlier), and he turned to the multisport scene, even winning the World Masters Duathlon Championship in 1989.

A lawyer who never practiced law, Shorter was 60 when he talked with me for *Run for Life* by phone from his home in Boulder, Colorado, on January 22, 2008. Busy, organized, and bristling with the self-confidence of someone who's done—and is still doing—all he set out to do, he discussed his past glories and his plan for staying superfit deep into the future with long aerobic workouts, intervals, crosstraining, and lots of weight lifting.

At age 11, I wanted to be a great downhill skier, and the best downhillers were the French. I was told that they did a lot of running as part of their training, so . . .

I said, "Okay, I'll do that." It was two and half miles to school and two and a half back. I'd run two or three times a week, maybe more. And I actually found a pair of basketball sneakers that I modified low-cut—that time they were sort of hard to find—and I convinced the principal of the middle school to let me wear these white sneakers, because at the time you could only wear black high-top shoes. Yeah, I actually convinced him, because I was, quote, "training." So that's when it started. I was the only kid at school wearing sneakers. In gym class, I convinced the teacher of the gym class to allow me to run laps around the field rather than do gym class.

I was pretty serious about skiing. And then when I was in high school—Northfield Mount Hermon prep school, to fast-forward—I had to make a decision about whether or not I wanted to be a skier or a runner. And I'd been having more success running. So, I decided to keep running into college.

I was the New England champion in both cross-country in the fall and the 2-mile in the spring. This is the league that has all the northeastern prep schools, like Andover, Choate, St. Paul's, Groton, Middlesex. That fall, I actually set a course record at every cross-country course I ran, so I guess I was doing pretty well.

I was born in Munich [on October 31, 1947] because my father was a military doctor in the occupation after World War II. He'd actually gone through medical school in three years. They were pumping the doctors through at the tail end of the war. He and my mother had grown up five houses apart on the same street in a little town in upstate New York called Middletown, about 15 miles from West Point. It was a coincidence that 24 years later I went to prep school there.

Running was one of the reasons I went to Yale. One, I wanted a very good school. I was pre-med. And also the track coach at the time, Bob "Gieg" Giegengack, had been the 1964 Olympic track coach. I got to Yale the next year, 1965. I knew I still wanted to run; it was more that I just wanted a place with the best resources for everything I was doing, whether it be athletic or academic. So from my perspective, Yale was the perfect place.

At that point, the longest race was two miles. And cross-country only ran 3½. My longest run was five miles in Van Cortlandt Park (in the Bronx) until my senior year in college, when I finished 18th in the NCAA cross-country, which was 10,000 meters, also in Van Cortlandt Park. That was sort of when things began to become apparent that I might have some ability beyond college. The top 25 were All-American. This was a big deal back then, because I obviously was the highest finisher of the Ivy League runners in the whole country.

Then it was literally three months later at the NCAA indoor meet, I actually finished second in the 2-mile national championships. So all of the sudden, I was getting really fast. Then, at the end of my senior year, another three months beyond that, I won the NCAA 6-mile and was second in the 3-mile a couple days later. I got really good—my curve sort of just took a steep rise my last year in college.

Since you couldn't make a living running back then, you did it for the true sport of it. The expectation was that you might stick around for a year or two and maybe make an Olympic team, and after that you were supposed to go on with the rest of your life.

I actually had a medical deferment (from serving in Vietnam) that occurred because I was training so hard. There was a meet against the Russians in 1970 that I won; this was a big deal back then. It was the Cold War—and I was on the cover of Sports Illustrated. But on that same trip, I started urinating blood. So when I got back home, I went to the doctor, had X-rays and stuff, and that was the basis of a medical deferment. Because the military didn't want to take me and take the risk of paying me disability for the rest of my life.

The effect: It allowed me to keep running. Because the goal was to try to make the Olympic team. Within a year, I won the 5- and 10000 at the 1970 U.S.

championships. And the next year, in June of '71, I won the Pan Am trials 10,000 and marathon. Later that year I won the Fukuoka marathon, which was the de facto world championships. So I improved very quickly.

I had run my first marathon in 1971, the national AAU championship, and finished second to Kenny Moore. That's the one where I turned to him and honest-to-God said, "Kenny, why couldn't Phidippides [the first marathoner of Greek legend] have died here?" I actually said that. I just knew I was going down. (laughs) I had just realized what "the Wall" was.

Kenny actually wrote an article for Sports Illustrated that appeared two weeks later, so that line appeared in print. Which also shows that I actually said it. He went on to a great career and wrote the screenplay for the second Prefontaine movie, the better one, Without Limits. He just wrote the book on [Oregon coach Bill] Bowerman, The Men of Oregon. He also was 4th in the '72 Olympic marathon.

The Olympics was about seeing how far I could go. I think I was lucky in college. I'd been coached very well by Geig and taught how to coach myself. [Shorter routinely ran twice a day for a total of about 17 miles a day in the seventies.] Actually, when I got out of college, I didn't have a coach. I was it. So I knew about incremental goalsetting, and for me it was just another step higher. If you think about the logical step, the steps were never too big. From NCAA championships, to national championships, to Pan Am trials, to Pan Am Games, to Olympic Trials, to Olympic Games. You always had the higher goal in the back of your mind, but it's the incremental ones that are more important, because from my perspective, I didn't know if I was going to level off. But the whole point was, the way I set the goals, that was as far as I was going to go.

GOLDEN IN MUNICH

Although I might have been the favorite, I did not assume I'd win in Munich. For the Olympics, I didn't assume anything. All you do in a marathon, the way I've always run the marathon, is—at the highest level—I always said, look, ten people have the training to win. Then you get into the mental part, and three of those people are going to have a good day. There's a 30% good-day rate, I think, in a major marathon—if they're drug-free. And at that time, they pretty much were. So my goal was just to be one of those 3. So even just going into the Olympic Games, all I wanted to do that day was run as well as I could and try to be one of the three that had a good day.

You see, in the marathon, you don't run against any other individual; your competition in the marathon is whoever is running next to you. (laughs) That's your competition. And it doesn't matter what point in the race it is. If they're there, they're a competitor, and they're a threat.

[Running on the last day of the Olympics, Shorter and the lead pack passed through the 10k mark at 31:15. He pushed the pace in the next 5k to under 15 minutes, establishing a 5-second gap by nine miles. Then he relentlessly stretched the lead.]

The old coach's advice is, "You run through the tape." I had backed off. And I knew I was going to—and again I use the words "most likely"; I never said "I'm-gonna-win-this"— I knew I would most likely win if I kept pressing and nothing happened. See the difference? You don't start celebrating until it's over. Anybody who runs track and field will tell you, if you do, you'll get nipped at the tape." (laughs)

[Shorter entered Munich stadium 2 minutes ahead of, in order, Belgian Karel Lismont, defending Olympic champ Mamo Wolde of Ethiopia, and Kenny Moore. He won the marathon in 2:12:19, the then-second-fastest Olympic marathon time.]

On the bus back to the Olympic Village after the medal ceremony, I ran into my old coach [Geigengack] who I hadn't seen in two years. Geig said to me, simply, "Your life will never be the same." He was right.

But at the time, I didn't think my life was changed. In a sense, I had kind of a negative example of what I wasn't going to do: Mark Spitz, who basically tried to instantly capitalize on his fame [with his appearance on the Bob Hope show and numerous commercial endorsements, forfeiting his amateur status]. And that's fine. That was good for him because that's what he chose to do. But it was good for me that I could decide for myself, "no, that is not what I'm going to do." My feeling when I won was to say, "okay, I'm going to let this all settle in for a while." And to do that, I'll just go back to my life before the Olympics, which was law school. I'd been going to law school full-time at the University of Florida the two years leading up to the Olympics. I went back, finished, graduated, came out here to Colorado and took the Bar, and then started training again for the 1976 Olympics in Montreal.

So, no, I never really thought my life would change in terms of leveraging it or capitalizing on it. Because it wasn't—again, you didn't earn your living doing this. My perspective was, it's only going to be limited, it's only going to be for a short period of time, and it's not what I want to do anyway because I feel I could do other things. My view of capitalizing on that time was that you did it if you really didn't have anything else and you're really going to have to make your retirement within two or three years after the Games. Because there wasn't going to be anything else you could do to make a living. That wasn't my view, because I could do lots of things.

I ran the second Olympics with a broken foot. I'd broken what's called the navicular bone inside my ankle, but I had to run on it. I couldn't take time off to let it heal because it was late February, which meant I'd have had to take off until the first of April, and the Olympic Trials were the end of May. So I couldn't do that, and kept running on the broken foot through the Olympics. Which is why I didn't run the 10,000 meters in Montreal [even though he'd won the trials 10k]. I wanted to make sure my foot would last.

As for [marathon gold medalist Waldemar] Cierpinski, the entire East German team was on the drug program. You had to be [on the program] to be on the team. It wasn't as if they had a choice. Again, my reaction to that was not to say anything at the time, and then when it came time to help form USADA, the U.S. Anti-Doping Agency, I saw that as a window that was not going to open in that way. I worked with President Clinton's drug czar, Barry McCaffrey, to set up the U.S. Anti-Doping Agency. It was set up by the U.S. Olympic Committee in 1999. We took over after 2000.

My feeling on this has always been, "don't complain, don't sound like sour grapes, do something." I think I've taken what was obviously a disappointment that shouldn't have happened and turned it around to now know that I had a big part in what's going on with Marion Jones and Barry Bonds and Roger Clemens and testing kids in high school and the Tour de France and everything else. I think it's worked out well. Because rather than to try to remedy my own situation, I felt I should try to put my effort—because of the unique situation I had, with regard to the notoriety and the ability to speak and have people listen—I would do it to try to change the system so that it most likely wasn't going to happen again.

NEW BUSINESS MODEL FOR RUNNERS

I got my law degree, but never practiced; I just went into a business. I started my own businesses so that I could put my name on them and gradually erode the rule that didn't allow athletes to endorse products, so essentially earn a living. You see, when Mark Spitz did the commercials, he became a pro. Ironically, because of the work I did in the opening up of the sport—I'm the person who came up with the idea of the trust fund that allowed athletes starting in 1981 to win money and put money into their own individual trusts, and take it out for education, living, and medical expenses. Because we knew the Eastern Europeans—the East Germans—were doing the same thing, and the international federation passed it. Eventually, it just sort of just eroded away, and now the sport's open—you can win money. But the irony is when Mark Spitz decided he wanted to try to swim again, he got the benefit of that, you see what I'm saying? At age 47 (when Spitz tried to make the Olympic team)—it didn't work, but that's okay.

The thing is, I decided to make my living not from the sport or from doing endorsements, but working what I call ancillary—close to the sport, involved in the sport, but actually actively working. In 1978 I started my store and clothing line. I came up with the trust fund idea in 1981.

I actually did the first TV commercial for Hilton Hotels in a 3-way deal with the U.S. federation. That's what allowed

RUN FOR LIFE

athletes to do commercials. I worked out a three-way deal where the U.S. track federation got $25,000 a year in an agreement with Hilton to have a commercial made with an "amateur athlete." Well, I volunteered to be the athlete. And then I had a side agreement with Hilton to actually work for them. For those 2 years, I helped establish running courses around some of the Hilton Hotels, and believe it or not, we worked on the first Health Mark Diet. The Hilton Hotel restaurants were the first to have healthy diets with the little logos by them.

This was in 1978—before the trust fund idea. You can see that was sort of halfway. I wasn't in any jeopardy with this agreement because the federation agreed to it. They just agreed to supply an athlete; I volunteered to be the athlete on behalf of the federation. Me and Hilton came up with the idea, and I had Hilton approach the federation.

So I stayed in the sport. You can fast-forward to my involvement in the drug agency and see that it's a continuation of what I've always done.

[In 1977, Shorter was forced to take a break from competition because of his bad ankle, which was operated on the following spring. The long rehab had a silver lining: time to practice his cycling and work on his store and clothing line.]

After that, I lasted two or three more years, taking 3rd in the 10000 in the '79 PanAm games. And in 1981 and '82, I won a couple of big road races in the U.S., but that was pretty much the end.

FIT FOR LIFE: WEIGHTS AND CROSS-TRAINING

At that point, it becomes a matter of staying fit. I still do interval training, the same routine, but I don't run for all of my exercise. I still work out sometimes twice a day, but in the morning I get on an exercise bike and ride, and in the afternoon either run or do the intervals on an elliptical machine using my pulse rate. And then I also do a tremendous amount of weight training. I probably do some weight training four days a week. Some for the upper body, some for my legs.

I'll do the hamstrings and quadriceps with the machines, and calf machines and toe raises. I do two separate workouts for the calves, quads, and hamstrings, then I do some core work, which is sort of torso training along with a lot of sit-ups. The upper body, I use dumbbells. I got away from barbells because I was getting too competitive. I got my bench press up to 190 pounds; I weighed 138 at the time, and I figured, well, maybe I'll just back off. I do dumbbell curls, presses, and lat pull downs, dips, and chin-ups.

I think once you get past 35, you can stay as strong, or actually stronger than you were when you were younger. And if you don't, you lose muscle mass at about three to five pounds a decade, even if you're very active. You have to do the weight training to even maintain muscle mass. I've been doing this for 25 years.

And I've been riding the bike—now I'm 60—when I first turned 40. In fact, for two years in a row, I was the world champion in the Masters division of the duathlon, The Desert Princess series. I started cross-training 20 years ago, and it came in very handy in 1998. Because it turns out I had a broken back, and the nerves in my legs were getting impinged, the L-5 and the S-1 nerves, and so after I had the back fusion and they cleared up the problem, I was all set. I'd already done so much cross-training, it was already engrained in me. I did a lot of cross-training. I probably work out an hour and a half every day.

That's just aerobic or anaerobic. It doesn't include weights. The last 25 years, I probably spend as much time working out as I did when I was running 20 miles a day, it's just that I'm not running all that time.

I enter races but don't compete. I'll jump in a half marathon and see how close to an hour and half I can come. I don't run marathons anymore, but I've run four half marathons in the last 6 months. That's typical. I run them slowly and have fun. Again, for me, it's to stay fit and not look as old as I am.

All I've really done is substitute cross-training into the same kind of routine of easy aerobic conditioning and once or twice a week hard anaerobic training, which is a very small percentage of the overall training. It's just that now, instead of doing it all running, I'll mix it up.

DON'T GO HARD

If older runners are doing anything wrong, I think it's—I call it "The Myth of Overexertion." People think you have to go too hard to get the training effect. Actually, you have to go what I call "conversational pace." You and I are talking. And if we were running, we would want to be running at an effort to where we could still be talking like this. And if we couldn't, because we sort of had to pause to catch our breath, we'd actually be going too hard. You can stay fitter by going at 70% of your max effort than you can by going harder than that. You do the other training to race. But any aerobic exercise you do to be fit can be done at conversational effort.

A lot of people are going too hard. The effect is diminishing returns. You get hurt, get tired, you get in a downward spiral from workout to workout.

I wore my knees down, but anybody—if they live long enough—gets osteoarthritis. You wear out your joints. They're wearing out, but they're still working. Yeah, it hurts.

I actually inject with a product called hyalgan; it's purified rooster comb. It's absorbed by what you have left, and it stimulates synovial fluid so that you can basically have the knees of an 18-year-old for 8 to 10 months. And I've done this for about 5 years. I had no meniscus left in my right knee, and very little in the left. And when I use this stuff, I can run without pain for about 8 to 10 months. It's much better than getting a new knee.

It works for me. It's like anything. Glucosamine and chondroitin works for a certain percentage of the population. This works for a certain percentage within that percentage. You see—it's not a guarantee, but it's worth trying.

I don't do any supplements. Because as former chairman of the United States Anti-Doping Agency, I have to tell every Olympic athlete—and now triathlete—in the Olympics, that they take supplements at their peril because there's not enough oversight by the FDA to ensure that what they're taking isn't tainted. In other words, you have no idea with a supplement whether or not it's working because what they say on the label is making it work or what's not on the label that's illegal is making it work.

VEGGIES, FISH, WHOLE GRAINS

Whether it's the pyramid or food groups, I eat a lot of vegetables. I don't eat any refined sugar anymore, and I found that increased my desire for fruit. Eat a lot of granola and whole grains, and lot of fish—lot of salmon. I eat meat maybe once every two weeks. Because I think there are some essential amino acids in meat that you just need. In other words, I eat meat to craving. I crave some red meat maybe once every two weeks.

I'll have a lot of complex carbohydrates. Lot of granola, lot of wholegrain bread. The Atkins (low-carb) Diet is great if you never want to contract a muscle again. Because you need complex carbohydrates for the gly-cogen that's the fuel source, and you can't fight Mother Nature. We knew, when we did the carbohydrate deple-tion diet in '76—you were supposed to just eat protein and very little carbohydrate the first part of the week, and then carbs the second part, and it would super-saturate you with glycogen—and you know what?—we found out that in the depletion phase you have no energy at all. And why many people go off the Atkins Diet is that you have no energy. Now, if you want to be in bed, totally sedentary, on an IV, eating nothing but protein, you'll lose weight. Fine. But if you want to be an active person, you're not going to have the energy.

Actually, hate to cut this short, but you know I'm going to have to go. Got to meet someone I'm working out with. We're doing intervals—interval training. And I'm not going to let this person wait. Bye.

RUN FOR LIFE

RUN FAST

Extremely hard efforts are uncomfortable but essential for longevity because they cue your body to get stronger.

One day in the fall of 2005, while making phone calls to fitness machine manufacturers looking for new products to test for my *Los Angeles Times* fitness gear column, I was told about a "hot, new interval program" on a Vision Fitness treadmill. It was called "Sprint 8."

"I read about it in a book written by a coach in Tennessee who has you do a 20-minute workout with eight all-out, 30-second sprints that leave you gasping, with easy recovery jogging in between," Vision President Nathan Pyles told me. "The sprints give you phenomenally fast gains in fitness. I lost a lot of weight and got in the best shape of my life—all while working out less." He was so impressed that he licensed the name Sprint 8 from the author, Phil Campbell.

I called Campbell, and he had an interesting story. He was a superfit 54, a coach and author of the book, *Ready Set Go! Synergy Fitness*, but a decade before he was a doughy hospital administrator who jogged 45 minutes a day but never lost weight until he started training for his family's annual Thanksgiving flag-football game. Busy workloads gave him less time to run, so he figured he better throw in some intervals to burn additional calories. Soon, he got a shock: for the first time in years, he was dropping weight. He sped up the intervals; more weight fell off. He sped up the intervals to all-out pace that left him gasping—and lost more weight, all of it on half the workout time as his old runs. Of course, he had dozens of cases more dramatic than his to tell: People he'd taught Sprint 8 to who'd lost 50 pounds, lost 8 inches off their waist, you name it.

Now, I hear impressive stories and claims all the time. And I know that interval training has been a proven training method for a century. What runner hasn't done it? What athlete hasn't done it? I ran lots of what we called "wind sprints" while playing football and basketball in high school, and on the wrestling team in college. But these short, super-high-intensity, lung-heaving, to-the-edge-of-passing-out Sprint 8 intervals of Campbell's were something new. If a short workout like this could have such a rapid and pronounced impact on weight loss and fitness, was it a true breakthrough?

And let's take it further: Could Sprint 8 also be a boon for running longevity, the focus of this book? After all, a 20-minute workout would allow you to run less, which is essential for preserving your joints. And could it address another key downside of athletic aging: The relentless decline in VO_2 max (oxygen processing ability, the maximum amount of oxygen that your lungs, circulatory system, and muscles can take in, deliver, and use in one minute)? Like the decline in muscle mass, VO_2 max is thought to drop roughly 1% a year after age 35 or so. Even lifelong fitness can't stop the decline; one study found that highly trained athletes age 55 to 68 had 10 to 20 percent less blood flow to their legs than athletes in their 20s.

But what if those athletes consistently did hard sprints—hard to the point of making you uncomfortable? Can Sprint 8 do what normal training can't?

After spending a lot of time hunting for an answer, I concluded maybe it can. The hunt started with Campbell, who lacked a PhD in exercise research, but had results and a growing list of believers.

"Why are your sprints 30 seconds long?" I asked him. "Because that's about as long as you can go at all-out pace before you pass out," he said. "In fact, if you go for more than 30 seconds, I'd say you aren't trying hard enough."

"Why eight sprints?" I asked. "Because it's about all you can do before you get too exhausted," he said. "Besides, Sprint 8 sounds good."

"How does it make you a lot fitter and a lot leaner so quickly?" I asked. "Because it gives you a big spurt of human growth hormone," he said. "It's there in the research."

Whoa. Wait a minute. HGH?

Talk about déjà vu. Didn't I hear this same HGH story line from Dr. William Kraemer of the University of Connecticut a few years earlier about rapid-contraction weight training?

I felt like I'd stumbled upon a unified theory of fitness, power, and longevity. What rapid-contraction, go-to-the-limit weight lifting is to muscles, ultra-intervals are to the cardiovascular system—the lungs, veins, metabolism. The benefits are the same. Whatever fitness activity you do, doing it with bursts of all-out anaerobic insanity has good effects on lean muscle mass, fat loss, bone density, and more.

The "more" includes VO_2 max, the Achilles heel of older athletes. In the next chapter, you'll read about how a wild, all-out Japanese workout called "Tabata intervals" raised VO_2 max. Why it happens is simple. In a 2007 *New York Times* article, Dr. Hirofumi Tanaka, an exercise physiologist at the University of Texas, explained that that the act of repeatedly going all-out, then easing up to recover, then going all-out again, trains the body to increase its oxygen consumption. In other words, if you take yourself past the limit, you can initially raise the limit. Then, when you hit the ceiling, going to the limit can keep you there longer.

VO_2 max rises not just because the body was "trained," but because it was made stronger. HGH enters the picture because it's the hormone that makes muscles grow.

In articles I wrote for *Outside* magazine and the *L.A. Times*, I ran across a number of medical journal articles that linked high-intensity interval training with HGH spurts, as Campbell had said. The hormone doesn't last in your body for more than two hours (I had a blood test done 12 hours after a workout to search for long-term elevated levels, and it wasn't there), but apparently that 2 hours is enough to repair and strengthen muscles and speed recovery. And as I was told by

Dr. Mike Joyner at the Mayo Clinic, if it isn't the HGH that is making you strong (they couldn't be 100% sure), something similar is—because a whole basket of good hormones is released when you push hard.

In fall 2005, with an article assignment in hand and my 50th birthday in sight, I was highly motivated to use myself as a Sprint 8 guinea pig. I did it every day in different sports, and despite being quite fit already, immediately felt even fitter. I used it on my bike trainer for 20-minute workouts during the week and started hammering past my buddies on the climbs on the weekend. I used Sprint 8 in the pool and my terrible swimming immediately improved to merely bad. I used it on my elliptical machine, up hills on the tandem bike with my son Joey, and while running 3 nights a week with my dog Bruce. I did the La Ruta de los Conquistadores 3-day mountain-bike race across Costa Rica on a third of my usual bike training, and had my strongest finish ever.

One day that fall, I ran into a woman at the gym who told me that she could never lose weight even though she ran every day; a month and 10 fewer pounds later, she saw me again, and I ended up using her for the lead of my *Times* story. I had my son and the other 11- and 12-year-olds on my AYSO soccer team do eight progressively longer sprint races every practice, and even had the other dads who showed up join in.

For several reasons, high-intensity intervals are ideal tools for aging. Done right, you can run much less (thereby saving your knees) than steady state running but get the same benefits. In fact, you'll get more: gains in VO_2 max and muscular power, danger zones for all older runners and non-runners alike. The advantages of ultra-intervals are striking—if you can handle them.

I interviewed a lot of runners and researchers on this subject, and even conducted my own not-so-scientific study: My soccer team dads. Even though we came in last place under my management (hey, I never played the game growing up), several fathers told me that they hated for the season to end. Those 4 minutes of sprinting each week made them feel fitter than they'd been in decades.

CHAPTER 10

THE ULTRA INTERVAL

*Going all-out for 20 or 30 seconds can melt fat,
save your joints via reduced workout time,
stop your V0$_2$ max from declining, and increase muscle
power and longevity. If you can handle it.*

For years, Michelle Cuellar exercised five days a week. "But you wouldn't have known it by looking at me," says the 35-year-old mother of two from Centennial, Colorado. "I felt fit—but I was still fat."

In fact, no matter what Cuellar did—run on the treadmill for 30 minutes five days a week and take the occasional spinning class or boot camp—her weight rose. By last summer, she'd grown into a size 10 dress and carried 176 pounds on her 5-foot-6-inch frame.

But by the fall, for the first time, Cuellar started shrinking. "I tried on a pair of size 8 pants that hadn't fit since 1998—and they fit!" she says. "In 8 weeks, five inches came off my butt, two inches off my stomach. The weight—7, 9, 12 pounds—just started falling off."

Was her breakthrough a new diet? "No," said Cuellar, "I started doing intervals."

Jeff Mitchell, a 42-year-old business consultant from Jackson, Tennessee, can relate. He cut 2 seconds off his 100-meter-dash time, lost 40 pounds, and shed 6 inches from his waistline—all in just over a year. His muscles bulged, his skin looked smoother, and he hadn't felt so good since playing college basketball.

"'You on steroids or something?'" he says a friend asked. "'No,' I said. 'Just intervals.'"

Not just any intervals. High-intensity intervals—20-minute workouts peppered with eight 30-second, lung-heaving, all-out sprints that left them both gasping for air. Cuellar, who runs 10 minutes fewer per day now than she did before, ramps up from her normal steady-state 6-mph jog to an 8.5-mph interval. "Sometimes I almost feel like I'm

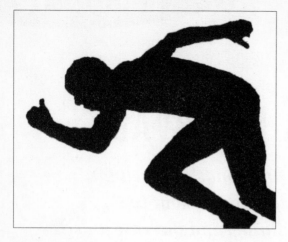

going to pass out," she says. "But Sprint 8 is worth it."

Sprint 8, the centerpiece of Phil Campbell's "Ready Set Go Synergy Fitness," is one of the new breed of super-intense, super-short interval workouts that are making believers out of athletes of all ages and abilities. And it's not just runners. Top Masters road and cyclo-cross cyclist Tom Gee, 56, says his Sprint 8 workouts helped him do a 40-kilometer time trial in 57 minutes, 30 seconds two years ago, the same time he rode as a Category 1 rider at age 24. Internet marketer Robert Burns of San Diego, 43, says he lost 25 pounds in six months doing three Sprint 8 swim workouts per week.

If you want to be as fit as possible at any age, the experts say, train hard and train often. But if you have to choose one, do what those people did: choose hard. High-intensity is better for you than long and slow. Here's why:

HOW INTERVALS WORK

The key to improving your level of fitness, trainers and sports scientists agree, is shocking yourself. "After a certain period of plodding along doing the same steady-state jogging and cycling, you don't progress—your body gets used to what you're doing," says Christopher Drozd, a Santa Monica strength and conditioning coach and Ironman triathlete. "You have to literally shock your body off the plateau. If you push yourself to the limit (with intervals), you're going to get a new limit."

The phenomenon is known as the "stress adaptation response," says Leonard A. Kaminsky, director of the clinical exercise physiology program at the Ball State University human performance lab, and editor of the exercise guidelines manual of the American College of Sports Medicine.

"The human body adapts to the stresses placed on it," he says. "Challenge it, and it improves. To affect change, you need to overload your system beyond what it is accustomed to. When you go beyond your aerobic threshold (the point at which you are unable to bring in enough oxygen to support the exercise)—to where you perceive that you're getting winded—you initiate a chain of positive events that work for everyone. Even nursing-home populations can improve."

Intervals improve fitness by upgrading your oxygen-processing system with new capillaries and stronger lungs and heart, adding more mitochondria (tiny cellular motors) to muscles, and developing a higher tolerance to the build-up of lactic acid, a waste product associated with going anaerobic (into oxygen-debt). It works for everyone, every ability, even the already superfit. A 2005 study of competitive cyclists at New Zealand's Waikato Institute of Technology even found that intervals can speed up serious athletes in mid-season form; 8 to 12 sessions gave test subjects power gains of 8.7% for 1 kilometer and 8.1% for 4 kilometers over a control group of non-interval trainers.

But it is the unexpected weight loss, time savings, and sense of "feeling younger" that have average and aging exercisers most excited. The latter may come from a temporary increase in the release of human growth hormone, a powerful substance which declines to just 20% of your teenage levels by age 60. A 2002 University of North Carolina–Greensboro study published in *Sports Medicine* found that all exercise, both aerobic and strength training, stimulates the release of HGH, and that greater exercise intensity—as with interval training—stimulates greater release.

HGH, produced episodically in the pituitary gland, gets a lot of attention these days. That's because it might be the closest thing we have to a fountain of youth.

HGH is known for many youthlike effects, including development of lean muscle mass, enhanced sexual desire, stronger connective tissue, reduced fat, thicker skin, reduced wrinkles, and improved sleep. HGH improves recovery and protein synthesis throughout your body. Better trained people also maintain heat tolerance, and get sick less. The HGH effect works for all ages and both genders.

This pronounced anti-aging effect, first documented in a landmark HGH study by Dr. Daniel Rudman at the Medical College of Wisconsin in 1990, has led an estimated 500,000+ Americans to line up at anti-aging clinics and pay $500 to $1,000-plus a month for HGH therapy, which was approved by the FDA in 1996. The promise of age reversal makes them willing to tolerate potential side effects like joint pain and stiffness, carpal tunnel syndrome, hypoglycemia (low blood sugar level), necessary insulin injections, and remote possibilities of diabetes, high blood pressure, or heart and kidney enlargement.

Campbell wonders why anyone would inject artificial HGH when they can quickly produce a safer version in their own bodies. It turns out that anaerobic activity provokes the pituitary gland to radically crank up HGH production.

"It's simple: The harder you work, the more HGH you make," Campbell says. He likes to point out that he didn't invent this idea. In the past 15 years, the connection has been documented in dozens of research studies, such as an article in

RUN FOR LIFE

the August 1999 issue of the *Journal of Applied Physiology* which concluded that "the HGH secretory response is related to exercise intensity in a linear pattern."

And that's not all. Intervals' time-saving effect was documented in a 2006 study at Canada's McMaster University published in the *Journal of Physiology*. The test found equal increases in fitness between six short bouts of interval training over two weeks (20-minute cycling workouts, consisting of repetitive 30-second all-out efforts each followed by 4 minutes of recovery) and 6 longer moderate-paced sessions (90 to 120 minutes a day) over 2 weeks.

Surprisingly, the weight-loss effect of intervals does not mostly come from the real-time interval training itself (intervals are mainly fueled by fast-burning glycogen, not slow-burning fat), but from its long-known aftereffect: It ramps up the metabolism.

Back in 1985, a study in the *American Journal of Clinical Nutrition* found that high-intensity training ramps up your metabolism for 24 hours afterward, whereas low-intensity training does not. A 1991 study in *International Journal of Obesity* found that more exercise intensity, not more duration, provoked increased postexercise oxygen consumption. The result: Intervals zap more fat all day long, according to a 1994 skin-fold measurement study in *Metabolism*. A study conducted by a team at Canada's

University of Guelph and published in 2005 in the *Journal of Applied Physiology* found that just two weeks of alternate-day interval training increased moderately active women's fat-burning ability by 36% and muscular capacity for work by 32 to 20%.

All this may help explain why Michelle Cuellar gained weight with regular exercise—until she added intervals.

"Given that resting metabolism does decline as you get older, it is not uncommon to see regular exercisers add a pound or two per year over time," says Ball State's Kaminsky. "Either that, or Michelle was stopping at Starbucks a couple times a week" (a charge she denied).

CAN YOU HANDLE A 4-MINUTE WORKOUT?

What type of interval is best? All-out, lung-heaving efforts for 30 seconds followed by low-intensity recovery for two minutes, à la Sprint 8, or longer-lasting, less-intense efforts with shorter recovery periods in-between?

The latter have plenty of success stories, too.

Chad Kolakowski, a 27-year-old golf company executive from Austin, Texas, dropped from 290 to 230 pounds in 8 months by using Momentum, a 3-day-a-week, 25-minute workout program that features 3-minute intervals followed by a minute of recovery.

Designed by Broomfield, Colorado–based Breakthrough Health & Fitness, the program requires the user to wear a heart-rate monitor to help gauge perceived levels of exertion.

"The cool thing is that you only need to push hard for three minutes at a time before you get to rest," says Kolakowski, who mixes some cycling and swimming in with his running workouts. "Anyone can push for 3 minutes."

Maybe so. But can anyone push it to the limit for 20 seconds, rest 10 seconds, then repeat the sequence a total of 8 times? That's a total workout of 4 minutes.

Welcome to Tabata intervals, which refers to a 1996 study led by Dr. Izumi Tabata at the National Institute of Fitness and Sports in Tokyo, Japan, "Effects of moderate-intensity endurance and high-intensity intermittent training on anaerobic capacity and VO_2 max." The six-week study, published in the journal *Medical Science in Sports and Exercise*, used test subjects who were anything but couch potatoes: members of the Japanese national speed-skating team. The moderate intensity group rode a stationary bike at 70% of VO_2 max for 1 hour, 5 days a week. The high-intensity intermittent group did just 4 minutes of cycling 5 days a week, but at a mind-blurring level: 8 20-second all-out rides at 170% of VO_2 max with a 10-second rest in between.

After six weeks, the moderate-intensity group's VO_2 max increased 10% while anaerobic capacity was unchanged. The high intensity intermittent group's VO_2 max increased 14% while the anaerobic capacity increased by 28%. So these athletes, already trained, gained *more* aerobic capacity from the high intensity training in addition to their increase in anaerobic capacity!

Phil Campbell makes the argument that to do each of his Sprint 8s at full speed—and thereby reap maximum HGH and other benefits—you need to be rested for 90 seconds or 2 minutes between intervals. But the 10-second rest of the Tabatas would seem to debunk that.

Many people who see the amazing improvement in aerobic and anaerobic fitness of the crazy Tabata 4-minute workout think it would be of best value to athletes who participate in high-intensity sports such as boxing, mixed martial arts, or wrestling.

But I think it is of equal or greater significance to athletes over age 50. It reinforces in a very dramatic way the key role intervals should play in anyone's anti-aging fitness strategy. The bottom line is intervals do work—certainly the more intense the better to rebuild depleted power and fast-twitch muscle fibers. And they do so without beating up your knees and hips and requiring a lot of rest, recovery, and healing time, like a long run does.

The small time commitment and the big payoff also take away excuses. If you have 20 or 15 or even 4 minutes,

WHY HIGH-INTENSITY INTERVALS BUILD RUNNING LONGEVITY

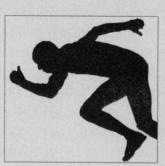

You can jog 5 or 10 miles a day at a consistent "Runner's High" pace, and you will burn plenty of calories and float on a lovely cloud of endorphins, but you won't really make your cardiovascular system much healthier. You can do mile-long interval repeats and they will make you faster and fitter. But the safest, most effective, most time-efficient way to keep yourself young is 20 or 30 seconds of all-out intensity that floods you with fountain-of-youth chemicals, takes your cardio and respiratory systems to a new level, and teaches the arteries to open wide when your muscles really need a lot of blood.

The Benefits of Ultra Intervals

- They reduce running time, which reduces oxidation, cumulative pounding on your joints, and the potential for long- and short-term injury.
- Sprinting's body position places you on your forefoot and toes, so you can't heel strike while doing it.
- They maximize HGH and build fast-twitch muscle, which gives you power.
- They increase or — at worst — slow the decline in VO_2 max.
- The HGH and ramped-up metabolism burn fat.
- Ultra-Intervals can be done with any aerobics — running, swimming, elliptical, biking.
- They're simple. No complicated 5-by-1000-meter interval sessions one day and six miles at mid-tempo pace the next, like in other "Run Less" running programs. The Sprint 8 program is always the same: Eight sprints. As you get fitter, do them faster.

Warning: Periodization has a Place

- For training for a lengthy race, intervals can help, but can't fully replace traditional Periodization (Chapter 26). Twenty minutes a day can't get a body ready for a 4-hour marathon, or teach you to plan for hydration, nutrition, and other issues of race strategy.
- Intervals won't give you the Runner's High. You need a steady rhythm for that. You will have to seek other methods of therapy.
- Intervals of any duration risk injury due to their intensity, so take them slow the first couple weeks to build up your superstructure.

How to do it

- *20 to 30 seconds, all-out.* Recover 90 or 120 seconds, and do it again. On a treadmill, ramp up 2 mph initially from an easy steady-state pace. If you can handle that, ramp it up 2.5 mph next time. On the road, just go all full-bore. Do the first sprints easier to warm up. By the sixth, you should hate life. By the eighth, done right, you're completely wasted.
- *Don't do Sprint 8 two days in a row* (as with any land running). Muscles need 48 hours of recovery time after a strenuous strength workout, which sprinting is. The next day, crosstrain for recovery.
- *Try an alternative.* If high-intensity interval runs bother you, do them in the pool, up hills, or while cycling uphill. Dr. Tom Miller, coach of octogenarian star John Cahill (see his interview) says standing bike climbs do a great job of training running muscles.

Bottom Line

For fit aging, short and fast is far better for you than long and slow. That goes for weight training as well as aerobics. "High performance is really determined more by intensity than volume," Steven Hawkins, an exercise physiologist at the University of Southern California, told the *New York Times*.

So when you have to choose between hard and often, choose hard.

---

you can do yourself a lot of good. "It's perfect for the executive suite, too," says John Lindahl of Boulder, Colorado, 45, a corporate program manager who lost 50 pounds and 9 inches off his waistline in 8 months with Momentum. "We all have less time nowadays," said the former high-school 400-meter track champion. "On the road, you answer e-mails at night instead of working out. This workout is bang-bang-bang—no wasted time. If you have an hour, you can do it and shower."

On the other hand, if your intervals are so intense that they leave you lying on the floor gasping for breath, like the Japanese students in Tabata's study, back off on the intensity a bit. Otherwise, you probably won't do them very often.

Here's how to address that problem:

THE PLAN: MIX UP YOUR INTERVALS

The fact that super-intense Sprint 8, moderately intense Momentum, and crazy-hard Tabata intervals are all effective is good news.

"Ironically, you can't do the same intervals all the time—you'll stagnate," says Drozd, the Santa Monica trainer.

125

"You need variation—for your body and your mind. For best fitness, mix short intervals and long intervals. Whatever you choose to do, do it hard."

He's right. The aforementioned New Zealand study showed that the cyclists' performance gains plateaued after 8 to 12 interval sessions. "To keep increasing your fitness after 6 weeks of intervals," says Joseph Grassadonia, publisher of the fitness-trainer magazine *OnFitness*. "Be creative: push it even harder or longer, add hills, stairs, crosstraining. I'm a 55-year-old big-wave surfer, but I can hang with 20-year-olds because I do very intense 10-mph sprinting on the treadmill, all-out sprints in the pool—constantly mixing it up, shocking my body."

"Going hard, however, may be a problem for some," says Dr. Chet Gentry, a Sprint 8 runner. After the 46-year-old family physician from Sparta, Tennessee saw significant fitness gains and a 55-point drop in his LDL—the "bad" cholesterol—(from 130 to 85) he began prescribing Sprint 8 to all his patients "But it's hard to get my patients to do Sprint 8, because it makes you so uncomfortable," he says. "But those that do, get very good results."

Gary Green, a 47-year-old Internet businessman from Tustin, California, who halved his workout time and cycled off 25 pounds in 7 months, is one of those. "I find Sprint 8 invigorating, but I don't know if it's for everybody. It's a pretty hard workout—mentally and physically."

Physically, although interval training can often be safer than regular steady-state aerobics because it eliminates the repetitive motion of long workouts that often lead to injury, it can also initially be risky for joints, tendons, and muscles used to less intensity.

Advice? Ease into it. "Ramp up slowly over 2 or 3 weeks," says Breakthrough founder Jonathan Roche. "Guys, in particular, will go all-out and waste themselves." Properly done, a high-intensity work interval should be followed by a low-intensity rest interval that allows your heart rate to recover or come down to a level where you're breathing comfortably. Generally, the more intense the work interval, the longer the rest interval. And to allow recovery and strengthen, follow the same 48-hour rule as weight lifting: Don't do intervals in the same sport 2 days in a row. Follow running intervals with cycling, rowing, or swimming intervals. The elliptical machine may or may not be too close to running to allow recovery, depending on the machine and your physiology—same with water running.

The biggest challenge of intervals may be psychological. This is anaerobic agony that most people would rather avoid. You really need to get psyched up. Intervals are a whole different ball game than blissful, steady-state, endorphin-high, long-slow distance.

"Intervals can be more fun because we like to be challenged to do better, but they are more gut-wrenching and grueling." says Ron Jones, an Atlanta- and L.A.–based corporate wellness coach and champion age-group cyclist. "Although we know that lukewarm goals don't work very well, too-hard ones can frighten you away."

Like Roche, he advises taking it easy at first with slower, shorter efforts. "I've had people do 5-second intervals," he says. "Then slowly—*slowly*—build on that success. Remember that it takes 3 weeks to psychologically form a new habit, and 6 months to change a behavior. Even seeing the physical changes [i.e., weight loss, increased muscle mass] that come with interval training may not be enough to let you stick with it. You have to feel good about what you are doing."

Michelle Cuellar got to that point when she lost 20 pounds in 6 months with Sprint 8. "My husband offered to buy me a whole new wardrobe," she says, "but I told him to wait until I got down to a size 6."

THE RADICAL "PRIMAL BLUEPRINT"

"Evolution," says a reformed run-aholic, "dictates that we do two things runners may not want to hear: Throw out most carbs and do no hard, steady-state running at all."

I yawned. "Too Much Exercise Can Damage Heart" read the headline in the *New York Times* on January 22, 2007. Ho-hum. After all, Jim Fixx died running. And reports of runners training themselves into weird hormonal imbalances and potentially deadly conditions like ventricular arrhythmia, in which the heart beats erratically, crop up all the time. When I worked as an editor at *Triathlete* magazine in the '90s, tales of competitors whose "adrenal glands were shot" were legion. But these stories only apply to extremists who train five hours a day, not you, right? Regular steady-state running, 30 to 60 minutes a day, is all good. Yes?

Mark Sisson says no. He says regular old steady-state, high-heart-rate running, the kind you would do in training or a race itself, is not good for you, is not natural, and certainly will not help you live to 100, much less be in running shape when you get there.

Mark *who*?

Sisson, a former 2:18 marathoner who finished 4th in the Hawaii Ironman in 1982. He rose to a position of prominence in establishing the International Triathlon Union and getting the sport into the Olympics, serving as its antidoping commissioner for many years. As I write this in 2008, he also is in freakishly good shape at age 55, as the accompanying photo of the buffed, teenage-looking body will attest. That can't be all due to the anti-oxidant vitamins he sells for a living.

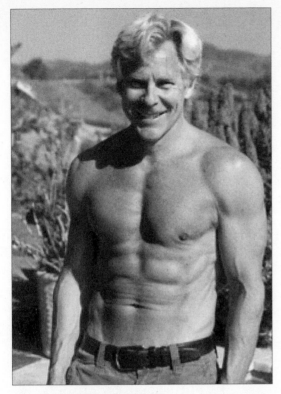
Anti-runner Mark Sisson flexes at 55.

and biking for hours alongside his clients. That left him on his own, with time only to do short, intense sprint workouts at the track or hill repeats on the bike.

"And lo and behold, within a year, my injuries were healing, I was rarely sick, and I was even back to occasionally racing—faster than ever," he says. "Something 'primal' was happening. I got healthy because I was training like a hunter-gatherer."

Analyzing his situation, Sisson became convinced that his carbo-fueled high heart rate aerobics were burdening his body with "continuous systemic inflammation that was severely suppressing my immune system ... leaving me soaking in my own internal cortisol (stress hormone) bath ... [and causing] increased oxidative damage that was tearing apart my muscle and joint tissue."

Building a fitness program around what he calls "our primal DNA blueprint," Sisson now observes a fitness lifestyle that includes strength training and no steady-state, high-heart-rate running or other lengthy, high-respiration aerobics—just short, hard sprints and aerobic activities done at a slow, low-heart-rate conversational pace. His diet includes animal protein, colorful vegetables, fruits (mainly berries), healthy fats (nuts, avocados, olive oil), very few sugars, and whole-grain–based carbs. He outlined the plan and the logic behind it in an article he sent me called "A Case Against Cardio

Sisson used to be a run-aholic, running up to 20 miles a day during two decades as a competitive athlete. "I read Ken Cooper's 1968 book *Aerobics* and celebrated the idea that you got to award yourself 'points' for time spent at a high heart rate. The more points, the healthier your cardiovascular system would become," he said. "Then my body began breaking down."

Debilitating osteoarthritis in his ankles at age 28; chronic hip tendonitis; recurrent upper respiratory tract infections. Sisson retired from pro racing and became a personal trainer who did weight training and low-intensity hiking (from a former mileage king)" that he posted on his website, MarksDailyApple.com and elaborates upon in his upcoming book, the Primal Blueprint.

I found it intriguing because it takes what I've written here in *Run for Life* a step further. No endorphin-high running *at all*? Sisson's view is that human physiology, calorie-processing, and energy systems are not designed for the running we do today. His view is supported by academics like Northwestern University anthropologist William Leonard, quoted back in the intro to the Soft Running section as saying that Homo erectus did sprints and long-distance striding (fast walking), but not running, indicating that modern man indeed may have to "learn" how to run.

The question then is: Have our bodies, in the 20,000 years removed from the cave, "learned" to handle unnatural hormonal, oxidative, impact loads, and the refined, high-carb foods that go with steady-state running, a fitness activity only done for the last 40 years? Sisson says they haven't.

His analysis starts with the way the body uses different fuels for different tasks. Since ancient man moved slowly and steadily most of the time, he primarily used fat as a fuel. Fat is quite efficient. Loaded with 9 calories per gram (twice that of carbs and protein, the latter being primarily a muscle builder) and found in abundance even on slim people, it fuels us while at rest or sleeping and during continuous, low levels of aerobic activity for days without food. For the occasional bursts of short fight-or-flight speed, running from or to a lion (or swinging a golf club), we use ATP and carbohydrates as fuels. ATP (Adenosine triphosphateis) is a high-octane fuel our body creates for intense, life-or-death workloads. The muscles can only store about 20 seconds' worth of it. Carbs, stored in the muscles as fast-burning glycogen, do double duty, helping fuel the muscles' fast bursts *and* fueling vital bodily organs like the brain. But at only 4 calories per gram and limited to 2,000 calories in a male adult, carbs aren't set up for all-day hammering.

"Fortunately, our hunter-gatherer ancestors didn't need a lot of carbs because they didn't regularly ramp their heart rates up for over an hour a day like we do now," says Sisson. "Fat fueled the all-day tracking [fast walking pace] that let them chase down their prey. They didn't run. In fact, hours of running would have likely hastened your demise if you'd failed to catch—and eat—an animal, leaving you empty, exhausted, and some other animal's prey."

That's why heart and skeletal muscle evolved to prefer fat as fuel over glucose, says Sisson, and why the high-carb/sugar foods that fuel today's high-intensity aerobic activities are a problem. The sugar promotes overproduction of insulin, the aerobics multiplies normal oxidative damage (free-radical production) by a factor of 10 or 20 and generates high levels of the stress hormone cortisol in many people, leaving them susceptible to infection, injury, loss of bone density, and depletion of lean muscle tissue—all while encouraging their bodies to deposit fat.

"So carbo-loading and running hard for 45 minutes is far from that healthy pursuit we all assumed it was!" says Sisson. "The answer? Go back to our DNA blueprint. You get stronger and healthier the more you use the fat and ATP systems."

That means walk, hike, bike, swim or other low-level aerobic work at no more than conversational pace for 45 minutes or an hour a few times a week. "That's healthy," he says, "because it will maximize our true fat-burning systems, increase the capillary network and muscle mitochondria." To get strong and lean, add weights and a half-dozen all-out "life-or-death" sprints of 20 to 40 seconds each every few days, à la Sprint 8.

"Add some easy stretching afterward, and you'll do more in less time than you could ever accomplish in a typical 80–85% Max heart-rate cardio workout," says Sisson.

Sisson's take may seem extreme, but it not only dovetails with Chapter 10's Ultra-Intervals, but, counterintuitively, Chapter 26, Periodization. Although Periodization embraces the kind of steady-state pace that violates the "DNA blueprint," some believe that it is possible, through a disciplined progression, to teach your body to both burn more fat at higher speeds and to clean up excessive free-radical production.

Mopping up free radicals is speculative, but training-enhanced fat burning is a fact. Example: 6-time Hawaii Ironman winner Mark Allen had great success with a low-heart-rate program devised by his coach Phil Maffetone. While running, Allen was not allowed to exceed 150 beats per minute. At first, he had to walk to keep it below that threshold. Over time, he biked 112 miles in under 5 hours and ran 2:40 marathons in Kona at 150 bpm, in theory staying better-fueled than his rivals by sparing carbs and burning a higher percentage of high-calorie fat.

The take-home message? Low-exertion aerobics, weights, a diet of meats, good fat, fruit, and complex carbs (e.g., wholegrains), plus short, all-out intervals are good for anyone's health and longevity. Long-distance, moderate-to-high level aerobics probably aren't, except for the mental bliss. Don't let the endorphin high brainwash you into destroying your body. Yes, if you feel great all the time, keep doing what you're doing. If you push hard all the time, beware. Back off if your body starts doing strange things like Dr. Cooper's 20 symptoms of overtraining (see sidebar in Chapter 26).

RUN FOR LIFE

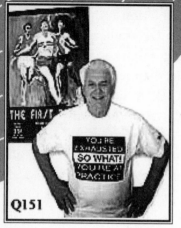

LASZLO TABORI

The Third Man to Run the 4-Minute Mile

The white-haired old man on the USC track with the three stop watches, thick goulash accent, and smooth, muscular legs constantly shrugs his shoulders, gesticulates like an acting class teacher, scribbles split times in his overstuffed black-leather logbook and rains his students with gruff and shrill exhortations ("you can do better than that!" and "don't waste my time!"). The college kids don't care that the man they call the "Mad Hungarian" made history on May 28, 1955, in London. That's when Laszlo Tabori, a little-known runner from Hungary, became the third man, after England's Roger Bannister and Australia's John Landy, to run a mile in under 4 minutes. The 3:59.0 he ran that day was the beginning of a remarkable, yearlong assault on the record books that would eventually leave him with the then-world 1500-meter record (3:40.8, set in Oslo that fall) and national records in three different distances in three different countries: the English mile, the American three-mile, and the 1500 meters in his homeland of Hungary.

Tabori's training methods, taught to the many great Hungarian runners of the fifties by legendary middle-distance coach Mihaly Igloi, came to this country in 1956. As Soviet tanks were crushing his country's anti-communist revolution, Tabori defected while at the Melbourne Olympics. After racing as a man without a country for several years, he struggled to learn English and rebuild his engineering career in southern California, where he married a Hungarian émigré in 1962, fathered two daughters, and began coaching. By the seventies, he'd gained a worldwide reputation that won him the New York Road Runners' Award for Outstanding Contribution to Women's Running, and the prestigious Paavo Nurmi Coach of the Year Award presented by *Runner's World* magazine.

Claiming that he learned how to run by stealing food from German soldiers in World War II, Tabori coached at Los Angeles Valley College from 1968 to 1974 (winning seven individual national

RUN FOR LIFE

junior-college titles and three team state cross-country titles), and founded a running shoe shop and the San Fernando Valley Track Club in 1973. His athletes have won New York and Boston Marathon titles and have included Jackie Hansen and Miki Gorman, the first women to break 2:40 in the marathon.

Known for his intense, irascible, gruff "old school" manner, "he pushes top athletes to do things they never thought that they could achieve," says Ryan Lampa of USA Track and Field. "He has left his mark on the sport."

Born July 6, 1931, Tabori was 76 when he was interviewed on November 9, 2007, and again on April 18, 2008. Speaking with a pronounced Hungarian accent, he has a vivid, entertaining storytelling ability that left me begging for more.

Growing up, I was labeled. Everybody was telling me that I'd be like my old man, a railroad worker. I hate to say this, but he pretty much liked the booze. I never had an alcohol problem, because my old man had the problem—and I hated it. Everybody was saying, "The old man's a boozer, the son's going to be a boozer." Matter of fact, it happened about 10 years ago, the first time I went back to Hungary. I was walking with my sister in the town with the long name. My sister was talking with an old guy, and I overheard their discussion. "Oh yeah, that so-and-so had a son, but probably he's the same as his old man was, he's probably an alcoholic." I walked around behind him and turned him around I said, "Look at this face. You see this face? I'm his son and I'm not alcoholic like you said. You are just a fool ..." Then I told him something nice (i.e., cussed him out). Then I told him, "Many, many places worldwide know me as an athlete."

RUNNING FOR FOOD

I was born in Kassa, in what is now Slovakia. I was a Slovak-Hungarian. Remember, the border changed a lot of times between Czechoslovakia and Hungaria. Tabori is a Hungarian name that means "Camp." We left Kassa in 1941 when I was 10. My dad was working for the railroad, and was moved to Ebauyszanto, northeast Hungary, near Hungary's winery/grape-growing area. Budapest was 200 miles away.

Everybody was affected by World War II. My dad was taken away; all the railroad guys had to go on the German side. The Germans came first through Hungary, then invaded Russia. The front line changed with the Russian counterattack in the winter of '42 or '43. I was pretty young, so I don't remember it exactly. My father didn't get killed. He was a pretty skinny man, born in 1900, 44–45 years old. He hitchhiked back on the trains from Germany.

I remember when the Russians pushed away the Germans from Hungary. I saw lots of things. The bombs were coming straight for 24 hours—boom! boom! boom!—and the planes were coming, and the soldiers. All of us in the family lived through the war.

I was not athletic in school. We just chased each other around, listened to the radio, or stole fruit from somebody's backyard. (Laughs) I was not running until I was 18 years old.

I was an average student, just getting by from grade to grade. From 1940 to '45, there were no books. When the Germans came, we were forced to learn German. When the Russians came they forced Russian on us. I can speak Slavic, which lets you speak the language of five different countries, like Ukraine and Russia.

In the Second World War, food was very rare, so it was our first concern. And I knew at the railroad station they had the barracks for the soldiers which had a different type of dry food there—corn, rice, dried beef. You cannot say stealing—that's not a nice word. My mother said, "They'll shoot you if they catch you stealing food." And I said, "They'll have to catch me first." So I'd say, "I'll go there and borrow some food. God told me I can borrow some food."

I learned how to run when they were chasing me. True—it happened a couple of times. (laughs)

Anyway, bottom line: When the war is finished, I went to the technical school. That was the only thing available for the poor guys like I. In the morning, we work in the factory, we got paid, then we go to the school. The school would teach us about footwear, how to work in a special factory with machines, like they have now in China. The brand was Bata Shoes from Slovakia; we worked at the branch called Cita in Hungary. That was going to be my career—shoes. You needed money to go to college.

In that school, we had physical education twice a week. You tried every sport, and tried to find something you were good at. I went to play soccer, I went to play boxing. None of them I excelled at.

One day, in the spring of 1948, when I was 17, I did a 2-mile race—3-kilometer. It was a run on boat docks, on a riverbed, on the streets, and on the dock again. There were 50–60 people in the race. I didn't train. I'd been training my whole life.

And I beat the second place by like 400 meters.

It was a surprise for me. After the first kilometer, I found myself alone, and I was so scared. I was scared somebody would catch me and I'd be losing, so I ran faster. I didn't know nothing about running.

By the second kilometer, some of my classmates were cheering me on. I don't remember what time I finished in.

Prior to this, I had looked in one of the windows at the store of the town and saw the medals for the race. The first place was a silver, shining little medal, about the size of a 50-cent piece, maybe the size of an old silver dollar. It was on a ribbon—I can't remember the color. And I thought, "Boy, it would be nice to have that medal." That was in my mind during the race.

I didn't feel that that day changed my life. I had two years left to go to school. I was a beginner. I would go run five laps around the football field. That's it.

Two months later, there was a big meet, and I did another race. There were more runners. I won by about 15–20 yards. After that, I still didn't feel serious about running, but my P.E. teacher began to push me, encourage me to race more. "You have to go run more races. There is another race over here and over there," he said. His name,

by the way, was Laszlo Frank—his first name was the same as my last name, which in Hungary was Tabori Laszlo, the last name first. Now, I go to see him every time I go back to Hungary. Anyhow, he sent me a few more places to run. Later, like May and June, was the cross-country season there. I trained on the riverbed—two kilometer up and two kilometer back.

A year later, in 1949, my teacher sent me to a national cross-country race and I came in third in the Junior class (under 19).

By now, I know I'm a good runner. So in the end of August, they sent me to the national track and field championship to run the 1500-meter. I came in third again, and I ran a 4:11.0. It was good. At the time the world record was 3:48 for the 1500-meter. We were dreaming of running a 3:48.

I don't know if that motivated me. I looked at the other guys and compared myself. He's got a pair of legs, two arms, and a torso—he's no different than I am. Why is he better than me? I began to compare myself to others physically. I could not be a basketball player because I'm not tall enough. But I could run. And I was hungry.

In the late 70s and early 80s when the Kenyans and other Africans began to come over here and get good results, some guy came to me and asked, "Gee, Laszlo, why those Kenyans and Ethiopians running so well?" I said, "I know the reason. One word: hungry."

If you go to Kenya with a couple hundred dollars—I have some friends who were there—they say on 400 bucks a family of four can live like a king. They are coming in here, picking up some money, and go home and become rich people. I saw a show about Haile Gebreselassie, the 5- and 10k gold medal runner for a couple of Olympics (and world marathon record holder, 2:04:26 in Berlin, September 30, 2007) , and they showed mansion he has in Ethiopia. He's a rich guy. Take the other one from Africa, El Guerrouj (of Morocco), who won the 1500-meter last Olympic Games. They say his yearly income is 7 million bucks.

At the time I was running, there wasn't money. One day, I was teasing my wife—she passed away a few years ago—"You see these pair of legs [his]—they're only worth a penny." If I'd been born later, they'd be worth a couple million bucks. Last couple of years, go to the European circuit, if you win five races, you're eligible to split a million bucks. In my time, we got three bucks for food. If they give you four bucks, you're a professional.

After I came in third in the 1500 meters, I had one more year in school. I turned 21, and I had to go into the military. That time it was mandatory that every young man go in for two years to the army But just before I went in, I went 3:57 in the 1500 meters. The world record was 3:48.

After six months of training, they pulled me into the Hungarian Army Sports Group. They looked at us—me and [other top runners there] Istvan Rozsavolgi and Sandor Iharos—and says, "It looks like you will fit nice together. You will get to work with the great coach, coach Mihaly Igloi."

And in 1954, we began to run at all the world records. In the next two years, we broke 22 world records.

THE THREE MUSKETEERS

From 1500-meter to 10,000-meter, just about every distance belong to us—except the mile. I set the European record, not the world record: 3:59.

What was the secret of coach Igloi? He had three guys like us—and all three of us had a different temper.

We trained in a circuit. We pushed each other. All three of us were hungry, and we wanted to be good. If we were good, our life began to get a little bit better under the communism—because we got a little bit extra money. We got the job, we got the conditioning money, we got the regular paycheck, we got some special money so that we get enough food to eat to train hard.

They called us "The Three Musketeers." We had a fourth man, Ferene Mikes, when we needed a relay. All of us were good in the 1500-meter. Mikes was the slowest one and he was 3:47; we'd use him in the 4-by-1500 relay. The other three would break the other's world records.

Iharos broke it first, then I, then Rozsavolgi. By 1954, the record was 3:42. The Australian Landy had something

like 3:42.6 Iharos went 3:40.8 in Helsinki. I ran the same time in Oslo two weeks later. Rozsavolgi was the fastest of all. He went 3:40.6 and had the world record in the 2000-meter: 5:02.

All total, Iharos had 12 world records, Rozsavolgi had 7, and I had 4, including my 1500 and three relays. One of those was here in the United States in 1959 or 1960.

The Three Musketeers were together four years, but 1956, the Russian Revolution blew us apart. Were we famous? Yeah. We were like that basketball player on the Lakers—Kobe Bryant. If you walk on the street, people recognize you, correct? You're walking down the street, and people come and stop you and talk to you and wish you good luck. I remember that an old man stopped and talked to me in Budapest. He said, "You know Mr. Tabori, I'm watching you on the track, then I'm watching you here on the street, and I don't believe that you are the same person."

I said, "Why?"

"Because I've never seen such a racer walking so slow like you are doing here, then you go on the track and blow the world record."

If you have to go somewhere, a movie, a theater, or restaurant, you walk in and they say, "We don't have any room." So I say, "Are you sure? How about you look around a little bit for Iharos, Rozsavolgi, and Tabori." He looks up and says, "Hold on." Two minutes later, we had the table. That's how it worked.

Yeah, that was a good part of it, when they recogize you. Definitely, they took care of us.

In the Hungarian Army, the general came in to tell us one day that every year each soldier has to offer to do something positive for the communist Army. Well, we offered them the 4-by-1500 world record. And when we did it, they took us out for pastries. (laughs) Run for food! Nowadays, you make a world record and you get a million bucks. Four years ago in the track and field world championships Helsinki, one of the Russian woman high jumpers set a world record by 1 centimeter and got a $100,000 bonus. We got a piece of pastry. (laughs)

NO SECOND-RATE RUNNER

I did not expect to run a 4-minute mile.

If you are a middle-distance runner, you run a mile or 1,500 meters, it doesn't make any difference effort-wise. I did not have any goal of breaking the 4-minute mile that day. My best time was 4:05.2 prior to that race.

It goes further back. The previous year, 1954, when we (Hungarians) started to run our world records, Iharosh, who had the 3000 world record of 7:55-something, was invited to England to run against Ken Woods in the 2-mile for the world record.

So the Hungarian coach said, "Why don't you also take Tabori?" And the answer came back reading: "We ... do ... not ... want ... second-rate ... runners."

Igloi told me that as we were later on flying to England. Yeah, I got angry. I got pissed like a young man should get pissed.

Later on, I couldn't figure out why they accepted me. Anyway, the old man told me, "You may run in the mile behind Chataway, Iburtson, and Hewson, who all want to break the 4-minute mile."

The race was in White City stadium—a dog-racing stadium (laughs) in London. It was an invitational. Bannister had broken the 4-minute mile May 6, 1954, exactly one year and three weeks before.

At the race, it was the typical English weather. The mist was foggy, the track was heavy and wet. About five minutes before the race, Igloi grabbed my spike shoes and ran away, and a couple minutes later came back and said (imitates a rough, angry voice), "Here, put it on."

I would tell you the secret. But he would jump out of his grave if I did. Later, Tabori said Igloi oiled the sole to keep mud from sticking, so "I ran lighter than the others."

Anyway, he gave me back the shoes. And I said, "What do you want me to do?" He said, "Follow the red-haired guy—Chataway. He wants to break the 4-minute mile."

I was second and third, second and third, behind Chataway and Brian Hewson as we were going by. At 250 yards to go, I pulled out into lane two and three and I began to blow. I began my kick. Because they pissed me off earlier with that, "I don't want the 2nd-rate Hungarian."

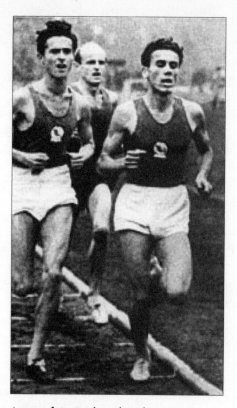

4-minute form: Laszlo on the right.

We reached the 1500-meter mark at 3:43. As we entered the home stretch, I was right between the two guys. At 100 yards, they were behind me, but 50,000 people were screaming, "Chataway-Hewson, Chataway-Hewson, Chataway-Hewson." When I broke the finish line, I heard "Bravo, Tabori!" and my coach ran over and gave me a big hug.

I said, "What?"

He said, "You ran 3:59!"

I said, "Oh, come on," thinking the old man was joking me.

Then I saw the photographers. A hundred photographers—their flashes were going off all around me, like a star was falling.

Everyone was saying, "Three runners had broken the 4-minute mile. The first time that happened in history. The Hungarian beats the British!"

I went to pick up the evening paper, and I hear the newspaper guy yelling, "The Hungarian beat the British! The Hungarian beat the British! Three men under four minutes!"

By that time, back at the hotel, was a table set up in the middle of the dining room, and the translator came to us and said, "You guys are invited to a dinner from the owner of the hotel." So we sit down at that table and a few minutes later—now I know it, remember at that time I didn't know what it was—they bring up a beautiful filet mignon steak and put it right in the middle of the table. Right in front of everybody. We all look at each other and say, "What the heck is this?" At the bottom is all this red-colored fluid—the blood of the steak. We had never seen meat like this.

Hungarians didn't eat steak back home. So we asked the waiter to bring some bread. He came back with a silver holder with one slice. We wanted lots of bread. Finally, somebody got an idea and they went out to a store and picked a loaf of bread with a big salami. And we were cutting big slices of salami in 2-inch-wide circles, and we begin to eat salami-and-bread, salami-and-bread all dinner, with a big, beautiful piece of filet mignon steak sitting there untouched. We didn't want raw meat! Who wants that, you know? (laughs)

Even now, 53 years later, I'm cracking up on it. Because I like it now—a good filet mignon steak, well-done. Nothing's better.

Anyway, after that we go next to the Hungarian Embassy on Sunday. And they were very, very happy. They gave me a plaque, and whispered in my ears, "Laszlo, you don't know what you done for us in here. You opened so many doors for us with that winning." And the meal this time we liked: a nice Hungarian paprika chicken, with homemade noodles.

Monday, we fly back to Budapest. As I look down to where we are landing, I see a bunch of uniforms down there. I look over to Iharos and say, "You will have to make the acceptance speech, not me. You are the older one."

We went through the ceremony, then got our orders. The next day we had to go before the general, the number-one soldier in Hungary. At 10 o'clock, we go into the general's headquarters. Roshavic and I were always the tailgaters, taking with the guards, shaking hands with them, joking with them. We go up to the general's office and line up like soldiers. The general steps in front of us and you say your name and your rank. I was the shortest between us, so was at the end of the line. He steps in front of me and I introduce myself, then he puts his arm on his chest and looks at me. We were almost the same height—he was about an inch taller. He goes around me, comes back front of me, then goes behind me again and comes back.

Then he says, "Well, Mr. Tabori, you are the shortest one—just like a black pepper. Small but strong." You know, a black pepper, the little round thing. You find it in a salad with cucumbers. And when you bite it, it burns your tongue like a big flame.

Meantime, the captain poured booze into the glasses, and when we finish with the introductions, the general says, "Okay, for a beautiful victory in the athletic field, cheers for everybody." And he zoomed down the booze. I don't know what liquor it was, but it was burning down to my stomach. I thought I was going dark. But it was very smooth.

So that's the 4-minute mile. The second-class Hungarian runner changed to a number-one-class runner in a four-minute period. I was the first non-British citizen, non-English-speaking person to run the four-minute mile. Bannister, British, and Landy, an Australian. Then me and Chataway and Hewson. Four English-speakers and a Hungarian. Also, I was the first to break Bannister's European record, but not the world record. By that time, Landy already run a 3:58.

That four-minute mile gave me much better publicity than a 1500-meter world record. If you tell people that you run the 1500-meter record, they give you a stare. But I say I ran a 3:59 mile, and they say, "Wow!"

GOOD-BYE, HUNGARY. HELLO, AMERICA

We were doing great. Except we got the Revolution, and it blew apart everything.

The Revolution started while we were in Olympic training camp [for the 1956 Melbourne Olympics], 100 miles away from Budapest. After a couple weeks it was difficult to train because the bullets were flying all over. So we packed up all our gear and went to Budapest, 100 miles away. It wasn't sure if we were going to Olympics. It was, "we're going, no we're not going." Finally, in the last minute, they pack us into 2 buses and take us to Czechoslovakia. We were there for a week or so. Then took us to Zurich, and then flew 5 days to Melbourne. By that time, I was losing 3 or 4 weeks training.

We get to Australia, and the Melbourne airport is loaded up with Hungarians and Jewish people who left during World War II. I came down from the plane and I put my arms extended out from my sides, and a bunch of them came and tried to touch me. "Are you okay? You didn't get shot?"

"I'm okay—it's no problem."

Anyway, we got that far. They take us to the Olympic villaige and show us the places where we are supposed to be. And we tried to catch up with the training, but it didn't work very good. After the opening ceremony—that was a big deal over there—I started competing. I said, I'm here; I may as well do what I can. Monday, when the track and field competition begins, there was a 5000-meter prelim. So I begin to go. Last 120 yards, I begin to count 1–2–3–4. I was 5th. The top four advanced to the final. I see the guy about 15 yards ahead of me, and I said, "oh shit." I go and I catch. So I kicked—and made the 5000-meter final.

In the final on Wednesday, I tried to slow down Kuts, the Russian, but it didn't work—he ended up getting the gold medal in the 5000 and the 10,000. I wanted to make it a kicker's race, but he knew what he wanted. He went to the front and drove like a maniac, because he was slow. I came in 6th place, something like 14:06. He won in 13:40. Kuts was way ahead of everybody.

Thursday was the 1500-meter prelim. Same thing; with 100 yards to go, I just kicked and made the final. By the way, I just got a copy of film of the final. Saturday was the final; 110,000 people in the stadium, the newspapers said. I was in the middle of the pack, inside, with about 120 yards to go, when it got crowded up. Landy came up against me, but I was alert—I grabbed him, pushed him forward. That forced me backwards. It was a pushing match. If I didn't put my arm out, three or four of us would collide. I was against the curb when I started my kick. I came in 4th. The difference between 2nd, 3rd, and 4th was four-thousandths of a second. The winner was 3:41. The second was 3:42, and 3rd and 4th were both 3:42.04.

The lack of training and the jostling with Landy hurt. I think I could have got second.

After the races were over came the big decision: Should I go back to Hungary? I went to Igloi and said, "Hey old man, what do you think?" He turned around and walked away from me without a word. I had Hungarian Americans inviting me to compete in indoor races in the U.S. in the 1957 season. One day they gave me a permit, and the next day they revoked it. When the Hungarian team was going to fly home the next day, I just disappeared for 24 hours. Not just me—38 other Hungarians of the team of 135 did the same thing. The next day, when we are going in the airport to go to the United States, guess who is walking over there with the group? My coach!

But he would not talk to me prior to that day. I went up to him and said, "What happened?" He said, "Well, I'm going to America. Listen, I'm going there and you're going there. So why don't we stick together for a while?" And that's how we started our American adventure.

That was the end of the Three Musketeers. Rozsavolgi didn't go the Olympics because he had personal problems, was married, and his condition was lousy. I was the single guy.

I was sponsored by Sports Illustrated. So when I got to America, it was okay. I ran all over the East Coast, from Boston, New York, Philadelphia, Washington, D.C., down to Miami, then back Midwest to Milwaukee, Chicago, Des Moines, Cleveland. In May we had the Coliseum Relays in Los Angeles. So I came to California in May 1957. And in June, they dropped me like a hot potato.

No sponsor, no nothing. My English was perfect—I knew about 50 words by that time. No job, no money, no nothing. But, I'm here, I'm fine, thanks God.

But at that time, there was no money in track and field like they have this time in Europe. My coach Igloi stayed until 1962, then went to Greece, then to Hungary the last couple years before he passed away. He was a great coach. When he died, the New York Times did a big story about him and showed a picture of him and one of his runners, Jim Beatty, the first American who broke the 4-minute indoor mile in '58 or '59. Igloi's runners had 49 world records to his name between the U.S., Hungary, and Greece, and some 150 national records.

I, Beatty, and two others running for the Los Angeles Track Club were in the distance medley—all 4 laps different: 400, 800, 1200, 1600. I ran the 1600 in 3:59.6. It was on a dirt track, not a rubber track. We had five guys in that club who had broke the 4-minute mile.

I won the American 3-mile championship in 1960. That gave me three national championships in three countries: U.S., England—the mile, and Hungary—the 1500. 1961 was my last season.

THE COACH

From '61 to '68 I disappeared from Earth. I worked as an engineer for Everest & Channings making wheelchairs, making the design and the blueprints and everything else. I began coaching at Valley College in '68. I had Igloi's ideas and my ideas and tried to put them together. My philosophy: Have the guts to be honest with yourself and do the work. There is no other way to be good. It's like anything: If I wanted a good race car, I build a good engine and make sure I have a good tuneup in it.

I don't know if it's the same as the other coaches. I don't analyze the other people. My idea is if you reach good results, then the training was good.

I don't know why I did so well coaching women [he coached Micki Gorman, 1977 RRCA Runner of the Year and 2001 Long Distance Running Hall of Fame inductee, and Jacki Hansen, the first American women to break 2:40 in the marathon, as well as Liana Reinhart, who ran a 2:46

in 1977 to win the U.S. Marathon Chapionship.] I grew up with two sisters, and I have two daughters. So my house was always filled with females.

I founded a running shoe shop (Tabori's Sports in Burbank) in the early '70s that I just closed a couple months ago. But I'm still busy coaching. If I didn't, I would grow bananas, going crazy. I go three times a week to USC, I have the middle distance runners. I also still have the leftovers from my club.

I'm staying in shape as much as I can. I can't run because my second surgery won't let me. I have two hip replacements, 19 years apart, the last one 3 years ago. I can't run because my second surgery didn't come in right. So it limits me to walking my two little Dachshunds. I don't like the water or bike. Just walk. Don't lift weights. I use my own body—push-ups, pull-ups, chin-ups on the monkey bars.

The hip problems began in Hungary when I was 24. Two of us jump up, the other guy was heavier than me, and we hit hips. I was only 135 pounds, skin and bones when I was racing. The impact caused a 4-inch crack in my femur. I competed with a busted bone. I ran a 4-minute mile on it and set a world record on it. I didn't know it myself. Every day, I have a pain in my right hip and we didn't know it because we do not have the sophisticated instruments what we have now.

I don't know what is happening to this new generation. I go to USC and taught them to work. "You've got this scholarship, you have to give something in return." And they look at me and say, "I'm not a professional." Hell, according to the Olympics rule, you are professional, because you get money—tuition—for your studies. USC costs 40 grand a year. And they don't want to work.

The teenagers now growing up expect their parents to serve them like a silver plate. That's the problem. Athletes who were running with me when they were 50, 60 years old I like better than the younger ones.

A couple weeks ago at USC, I saw our team masseuse—a nice old guy like me—and he handed me an old book he bought for me in a book store called Moments in Sports, from the Associated Press, which had a bunch of pictures in it. One was of me. It was a three-mile run in London and I was as muddy as a pig, against Chataway and Ibartson. It was that kind of typical English weather—rainy, cinder, mud. It was a dual meet between England and Hungary. I followed because I didn't want to lead. Since I was behind, I got all muddy because the spikes just throw the cinder right on your chest. I looked like I jumped in a pig hole and came out. A great picture.

The book has all the unusual photos. There's a picture of Mary Decker laying on the ground crying after she was knocked down in the '84 Games. There's a shot of Bannister and Landy. Jessie Owens. Moho Medaly in his prime. Baseball players, football players. It goes way, way back.

Bannister and I know each other. I saw Landy two years ago in Australia at the 50th anniversary of the '56 games; There's a 50-year reunion at each Olympic Games. Landy was losing his hearing in his left ear when I was there. He's okay; he just retired from work. I never ran against either of them. Bannister quit when I was coming in. But I ran against Chataway, who was the number-two guy in England when Bannister broke the 4-minute mile.

I don't have so many regrets. A medal in Melbourne would have been nice. Not having to wait 25 years to return to Hungary also. But I really would have liked to coach Jim Ryun. He could have been the greatest of all time with the right coaching. He did not know how to warm up. You must break into oxygen—it's like a car engine warming up. Wait one- two minutes before you drive it. Ryun did not, so first lap, always dead last. Then second lap—moving up. Third lap—among the leaders. And fourth lap—he'd always say, "I got my second wind." But that wasn't his second wind. It was just that his body finally warmed up. My warm-up gets you into your second wind before the race starts.

I once asked his coach if Jim knew how to warm-up, and he said 'no.' Imagine, Ryun ran a 3:51 almost 40 years ago—just six or seven seconds slower than today's record. And his legs were still cold!

(See Laszlo's Race Day Warm-Up Rules in a sidebar at the end of Chaper 26, Periodization.)

RUN FLEXIBLE

One of the mysteries of the universe is why most of us don't stretch before and after we run. Maybe it's that we endorphin-addicted runners are so eager to get our fix that a few minutes of stretching seems superfluous.

But there's a problem with that: If you don't stretch as you age, your body naturally tightens up. Inch by inch, it loses its range of motion. To make matters worse for runners, running itself hastens the process, tightening the screws in your hamstrings, calves, and back. The result: corruption of your hard-won form, increased injuries as bones and ligaments get pulled out of alignment, declining performances, slower recovery, and odd pains that seem to have no rational explanation or origin. And then there's the worst part of it: You look bad. You walk stiffly, like old people do. Fact: If you're stiff at any age, you look old before your time.

Stretching is the antidote. So if you won't do it because it makes sense or improves your ergonomic efficiently, do it for the reason we all understand: Vanity.

This section gives you two different and complementary stretching routines. In Chapter 12, Bob Forster of Phase IV provides some functional runner's stretches, and an important reason for stretching that you may not have considered before: Stretching is the first step in good running form. If you don't care about how you look in normal life, you will surely care about how you look running.

Then there's the feeling. Some say a good stretching routine is part massage and part endorphin high. Joints relaxed, muscles open, posture and mood become suffused with chi, a healthy state of awareness.

Appropriately, Chapter 13 highlights the talent, creativity, and perfect proportionality of celebrated multisport star Steve Ilg, one of the rare trained yogis who is also a standout in endurance multisports, including running. The author of the best seller *Total Body Transformation* and the founder of High-Performance Yoga, Ilg designed a fun yet rigorous running-specific program for his upcoming book, *Age-Erasing Yoga for Athletes*. He agreed to share part of it with *Run for Life* if I agreed to print the phrase "suffused with chi." Ilg says it can be used anytime, anywhere, and as an ideal 7-minute warm-up for a run.

Ironically, that brings us back to where we started. If you still don't like to stretch, now you don't have to. Do yoga instead.

CHAPTER 12

RUNNERS' STRETCHES

Flexibility is the first stage of good form. Get it with these 11 warm-up stretches

I stretch my pecs.

That sounds a little weird, I know. I never thought I'd say that in public. In fact, I never even thought about doing it at all until I starting writing this book. But now that I know how good it is to do that, I cannot stop. It wouldn't make sense.

It seems that tight pectoral muscles—and apparently we all get them because we sit all day in a leaned-forward position and tend to favor front-of-body pushing activities over pulling exercises that work the back—are a problem. They wreak havoc with a vertical arm swing. They pull your arm toward the center. That wrecks the critical arm-as-pendulum part of running form that you've already spent too much time reading about.

Until I understood that, I didn't understand what phase IVs Bob Forster was talking about when he told me that stretching is more than mere stretching. To be technically accurate about it, *stretching is actually the first step in good form.*

"Stretching is a crucial part of your warm-up and cool-down," he says. "It gives you the flexibility to run with proper biomechanics and technique, and it will help prevent injury too."

The technical explanation: "Flexibility is defined as the range of motion of bones around a joint," Forster explains, "and bones must have the freedom of movement to be positioned *just right* in the sequence of sport motion. This is what we call 'proper technique.' When muscles have inadequate flexibility (i.e. they are tight), they will have to work overtime to put the bones in their ideal position."

It's not hard to see why that can be a problem. First, you may be so tight that you can't move your bones 'just right' without straining muscles and connective tissue. Extremely tight muscles can even pull bones out of alignment, torquing joints and potentially leading osteoarthritis. Next, tight muscles require more energy to get things done. If you are tight during a race, you'll use up extra energy and risk having fatigue set in earlier. Next, For longevity purposes, regular stretching gives you flexible muscles that allow you to safely push it harder and recover quicker, so you can tap the hormonal benefits of intervals and rapid-contraction weight lifting.

Interestingly, stretching doesn't mean that you are stretching muscle fibers per se. Red-blood-rich muscle fibers are elastic and will stretch without much resistance. You're actually stretching the white connective tissue that surrounds each muscle fiber and wraps groups of them into bundles as it controls and limits the muscle's range of motion. By the way, connective tissue is also the material of tendons (which attach muscles to bones), and comprises ligaments (which attach bones to bones at the joint).

According to Forster, connective tissue is not immediately elastic and requires the application of slow, sustained stretching to lengthen. Permanent lengthening of these structures equates to good flexibility and therefore puts you one step closer to good technique.

Here's an example of how poor flexibility can ruin good technique:

In good form, the knee rise in the front of the body must be high enough so that the foot will strike the ground moving backward, gripping and pawing the ground like a bull getting ready to charge a matador.

But if you have tight, inflexible butt and hamstrings muscles, that knee won't rise so high, and your foot won't have enough air time to land correctly. (If that example isn't sexy enough, just remember my pecs.)

STRETCHING RULES

- *Relaxed position:* Forster is against freestanding stretches that force you to brace yourself, like bending over and touching your toes and reaching back and grabbing your ankle. "You want to hit each of the major muscle groups while they are relaxed—not stressed," he says. "You want to be breathing easy.

- *Stretch before workouts and races:* "Ballerinas don't run around the room to break a sweat before stretching," he says. "They start the class at the stretch bar."

- *Stretch after workouts:* It aids recovery by "wringing" the waste products out of the muscle and returning the muscles to their normal resting length. This prevents you from decreasing your flexibility as a result of training.
- *Stretch at night:* It improves flexibility and your ability to adapt to strenuous workouts without injury. It will also help you relax for a better night's sleep.
- *Hold it a while:* Before and after the workout, stretch the target muscle 10–30 seconds, 3 reps. At night, hold for 60 seconds.
- *Start slow:* Follow the subsiding tension principle by moving slow into the stretch position and tuning into the tension you feel in the muscle.

PHASE IV RUNNER'S STRETCHES

1. Standing Hamstring Stretch: It is critical to monitor good flexibility in the hamstring muscle and the inner thigh to monitor good running form and prevent injury to the knees, buttock, and lower back. This stretch addresses the former. Notice that the model elevates the leg forward and hinges at the waist, but does not bend over and touch his toes. There is no need to stress the lower back.

2. Standing Adductor Stretch: This exercise addresses the inner thigh

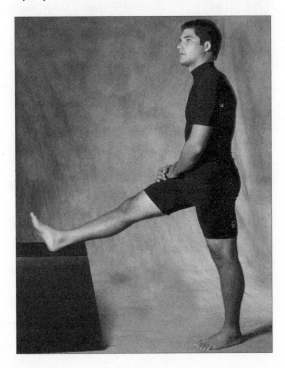
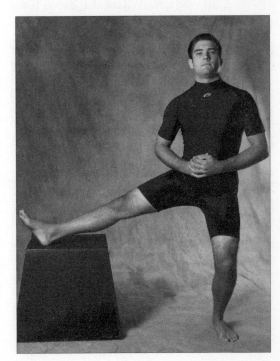

145

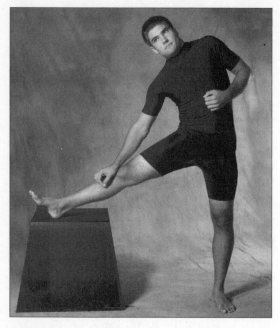

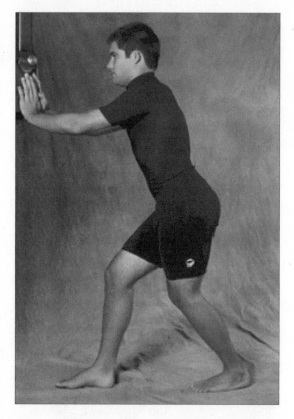

and the soleus, is essential to maintaining proper running form. Work the gastroc, the outside muscle, by keeping the rear leg straight and leaning forward.

4. Calf Soleus Stretch with bent leg: People often forget the soleus (the lower-inner muscle)—and pay the price

(adductors). Elevate the leg to side and hinge at the waist.

3. Calf Gastroc Stretch: Stretching the two muscles of the calf, the gastroc

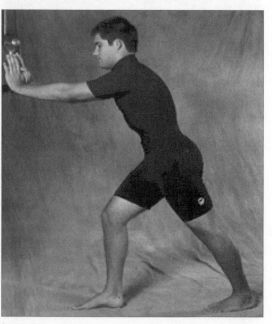

later in the race. Stretch it by starting with a bent rear leg, as shown, and lowering your body vertically by flexing both knees.

5. Kneeling Hip Flexor Stretch: The hip flexors will shorten with time and continued running, often causing lower back pain and injury. Keeping them

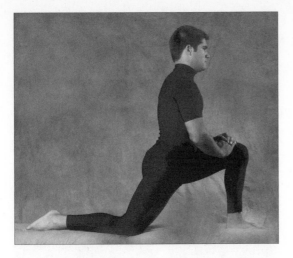

stretched out prevents groin injuries and spinal problems.

6. Standing Upper Trap Stretch: Narrows and restores shoulder blades, and stretches delts and upper pecs, setting up proper path for a vertical arm swing on the side of the body. Place right arm behind your back and grab your right wrist with the left hand and pull it gently down and to the left. Bring chin down to chest, rotate to the left, and look at your armpit. Repeat on other side.

7. Pec Stretch: Most of us have over-developed tight pecs that tend to disrupt a vertical arm swing, not allowing good backswing and pulling the arm across the chest. This stretch restores that flexibility. Make a fist and place your hand with thumb-side up on the wall or doorframe level with the top of your head. Step forward with the same-side leg to get a stretch at the front of the shoulder and chest.

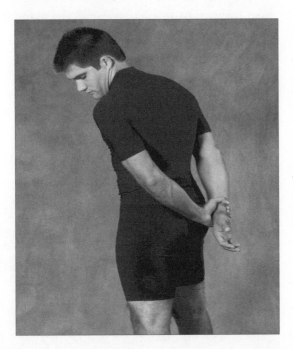

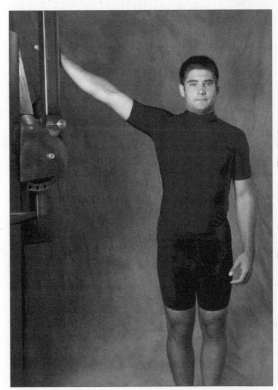

8. Advanced Pelvis Rotation: These next two stretches address the buttock muscles and are critical to avoiding injury. Over 50% of the running injuries we see are related to buttock and hip dysfunction.

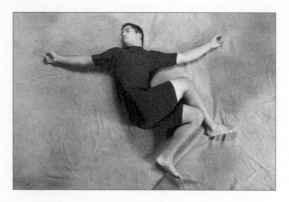

9. Pretzel Stretch: This one specifically addresses tightness in the deep rotators of the hip and "Piriformis" syndrome that commonly afflicts runners.

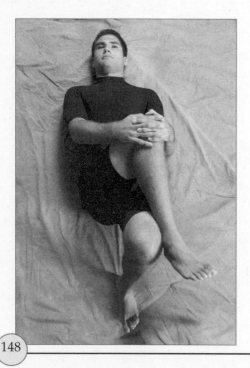

10. Supine Adductor Stretch: Raising knees to a 90-degree bend, place hands on insides of knees and apply light pressure, feeling the stretch at the inner thigh as the legs remain airborne.

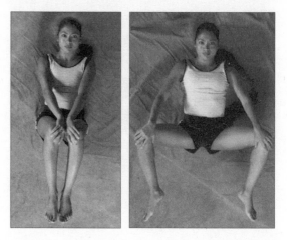

11. Side Lying Quad Stretch: Performing this stretch regularly is the single most important thing you can do to avoid knee injuries as you continue running. The quadriceps tighten over time and affect the knee cap and its ability to "track" properly between the condyles of the femur. If left unstretched, runners are susceptible to patella tendonitis or "runner's knee" and early arthritic changes in the knee.

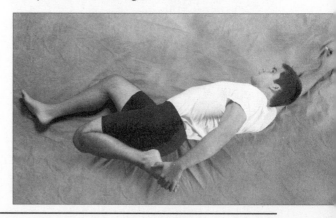

CHAPTER 13

YOGA ON THE RUN

Warm up with this exclusive High-Performance Yoga® for Runners plan by fitness guru/certified yoga instructor Steve Ilg

I f you know the name of one yoga position, it is probably Downward Facing Dog. With your body bent at a right angle, with feet and hands on the floor and butt high in the air, it looks like you're an "A" without the horizontal crossbar. Except, according to Steve Ilg, when you're a runner—then you look more like a backward question mark that's toppled over.

"Three out of four times, I can tell when a runner comes to class for the first time," says Ilg, the inventor of the highly athletic High-Performance Yoga and the author of the forthcoming *Age-Erasing Yoga for Athletes*. "Instead of straight lines, a runner's legs are bent and his upper body looks like a C. That's because the hamstrings, lower back, and Achilles tendons are so tight he can't straighten his legs all the way, and his skinny arms are fastened to scapulas that are virtually glued to the spine, so he doesn't have the flexibility in his shoulders to fully extend his arms."

Ilg has a good idea what athletes ought to look like because he is a rare combination: A full-blown yogi and elite-level athlete. In the eighties, he was on teams that won the run-bike-ski-snowshoe Mt. Taylor Winter Quadrathalon four times and was the 2-time course record holder at Colorado's 12,640-feet Pagosa Peak Run. In 1992, having gained a reputation as a trainer, peak runner, and multisport athlete, he was pictured on a cover of *Outside* magazine next to the headline, "This man can break you—and build you up again." I rode with him on a relay team at the 2004 Furnace

Creek 508 (mile) bike race through Death Valley (yeah, he's a great cyclist, too) and was astounded by a flexibility that allowed him to ride with a perfectly flat back while in the aerobar position. It turns out that rehabbing from an injury that left him temporarily paralyzed led him to yoga, and soon, to teaching it with a rigorous athletic spin.

Today, from his base in Flagstaff, Arizona, Ilg starts most days with a long snowshoe hike, mountain-bike ride, or a 9.6-mile run from 9,500 feet to the top of 12,633-foot Humphrey's Peak, the highest point in Arizona. Whatever he's doing, it's working; as you'll see by the photos we took in late April 2008, he's as limber as a yogi, as chiseled as a bodybuilder, and amazingly youthful for 46. On a bad day, he looks 35.

Sport-specific runners, however, don't look so good, says Ilg. "They aren't balanced. They arrive at a point where all they can do is run, and as you get older, that leaves you somewhat dysfunctional," he says. He believes that the repeated day-after-day impact of the femur jamming into the hip socket upsets what he calls "pelvic horizontal-ity," contributing to a host of problems: an imbalanced spine that cannot adjust; pinched spinal nerves that lead to glandular and organ disorders; weak midsections and hip flexors, undeveloped "internal flotation;" slumped shoulders; and brittle feet, ankles, and knees.

"Bottom line: Runners tend to get a compacted pelvic girdle. The wheels can't turn when they are jammed. This routine will de-compact you."

THE 12-MINUTE RUNNER'S YOGA WARM-UP

The following 12-minute "asana" workout (defined as "conscious breathing while sustaining postures") consists of moving deliberately, with little rest, between seven traditional, challenging, yoga poses. Ilg designed the workout to jump-start joint lubrication, align your arms and legs for vertical pendular movement, and warm the muscles up for training runs.

Pose 1: Yogi Squat into Forward Fold

"The squat returns the runner to his or her center," says Ilg. It restores mobility

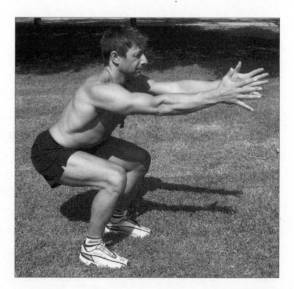

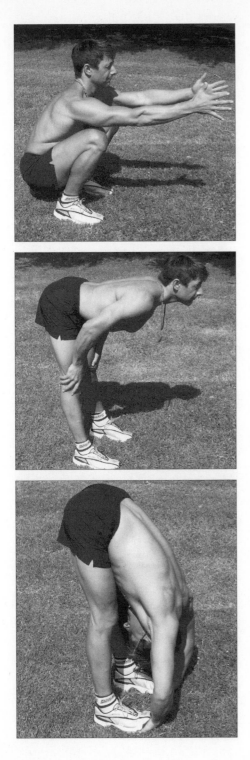

to dense skeletal and connective tissue. Starting with this exercise opens and releases the lower back (lumbar/sacroiliac) and hamstrings and straightens your upper body carriage-posture. The Forward Fold aerates and injects elongation to jammed-up lower back and hamstrings.

What to do: 3 to 5 reps.

Pose 2: Kneeling Warrior Pose

This prepares the spinae erector muscles to sustain the compression of running, lubricates the hip joint, and warms up the psoas, hip flexors, and quads.

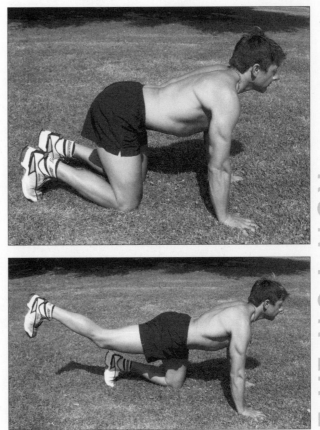

151

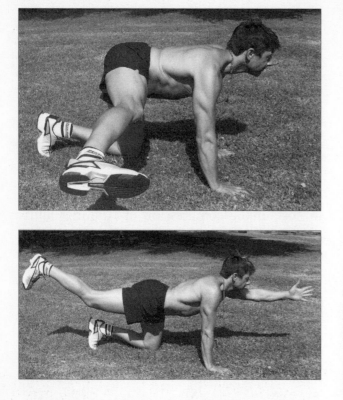

Kaplabhati, "The Skull Shining Breath," and make repeated sudden contractions of your abdominal muscles and diaphragm. This helps fire split-second breath "bullets" out of your nose (not mouth) like a wheezy machine gun. Try to contract your abs to your spine "like squeezing a toothpaste tube," says Ilg. The constant up and down of the diaphragm exercises your internal organs and muscles.

What to do: 3 to 5 reps of the 4-exercise sequence on each leg.

Pose 3: Hero's Pose with Breathing

This technical posture prepares the quads, pre-stretches and aligns the ankle, opens hip flexors, and, most of all, makes respiratory muscles more supple. It stretches the ribs, keeping them soft instead of brittle, and teaches the lungs to oxygenate more efficiently. "This will warm up the lung engine and permeate the body with prana (life force)," says Ilg.

Important: The arms and hands create a "skeletal brace" that keeps the spine erect, like the third leg of a tripod. Then, with mouth closed and chin down, you use a technique called

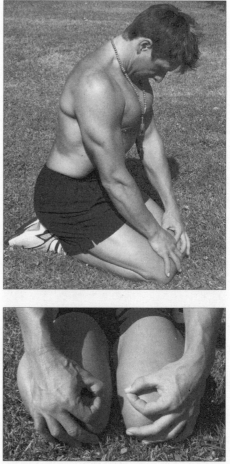

"Even well-known runners will find that orchestrating these subtle respiratory muscles is challenging," says Ilg. "What they need to tell themselves is that they are cleaning their internal engine, eliminating huge amounts of CO_2."

What to do: Start with 3 Kaplabhatis and move up to 21 as your ability improves. "Do *not* push through discomfort while doing these types of yogic breathing techniques," cautions Ilg.

Pose 4: Camel Pose/Backbend

This simple, effective pose rewires the proper sway in the back, opens up hip flexors, and expands the breathing cage musculature and aligning arm posture for a strong vertical arm swing. "The runner's upper body, like most of society, is kyphotic—too rounded—because the scapula (shoulder blades) are plastered to the spine and held in place by gluey rhomboids," says Ilg. "If I can free the rhomboids, they'll give the arms freedom of movement—and a warrior's grace will arise within their running." He believes that runners who run with a tight upper body tend to run like "robots," with no freedom in the shoulder blades. "You want your arms to be as free as your legs, with elbows higher on upswing and backswing. The arms drive the legs, if they can move freely."

What to do: Hold 30 to 60 seconds.

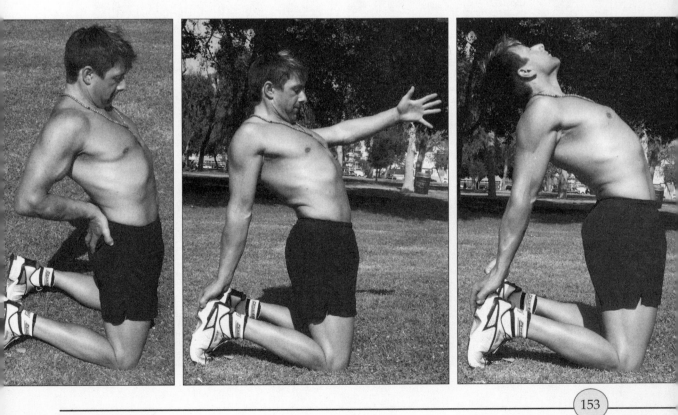

Pose 5: Adductor Stretch Spinal Twist

"The adductor muscle originates in the pubis and attaches throughout the femur," says Ilg. "If they are tight, it'll

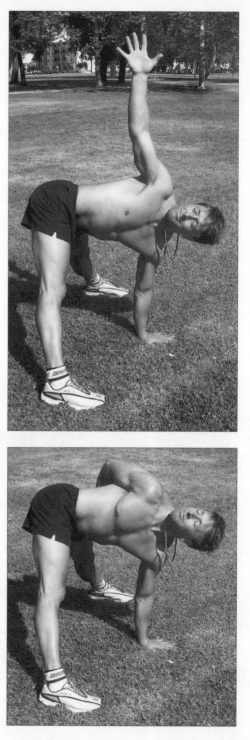

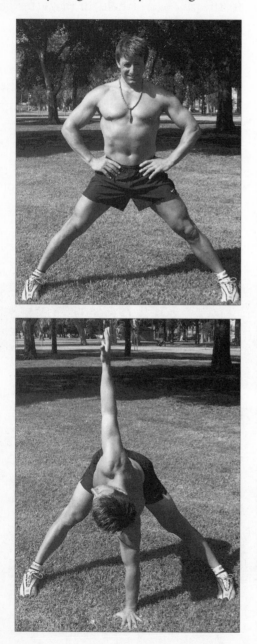

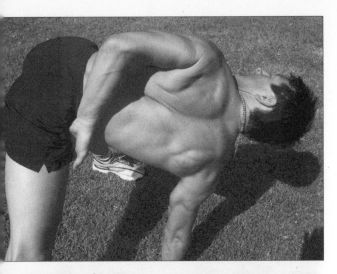

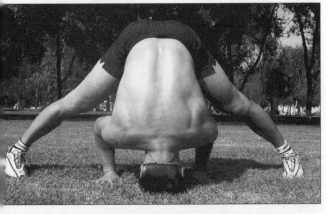

pull the leg across the midline, contributing to poor performance and longer-term health problems." You get tight adductors from sitting. Stretch them standing (not sitting), because runners stand, not sit.

The headstand option shown in panels 5–9 are done "solely to impress your friends," says Ilg. "Just kidding. A headstand is considered the 'most medicinal' of all yoga pose categories by the ancient yoga masters."

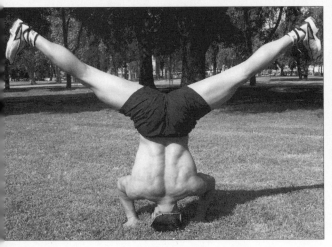

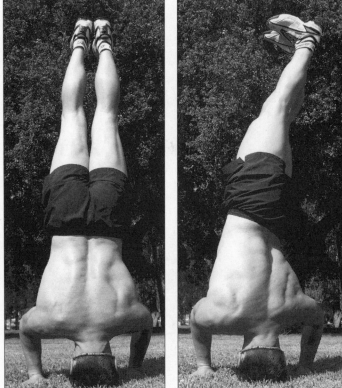

Pose 6: Crescent Pose with Twist

The Crescent loosens up ankles, stretches the quad, and frees up inner thigh/power chain musculature. It liberates stored kinetic energy within the hips—psoas, piriformis—all the deep pelvic muscles. Result: "A sensation of bodily lightness if done right before you run," says Ilg. The twist portion in shots 2–4 is difficult to do initially, requiring a

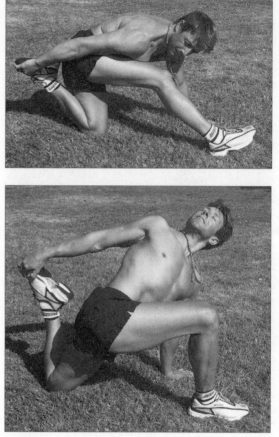

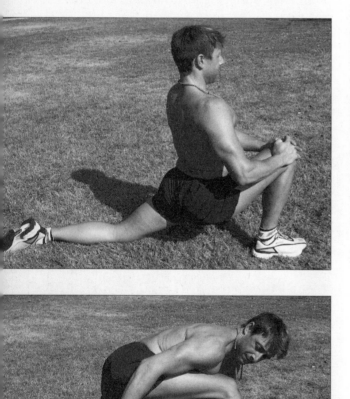

great deal of abdominal and lower back flexibility. It may take several weeks or months to get this.

Pose 7: Downward Facing Dog Knee Drives

The final step before you run, this classic yoga position is a very holistic, all-body warm-up, energizer, and stress reliever. It synthesizes the inner and outer architecture of all the previous poses, stretching arms, shoulders, hams, calves, Achilles tendons, arches of feet. It lengthens the spine and prepares core abdominals for better running mechanics. To get into it, start standing with feet flat on the ground, bend down, put fully extended hands flat on the floor, and walk back three feet. Send your butt high into the air. Let the spine lengthen by keeping the thighs firm, as if you are trying to lift the kneecaps up to the thighs. Lift your toes to lower your heels.

What to do: Hold the dog for three breaths then move to the second pose (with the leg up). This helps train the muscles to keep the hips in running position. The third pose, which drives the knee up and toward the chin, warms up the entire midsection and gets you motivated. "Running seems easy compared to this," Ilg says.

"This sequence is potent medicine, and should be taken every time you run," Ilg says. "It leaves you suffused with chi. Namaste, noble warrior!"

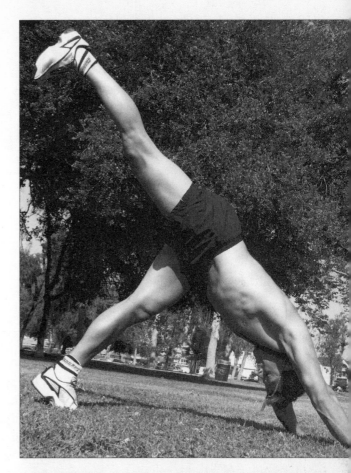

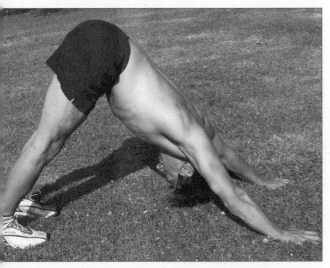

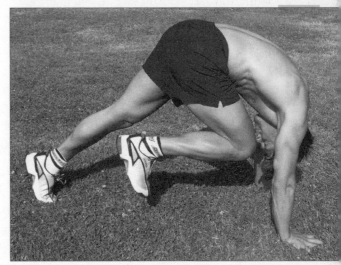

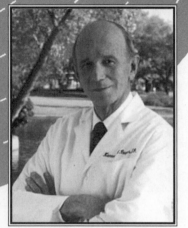

DR. KENNETH COOPER

The Philosophical Father of the Running Boom

Aerobics. Anti-oxidants. These words are part of our everyday language due to Dr. Kenneth H. Cooper, who introduced the former in his 1968 bestseller, *Aerobics*, which basically changed the way we exercised, and the latter in 1997's *The Anti-Oxidant Revolution*, which changed the way we eat. An Air Force physician with a Master's in public health from Harvard, the former Oklahoma prep track star provided the academic underpinnings of the coming running boom and the worldwide fitness revolution. He also developed the 12-minute fitness test and Aerobics Point System used today by the army, navy, secret service, and many schools and corporations; launched The Cooper Aerobics Center in Dallas, a now-internationally renowned research and treatment center; and has written 19 books. Having successfully fought weight gain and deconditioning in his late 20s and early 30s, and run 38,000 miles over the last four decades, Cooper is a good advertisement for his methods—superfit in his eighth decade due to weight lifting and power walking at an impressive 5 mph every day. He talks as fast as he moves, as I discovered in our interview on January 23, 2008, (when he was 77); the man spits facts and stories like a machine gunner on an adrenaline high. Here he outlines the telltale signs of overtraining, explains why he's backed off on *Aerobics'* central thesis of "more is better," why weight training is more important as you age, and why he feels so darn good.

I'm 77 years of age. And I feel 30.

I was a state champion at Putnam High in Oklahoma City, running the mile in 4:31 back in 1949. I was using the old-type of track shoes and cinder tracks like we don't have today so really it was pretty remarkable to run that fast. Of course, now they're running sub-4-minute miles in high school. But that got me a scholarship to the University of Oklahoma. I was there only three years—I did three years of pre-med with good grades. During that time, I kept running, primarily the mile, half-mile, and two miles. My times didn't drop that much. My best mile time was 4:18, my best half-mile was 1:56, and my best 2-mile was 9:40. But the reason for that, I became convinced, through my work in later years in exercise physiology, is that the training technique that was given to us by our coach, John Jacobs at U of O, was most inappropriate. We didn't train enough.

Jacobs felt that you needed to exercise in spurts. Like I ran cross-country in the fall, indoor in the winter, and outdoor in the spring. They were afraid back in those days that you'd take the spring out of your legs if you ran year-round. You never ran more than 25 miles a week. So when I ran against Wes Santee, a potential 4-minute-miler of that time who ran a 4:01, who some thought would be the first one to break the 4-minute mile, I of course never came close.

Now, when I was running in high school, I didn't have a coach. My coach was actually the principal, and I got written instructions from a Harold Mead, who was the sports publicity director at U of O—he sent me a routine every week to prepare for the meets. And I was undefeated my senior year in the mile and half-mile.

Mead encouraged me to go LSD—Long Slow Distance. It wasn't what the coach recommended when I got to college. But he felt, as I did, that the more I ran longer, the better I'd be at the shorter distances. So I concentrated on LSD. I was running 50, 60, 70 miles a week.

I wasn't doing much interval work. When I got to college, the reverse was, the coach felt, "if you're going to break the four-minute mile, then you better run the hundred-yard dash in 11 seconds." And so we did all these darn sprints. And we'd never run more than three or four miles at one time. It was so frustrating, because it was the exact opposite of what I'd been doing on my own in high school, and I'd done very well, and wasn't bringing my times down like I thought in my first three years of college. I recall on a Sunday I went out and ran 15 miles. And I got chewed out by the coach the next day. "What in the heck do you think you're doing? Coop, don't you realize that you're taking the spring out of your legs? Don't you realize you're going to ruin yourself? It's going to wear you out!"

So we would actually start training 6 weeks before the season for cross-country. We'd lay off between cross-country and indoors for about two weeks at least. We'd start back training indoors, then lay off after that until outdoors. We didn't run continuously at all. And then the summer we'd bike or something other than run. And I worked at a meatpacking plant, lifting weights. And that was our training program back in those days.

And we later found that the guys who were breaking the 4-minute miles were running 100 miles a week or more.

GOT FAT, CAME BACK, RAN BOSTON

When I was in college, I thought I was in great shape. I was able to get into medical school after three years because I made good grades—getting 4 hours of sleep a night. Keep in mind that obesity is the most common manifestation of stress. So ... I ate to keep awake. I was getting minimal sleep. My weight ballooned up from 168 to 204.

By the time I finished my medical school days on a one-year internship in Seattle, that lack of sleep was even worse. That's when I reached my peak of weight and de-conditioning. Getting married didn't help me much. I didn't lose any weight. And I told my wife, "I've got a 2-year hitch in the military and I feel like I'm dying of mental apathy." I had no interest, no desire, watching television, doing no athletic activity.

But in 1960, 29 years of age, after being totally sedentary essentially for 8 years, I went water skiing for the first time and tried to ski a slalom course. I'd skied slalom courses in my youth, doing jumps, and I was almost a competitive water skier in my early days. But I tried to ski this slalom course, and I ended up with an attack of tachycardia, skiing along and I feel like my heart is beating out of my chest. It went from roughly 120 to about 240. I didn't have an idea what happened—was I having a heart attack? They took me to the hospital. But by the time I got there, though, the heart rate had come back to normal.

So they checked me out. And they said, "Doc, the only thing wrong with you is that you are out of shape." I couldn't believe that. State athlete. National-class athlete.

159

All of that—in a very short period of time, I had completely deteriorated—what the majority of Americans have done, unfortunately—into massive obesity. It shocked me into reality.

At that time, I was going on to specialize in aerospace medicine and going on to Harvard. So I decided I was going to lose that weight. I lost it in 6 months, and I started running up in Boston. And I ran my first marathon a year later, the 1962 Boston. Never smoked. Got sadly out of shape. Gained that weight. Lost it all. And within one year ran that marathon in 3:54.

When I was at my peak, a sub-7-minute mile. I ran my second Boston in 3:20 in 1963—was trying to break 3:00. I maintained the pace for the first 21 miles, but I hit the wall at the top of Heartbreak Hill. I had 5 miles to go. But I averaged 11 minutes a miles from there so I lost 20 minutes. I never could break 3 hours for the marathon.

I ran steadily from 1960 to 2004. 38,000 miles. Several marathons—only two Bostons, a 40-miler once, averaging 50, 60 miles a week. I haven't run a marathon since 1969, but I ran a lot of 10ks, 5ks, but I didn't run competitively at all except for the 2-mile Tyler Cup here in Dallas. I did that until 2004. Then after 52 years on the slopes, I broke my leg skiing. Tibia plateau fracture of the right leg, required 2 surgeries, on crutches for 9 weeks.

ENDORPHIN TRAP #1: THEY MASK PAIN

I experienced firsthand the analgesic effect of endorphins caused by aerobic exercise that day at Beaver Creek in 2004. I ski all the black diamond slopes, and for some crazy reason I hit a rock or twig, or something, and fell. I didn't think I had a real problem. I skied a quarter-mile back to the lodge. I walked in to where my wife was having lunch and said, "I think I hurt my leg." I thought maybe I pulled a tendon or something.

She nodded and said, "Well, I'll see you at the bottom." She had compassion on me. I limped up to the chair lift, took the bus back to our home. By then, I was in severe pain. On a scale of 1 to 10, I was a ten. And boy, I called the hospital and they operated on me the next day.

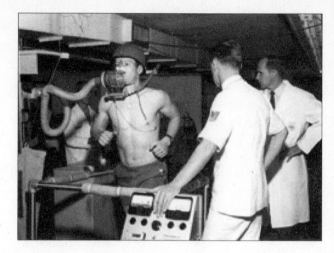

Again, the only reason I can figure that I coulda skied a quarter mile on a totally broken leg is the endorphin effect of exercise. Because it does act as an analgesic, we know that for a fact.

In fact, a true story happened in the 1982 Boston Marathon. A 39-year-old clerk from Salt Lake City qualified for Boston by running a 2:50. He started out in the middle of 9,600 runners. Seven miles into it, he stepped on a twig and heard something snap. Looked back, saw nothing, and was hit with severe pain—above the knee on the right leg. He almost fell, but he didn't. He kept his balance, kept going, his pain subsided, and he ran the next 19 miles, averaging better than 6:30 a mile. Crossed the finish line in a personal record time of 2:47. As soon as he crossed the finish line, his leg collapsed, he fell to the pavement, took him to hospital, in surgery for several hours, they put an intermediary pin through his fractured femur.

The big bone was totally broken through. And he ran 19 miles on a broken leg.

When people ask me, "How do you possibly do something like that?" I always say the answer is stupidity. That's how powerful the endorphins can be. The message: Don't let endorphins pull you into overtraining.

ENDORPHIN TRAP #2: THEY ENCOURAGE OVERTRAINING

In my first book in 1968, I said, "the more exercise the better." In my fifth book, in 1982, I changed that. What happened?

I'm smart enough to realize I've made a mistake. Over the years, we found that more is not better, more may cause you more harm than good. You may get detrimental effects from exercising too much.

I had people accusing me of changing my recommendation to sell more books; that made me nauseous when I heard that. I haven't changed a bit. Just modified my recommendations based on my personal experience and by undeniable research that we've done right here at this center.

It was just learning. Remember, we've been following 100,000 people, some as long as 37 years. Over 250,000 treadmill stress tests. You say how much exercise is enough, and the whole world listens. From 1968 to 1982, I used to say, if you run enough, forget about your cigarette smoking, your diet, your body weight; if you exercise enough, it's a panacea. Don't worry about anything else. Well then, I had too many times during that 14-year period that I had telephone calls from distraught widows.

They told me that their husbands followed my recommendations for running exactly but ignored his diet, ignored his weight, his smoking, and had a heart attack at 55 years of age.

That shocked me into reality. And that's why I coined the word "aerobics" in 1968 referring to endurance-type exercise. And I coined the word "wellness" in 1982, referring to total well-being. I said exercise is great, but there is nothing known to man that totally protects against coronary disease, whether it's medicine, surgery or marathon running.

Exercise helps, but it's not a panacea. Jim Fixx made that mistake.

I'm saying two things: We've done studies to find out how much is too much, because we've been concerned about the Lance Armstrong Syndrome. So many athletes—

Steve Scott, record-holder for the 1-mile run, comes down with cancer of the testicle; Scott Hamilton, cancer of the testicle; John Walker, first person to run the 4-minute mile 100 times, comes down with Parkinsonism; Marty Liquori came down with lymphatic leukemia, on and on and on. Far too many world-class athletes have come down with something they should have been protected against, whether it's heart disease or cancer.

So we feel that there may be a point of diminishing return. We're doing as much research in that as anything else, trying to find what is the detrimental point. It varies tremendously with the level of fitness of the individual, of which sex, whatever. We found two studies done in Germany in 1995 published in Mutation Research. They took world-class athletes and had them exercise to exhaustion on a treadmill. Then they measured DNA damage. Now, DNA damage is a precursor to cancer, most people feel. It's detected by free radicals, which cause the DNA damage. But what they found is that during and immediately after vigorous exercise, there was no significant increase in DNA damage. But they did find that peak DNA damage did occur 24 to 36 hours after the run.

When you finish the marathon, when are you the sorest—immediately after or the next day? The answer is the next day! We all are. You have to walk down the stairs backwards. Well, that's what they discovered: the DNA damage reaches its peak, related to your soreness, a day later. We always thought there was no damage from marathon running because we could detect none immediately after exercise. But then they found by putting these guys on high doses (1,200 units two weeks before) of vitamin E, a very strong anti-oxidant, they suppressed the DNA damage. That prompted a whole new field: Anti-oxidant therapy.

Hence my book, The Anti-Oxidant Revolution, in 1997.

That's been back in the news just this week. They've been criticizing vitamin E, beta-carotene, all the anti-oxidants in the "cocktail," saying that the levels of vitamin E in the blood relates directly to the onset of dementia. Can you believe that?

I'd predicted that from day one in my book. They've been talking about using vitamin E to treat heart disease. But you can't use anti-oxidants to treat heart disease—but to prevent heart disease. You can't use vitamins to treat cancer, but to prevent cancer. It's prevention all the way.

I tell my runners, if you listen to your body, the most important thing you can do is to watch out for overtraining. I have on page 96 of the Anti-Oxidant Revolution—you'll find 20 signs of overtraining. If you have any of those problems listed there, then you take 1,200 units of vitamin E—and run marathons, ultramarathons, Ironmans, I could care less what you run, as long as you listen to your body and you don't meet those overtraining requirements. I'm convinced then that you can run these great distances without damaging your body.

If you don't, you may be exercising too much.

The people who get injured by running aren't following those 20 signs of overtraining. I tell my patients that they are "straining, not training," You actually aren't conditioning; you're deconditioning your body.

That whole concept of "more is better" has been popularized by a lot of people. Well, that may be causing the dropout rate. Because they are overextending themselves; they think they aren't hurting themselves because that knee pain disappears because of the endorphin effect. I don't ask people if they exercise do they have pain at the end of the run; I ask them if they have pain two hours later—like my knee skiing. The endorphins mask the pain. You are masking the problem, and may be doing severe damage, but you aren't feeling it because of the body's system to control pain. That's why you have to pay attention to what happens a few hours later.

ZERO-GRAVITY TREADMILLS AND HIGH-ALTITUDE TRAINING

Of course, our (U.S.) marathoners have not done well until recently, being defeated constantly by the Kenyans and others. So one of the problems we have is that our guys are so heavy compared to them that they can't run 150 miles a week. They can't get down to that sub-5-minute pace for

26 miles, because they are too large compared to Kenyans and some of the Africans. So what (Alberto) Salazar is doing at his training camp—and we are experimenting with it too—is having their marathoners run 75 miles a week outdoors, and another 50 miles a week indoors on a zero-gravity treadmill. You heard about that? What you do is get into some shorts that tie around the waist. It's a balloon. You pump air into the shorts, and it lifts you off the belt. So you can reduce the body weight by 80, 60, 40, 20%—almost zero gravity. You can run a 4-minute mile with ease by doing that. So you still get your heart rate up for the aerobic training effect, without traumatizing the joints.

Another thing we're doing, too—I discovered this when I ran the Boston Marathon and was doing the Ph.D. in exercise physiology with some training in aerospace medicine thinking I'd go for the astronaut program—is altitude training. After I ran the first marathon in 3:54, I realized that you should run 26 miles before you try to run that; my longest distance was 18 miles. I was well-trained and in good shape, but I got to 18–20 miles and got the top of Heartbreak Hill and "hit the wall."

So the next year, I felt that if I could train at altitude, like they are doing in Kenya and other places, it might improve my performance. So we headed out to a chamber in the basement of the old 55 Shattuck Building at the Harvard School of Public Health in Boston that hadn't been used in years, and we got them to work it so I could exercise with a bicycle ergometer in the altitude chamber. I worked for nine weeks, starting at 9,000 feet and went up to 15,000 feet. Forty-five minutes, continuous cycling, had a monitor in there with me. We got so darn hypoxic, we were giddy.

But I could see that my red blood cell count increased. That was my thesis: Using continuous hypoxic exposure to improve athletic endurance performance. We tried to simulate at sea level there in Boston at least part of what they were doing in Kenya. That's progressed on to the extent that in Oregon they are having the athletes sleep in an apartment at 9-, 10-, 11,000 feet. They are spending 10 to 12 hours at that altitude. Which gives them a synergistic effect of training at sea level plus spending the night at altitude, and they claim they can improve performance in a short a period of time as 10 to 12 days. So both of those things are being used by Salazar and the group at Nike, or so I've been told.

We are doing the same thing here—we have now established the Michael Johnson High performance center. It's been moved from Bradenton, Florida, up here to our new facility at Craig's Ranch, Texas, which is a suburb of Dallas. We're putting in a 400-meter track, an indoor 60-yard track and a stadium with seating capacity of 6,000—a focal point here for world-class athlete to train. We're using the zero-gravity trainer, and also building a hotel across the street that will have between 10 and 20 rooms where you can adjust the altitude. Because we're not only just concerned with world-class athletes' performance, we're also looking at it as being of value for our clinical studies. People that have cardiovascular disease can't exercise enough to get an aerobic effect, but put them at altitude, even at rest, and they start getting some changes. You might see improvement, like I did at Boston, even with people who have disease. We don't know yet. It's all part of an ambitious plan that we have.

So what we were doing years back in high school and college, this is 180 degrees different. In retrospect, if I'd known then what I know now, I think I'd also could have gotten done to close to a 4-minute mile.

BEST TRAINING REGIMEN: BASE + SPEED WORK

What runners do now is actually combine what I did. First get the aerobic base, then (hone the speed with) interval training. In fact, in 1975, before the Montreal Olympics, we brought 25 of the world-class athletes here to test them for a period of five days—Frank Shorter, Steve Prefontaine, Don Cardone, Kenny Moore. We had people come from all over the country to evaluate these athletes, primarily to see if we could predict the winner of a race, a 6-mile event, based upon various factors. We knew the Russians were doing that, the East Germans were doing that, and we weren't doing that. We'd just train them and not worry about muscle biopsies and trying to increase aerobic capacity and all those various things. It was very

successful. We were able to show that we could predict very accurately the winner of a 6-mile race.

It was based on a whole series of things: Percent body fat, maximal oxygen consumption, and the difference between maximal heart rate and resting heart rate. The latter was a very good predictor of performance. Some had a resting heart rate of 44–45 and some maxed as high as 210 or 215. You wouldn't think you'd see that—these are world-class athletes. You'd think a world-class athlete would peak out at 190, 195—and in fact the average was 196. But for some reason, some of those guys were about to control the pain, or stress, whatever it was, and go beyond what we would have predicted for them to reach a maximal heart rate, but in conjunction with that, the oxygen consumption was increased. We found that was the best predictor of running ability.

In fact, we had about 20 guys in the group and—we published this in the New York Academy of Sciences—we were able to show that the best predictor was the delta—the difference between maximal heart rate and resting heart rate. The guys who had the biggest difference did best.

We did biopsies and, as expected, found that their muscles were 75% slow-twitch fibers. For the heck of it, I had a biopsy done and found that I was roughly half-and-half slow-twitch/half-twitch fibers. I was right in between a sprinter and a distance man. The highest was 96% slow-twitch fibers. There was one guy lower than I was, with 51% slow-twitch fibers—I was 55%—Don Cardone. His fibers were twice the size of anyone else.

So if you're wondering if most elite athletes are made, or are they developed, in most cases, it's who your parents are. Born that way. But once in a while, you get a guy like Don. He didn't have the genetic predisposition to be a world-class athlete, but apparently his training technique was enough that he had hypertrophied the slow-twitch fibers and placed fourth in the Olympic Marathon in 1976.

FROM RUNNER TO WALKER

After I broke my leg in the skiing accident, I kept myself in shape by exercising with the Schwinn Aerodyne bicycle. I'd rest my bad leg on the median, and exercising my arms

RUN FOR LIFE

and my left leg. So I didn't lose too much fitness. But it's been a slow recovery because I had multiple fractures that didn't heal well. One little piece in the center about the size of a half dollar that they tried to glue together didn't take. It left me with a divot in the plateau that resulted in constant pain.

I decided to tough it out. With my surgeon, Dr. Dick Stedman in Colorado, one of the world's authorities on knees, we decided that I should take glucosamine and chondroitin, which I do twice a day. Studies indicate that it stimulates growth of new cartilage and actually lubricates the joint. I don't think it was happenstance that I'd been recommending this to all my runners if they have any type of knee problem. I did the same thing. And lo and behold, that divot has filled in. I have no more pain. I even tried skiing again during the Christmas vacation.

I do no running. But I replaced it with walking. Walk 2, 3 miles a day. Work out 5, 6 days a week. I still maintain a high level of fitness. I do this by walking fast. As fast as 5 meter per hour, that's a 12-minute mile. Usually 13- or 13½-minute mile, done on a treadmill, outdoors, traveling around the world, whatever. That has allowed me to maintain a high level of fitness compared to people my age, which is 77 years of age.

I haven't cut out running completely. I do some interval running. I miss it. I'll run a quarter mile or a 220. That's because of the injury. I notice that I can walk fast for the last two and half years, and it doesn't hurt my knee. If I tried to jog two years ago, it hurt. Dick Stedman wanted me to do a lot of snowshoeing, and I did last year. I put a brace on my knee to go skiing, but I couldn't bend my knee and turn laterally without pain. I may give it up and concentrate on snowshoeing, an outstanding exercise. So I do the walking, the bicycle—did the ergometer for 30 minutes last night—and weight lifting. Try to get 12–15 miles a week in walking, and a little treadmill jogging. Might kick it up to ten-minute miles for a couple minutes. That doesn't hurt my leg anymore.

I probably am at the stage now where I could resume jogging without any problem, but I question whether it is worth it at this stage of my life. If I hadn't had the injury, I would still be jogging slowly—10-, 11-minute miles.

I did begin to have some problems with my knees from all the running over the years, but interestingly, Stedman found that my left knee was like that of a teenager, nothing whatsoever. My right, which I'd injured playing football in high school, had some osteo-condritis.

So I've said many times in my presentation: Jogging's not going to cause osteoarthritis, but can aggravate a pre-existing condition. We have studies to prove that in my new book, cowritten with my son: Start Strong, Finish Strong. It's my 19th book.

FITNESS CUTS JOINT PAIN

The new book should really be titled, Start Strong, Stay Strong, and Finish Strong—don't start, give it up, and try to start again. So you square out the curve, live your life to the fullest, and die suddenly, instead of suffering a long gradual decline. That's the goal for all of us.

On page 10, we have quality-of-life variables by fitness studies of 10,000 men and women: Fatigue. Snoring. Heartburn. Sexual function. Decreased sex drive. Impotence. Joint and muscle pain. Frequent headaches. Lower back pain. Difficulty sleeping. Depression. Anxiety. We classified people into three age- and sex-adjusted groups by their treadmill times. Low category is the bottom 20%. Next category, health and longevity fitness, is the middle 40%. Aerobic fitness is the top 40%.

We found the perfect correlation between levels of fitness and quality of life. The people in the bottom category had the most problems and the people in the top had the least problems—including less joint and muscle pain.

Of those in the aerobic fitness category, only 5.3% had joint problems, the middle category 29.3%, and those totally sedentary—34%. Bottom line: You have less joint pain at high levels of fitness than you do at either mid levels of fitness or low levels.

DO MORE STRENGTH TRAINING AS YOU AGE

As you find in my books, including Regain the Power of Youth at Any Age, in your 30s, you should be 80% aerobic, and 20% musculo-skeletal conditioning. In your 40s, 70–30. In your 50s, 60–40. In your 60s, 55–45. Because as you get older, you must do more strength training, otherwise you could be in great shape cardiovascular-wise, but you can't pick up a sack of groceries without pulling your back out. You learn that the hard way.

You need weights, but not heavy weights. You need toning-type weights, circuit weight training, that's what I do. I work at 65% of my one-rep capacity, 12 to 14 reps in 30 seconds, then go to the next station. Circuit weight training, 20 minutes. Do that at least twice a week. That maintains my muscle tone, protects my back. I've got a little degenerative disease in my lower back, as most people 77 years of age have, but I can compensate completely with my regular stretching, my Williams exercises, my lightweight training program. And I can do what I want.

CROSS-TRAINING: IT WORKED FOR W.

I have a lot of people using the elliptical trainer. One of them is POTUS—The president of the United States. George W. Bush has been my patient for 19 years. He's in fantastic shape. Sixty-one years of age. Ranks in the top 1% of fitness in his age-group. He was running with us for years before he became governor, and was running two miles in less than 12 minutes. That guy is a natural athlete, great athlete. Kept running, loved it, and started having knee problems. So he took glucosamine and chondroitin, which kept him running a while. About three years ago, more problems, I told him, "George, it's time to quit running." So he transitioned to cycling, mountain biking as you know, elliptical trainer, weight training, and his performance on the treadmill is just slightly below what it was when he was running 2 miles in 12 minutes. He's the most disciplined man I've ever met. Exercises for an hour six days a week. I've heard him say more than once, "I don't exercise for my heart. I exercise for my head. That's the way I can control the stress in my life."

I had the privilege on the 4th of August 2007, of spending 3½ hours with the president at Camp David. I spent about an hour with him by myself. And every year, I ask him, "What's the stress level in your life: low, moderate, or high stress?" He always says, "Moderate stress."

I always say, "George, you've said that for years. How could it be moderate stress?"

And he said, "It wouldn't be that way, except for my fitness and my faith."

6-STEP PRESCRIPTION FOR SUPER-LONGEVITY

One thing we just discovered is—and I've made a chart on this: We're reporting on 54,000 men and 22,000 women who have come to this clinic at least once a year for the last 20 years. And we're finding that the predicted life expectancy for a woman is 90.5 years and the men is 88 years. That's about 2 years longer than the average American man and woman. Unrealistic? An article published in the last week in the medical journal Lancet found huge longevity gains due to 4 simple things: If they didn't smoke, number two they exercised moderately most days of the week, number three they ate at least 5 servings of fruit and vegetable very day, number four, minimal alcohol consumption—4 things, meet those qualifications, and they are living 14 years longer.

That was a study of only 6,000 people—from 1970 to 2003—a 33-year follow-up. Pretty impressive. We've got 76,000 people in our study. Are they average? Now, we can't say. People come here from all over the world, corporate executives come back regularly, by and large they have a higher income, more educated, less likely to smoke and drink, may be more physically active, so I guess yes that's true.

I have a 90-year-old who can still run 2 miles in 20 minutes and 50 seconds—he did it in October 2007—he's been my patient for 25 years, and he had a 6-vessel bypass procedure in 1993. We now have a new CT angiography where in 45 minutes we can look at the angiogram, at their coronary arteries; we found that all of his native vessels were completely blocked and his 6 bypasses were completely open. That's just extreme. Another 90-year-old we're still working with set a world record a couple years ago when at 87½ she walked 3,000 meters at 11 minutes a mile. Set a world record for the 85+ age-group. One of the finest things I've heard from my patients all these years.

165

When she got back, she said, "Because of you, Dr. Cooper, I forgot to grow old."

I forgot to grow old. She's going to have a big dance on her 90th birthday. She's still dancing like a teenager. Ninety years of age. And I hear that all the time.

I've gone from exercise being a total panacea of a wellness program, to these six factors:

Number one: Proper weight, nutrition, and supplementation. We have an elite athlete formula for distance runners, with vitamin E, vitamin C, and beta-carotene.

Number two: Exercise, exercise. Proper exercise. How much is enough, and how much is too much? If you get 15 aerobic points per week, that'll give you health and longevity fitness that can increase your lifespan up to 6 years and decrease osteoporosis by 58%. And no one can argue with that statement. You do it by covering 2 miles in 30 minutes 3 times a week, walking. Or 2 miles in 35 minutes 4 times a week, or two miles in 40 minutes five times a week.

A study we published showed that people 60–79 years of age, if they walked 3 miles in 1 hour 3 times a week for 3 months, reversed their mental age by three years and increased the size of their brains. A new book, Spark, by Dr. Rady from Harvard, found that exercise actually builds new brain cells. If you want to prevent Alzheimer's, exercise, exercise, exercise, as he says.

Number three: Eliminate tobacco products in all form.

Number four: The control of alcohol and elimination of all habit-forming drugs. No more than 6 drinks a week for a woman and 10 drinks a week for a man.

Number five: Stress management. Not stress, but how you handle it. Exercise is nature's best way to control stress. Take it at the end of the day is the way I've been doing it.

Number six: The importance of a periodic wellness examination, the type we do at this clinic. Because a man's most common warning of heart disease is sudden death. That's what killed Jim Fixx—he refused to take a stress test.

So again, those are my six component parts of wellness. So I've really moved away from strictly using exercise as a panacea. And I'm convinced that the six I gave you is why a majority of our patients are going to be living at least 10 years longer.

TRYING TO SET A GOOD EXAMPLE

Fitness is the journey, not the destination. You've got to keep it up your whole life. What I'm hoping to do, at 77 years of age, is to screw up the curve.

Keep in mind that I gave a 2½-hour presentation this morning. And I'm not fatigued. But I work out at the end of the day to control the stress in my life. My race walking—I got my time down to a 10-minute average, let's see, my best time was two miles in 21:40.

I went to my 50th anniversary of my medical school graduating class in 2006, and out of 104 graduates, 35 have already died. And only 10 are still working. I'm working 60 hours a week.

I'm going to try to square off the (down-sloping morbidity) curve. I'm still traveling the world, doing 4 or 5 international trips. I just got back last week from 12 days on the road. We leave again next Saturday to go out to California to speak to a group of people out there, on and on and on. I weighed myself last night and I was 171. I graduated from high school weighing 168. I'm trying to set the example.

I tell my physician audiences, "If you want to get your patients to follow what you want them to do—your guidelines—set the example for them. If you want to get the troops involved, get the general involved. If you want to get the corporation involved, get the CEO involved. You want to get the country involved, get the president to lead the way. And if he has enough time in his day to find an hour to work out, to control the stress in his life, America, what is your excuse?

(Note: For Dr. Cooper's 20 Symptoms of Overtraining, see Chapter 26.)

RUN FOR LIFE

RUN LESS, CROSS-TRAIN MORE

Thus far, this book has suggested various strategies to limit the damage of running. Strength-trained muscles armor and cushion your joints. Intervals deliver spectacular fitness in limited time with limited foot strikes. "Soft" form, proper stretching, and perfect posture cut shock and wear by getting you off your heels and running balanced.

But no getting around it: all of the above can be overwhelmed by sheer mileage, as several of the stars interviewed in *Run for Life* illustrate. After 140,000 miles, Frank Shorter must inject Hyalene (purified rooster comb) into his knees every eight months to simulate the cushioning once provided by his now-eviscerated menisci; Sally Edwards runs in pain because 40 years of pounding pulverized the discs that provide cushioning between her lower-back vertebrae.

Simple logic would dictate that running less and filling in more with something else is the reasonable way to go. Yet we all know that running less is not as easy as it sounds. Its simplicity, weight control, superb cardio, and blissful endorphin high can lock you into a relentless left-right, left-right until you get hurt or worn out. But if you are serious about running for longevity, it's unavoidable: *You have to run less.*

How much less? It's obvious that regular megamiles in training and numerous marathons and ultras a year put you at risk of long-term damage. Some even believe that a single marathon is so traumatic that one a year is enough.

Fact is, any run is traumatic. That's why, while everyone is different, a good rule to follow is, *never run two days in a row.* Your joints, muscles, and connective tissue need a day off after a run to recover and heal. That means three or four days a week without running. And a great way to stay in running shape without running is cross-training.

The usual aerobic suspects—bike, swim, row, paddle, elliptical—are a good start because they'll let running-battered body parts heal even if you push it. Chapter 15 will even show you how you can use cycling in general and a specific "running on the bike" drill to make you a faster runner. To the cross-training list, add hiking, a bipedal action quite different than running that can be challenging and rewarding. Also, seriously think about adding in some multi-planal activities like tennis, boxing, rock climbing, and soccer that work the core, develop coordination, and rotationally exercise you in a way that linear activities like the triathlon sports can't.

All of the above will not only help make you a fitter, more well-rounded athlete, but radically reduce injuries. Using the "absence makes the heart grow fonder," theory, they may even help you appreciate your running even more.

And if you must run on cross-training days, you still can: Just do it in the water. Water running isn't just for the infirm or injury rehab anymore. Chapter 14 will show you how, with special gear, one of the world's best runners uses it to build running-specific fitness. If you aren't water running, you are missing out on a remarkable—and remarkably untapped—training method. It also gives you a great excuse to take a swim.

Bottom line: Beyond protecting you from running's repetitive motion injuries and aiding your longevity running goals, cross-training opens up the possibility of doing all kinds of fun stuff that can keep you excited about staying fit. The variety and excitement of triathlons, adventure racing, multi-day mountain-bike tours, and sea kayaking can add immeasurably to your photo album and your storytelling ability at parties. And if all you want to do is run faster, as the next chapters will prove, cross-training can do that, too.

CHAPTER 14

HOP IN THE POOL WITH LORNAH

A challenging, joint-friendly workout and cutting-edge resistance devices make water-running perfect for world champs and centenarians alike

In the early summer of 2007, Lornah Kiplagat of the Netherlands suffered a calf injury that knocked her out of the World Championships. Unable to run normally on land, she trained mainly in the pool for the next three months. On October 14, following two weeks of water running with no land training at all, she stunned the running world by setting double world records in the 20k and the Half Marathon at the 2nd IAAF World Road Running Championships in Udine, Italy. The 33-year-old defending champion, a native of Kenya, ran the 20k in 1:02:57, shattering her own record (set the year before) by 24 seconds. Continuing through the last kilometer, she took the gold medal in the Half Marathon distance in a time of 1:06:25, lopping 19 seconds off the previous mark.

How'd she pull this off without training much on land?

Although cardiovascular fitness declines quickly after two to three weeks without training, a number of research studies have shown that you can maintain it at almost the same level for several months with cross-training that is intense (above 70% of VO_2 max) and functionally similar. No activity is more similar to running than water running, which has the advantage of being impact-free, allowing injuries to heal.

"We started to use deep-water running when Lornah was injured and we still wanted to train," Kiplagat's coach and husband, Pieter Langerhorst, told me. "She was in the pool for two hours every day, and this worked so well that we decided to make it part of our normal training. When we got the special shoes from AQx, we use it more."

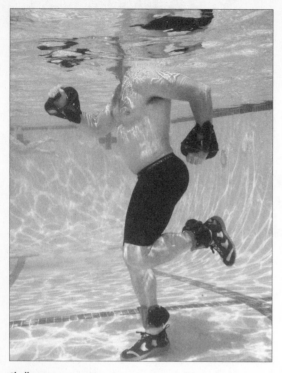

Shallow water running.

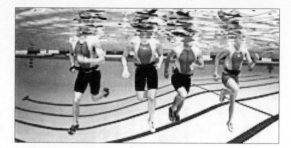

Deep water running.

AQx water-running shoes feature 3 cup-like plastic scoops on each side (6 in total per shoe) that increase resistance on the heel lift portion of the running stride. You need shoes in shallow water to protect your soles from the abrasive pool floor; you don't need them in deep water. Studies conducted by AQx founder Garry Kilgore, a professor of Human Performance and head track and field coach at Oregon's Linfield College, claims that the scoops increase resistance by 30% over barefeet and regular shoes and increase caloric burn and VO_2 max by 8%—which he calls "statistically significant." He may

obviously appear biased, but Langerhorst is convinced. "Lornah is always using the AQx shoes because it's coming close to the effort of normal running on land," he says.

Now, even when healthy, Kiplagat water-runs twice a week for 45 to 90 minutes each, doing both endurance and speed work. She uses an AQx vest, which she finds more stable than an Aquajogger-type flotation belt.

"All runners should be using water running as part of their normal training, even if they are not recuperating from injuries," says Langerhorst. "You can do extra training without having any negative impact on the legs."

The reason for the lack of muscle soreness at higher training loads than on land has to do with the unique properties of water, according to physical therapist Robert Forster, coauthored of *The Water Power Workout*. "Water eliminates the risk because it provides seven times more resistance than air," he says. "Along with ease on your knees due to the lack of the repetitive ballistic shock you get on land, harder workouts can be done at lower heart rates because the hydrostatic pressure helps force blood back to the heart. It's like using steroids." Generally, the water running heart rate is 10 to 15 beats per minute lower than it would be on land for same effort.

Forster knows first-hand of the healing and strengthening power of water. He was the physical therapist attending to Florence Griffith Joyner in 1987 when she injured her hamstring three weeks before the World Championships in Helsinki.

"She jumped in the pool and did intervals to match what she'd done on land," says Forster. "The result? She came out and set a personal record.

"If I had my druthers, my athletes would all do water running twice a week," he says. "There is a long list of benefits: Water running allows injuries to heal while maintaining and growing the aerobic base. It works you very hard. It can kick your ass in 25 minutes. It strengthens the core and hip flexors. It's a big time-saver, because you can work out two opposing muscle groups on the same motion. And it's a great recovery tool."

Pro football teams have noticed. In the NFL, HydroWorks pools with built-in treadmills, water jets, and TV cameras have become staples of training facilities of pro teams like the Philadelphia Eagles and Green Bay Packers. "You can increase cardiovascular fitness, running form, balance, and even some strength with less normal wear and tear on your joints," Eagles head athletic trainer Rick Burkholder told me.

Coaches like Marv Marinovich, former Raiders strength and conditioning coach, are beginning to use the pool for plyometric power training that builds speed, agility, and dynamic flexibility for superstar pro athletes (see accompanying sidebar). A recent study (Stemm and Jacobsen, 2007) indicated that there is no statistical difference found between land- and water-based plyometric training in terms of vertical jump height improvement. That is significant because you get the same benefits without the same injury risk.

"Water running reduces the incidence of stress fractures in runners," says Kilgore. "This is due to bone adaptation being driven by dynamic (plyometric) rather than static stimuli."

Conclusion: Water running is an ideal training activity for all runners, and is particularly relevant to those over 40, competitive or not, because it can simultaneously preserve joints and fitness. For those who have already had to cut back on their running due to injuries, it can be a godsend. Although it's not new (8-time Ironman triathlon champion Paula Newby-Fraser was well known for using it in her prime years in the eighties and nineties) water running has emerged as a true performance tool.

RUN FOR LIFE

Its effects are enhanced and multiplied, especially when paired with resistance shoes like AQx and resistance ankle collars and hand cages, like Speedo's Hydro Boxers and Hydro Kickboxers and ankle fins from AquaLogix. Using that ensemble tends to make you look like some sort of latter-day Roman gladiator racing in slow motion across the pool (I know—everyone stares at me; see the photos), but the workout is thorough, full-body, and as hard as you want to make it. In the water, the difficulty multiplies the faster you move, especially with the resistance devices.

When Sally Edwards told me in her *Run for Life* interview (starting after Chapter 21) that a painful lower back had forced her to seriously cut back on her running, I immediately asked if she'd tried water running. She hadn't—and sounded surprised by the suggestion. That was another sign to me that water running is vastly underutilized. If someone like Edwards, so connected in the running and triathlon worlds, isn't doing it, then a lot of us regular running folk are probably out of the water-running loop, too. And I like it for another reason besides the fact that it can keep you running stronger and longer for decades: it'll get you swimming, too. Since I'm right there in the pool, I almost automatically go for

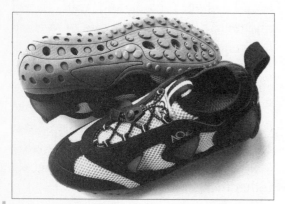

AQx water resistance shoes.

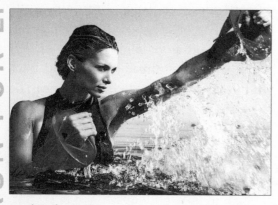

Speedo Hydro Boxers.

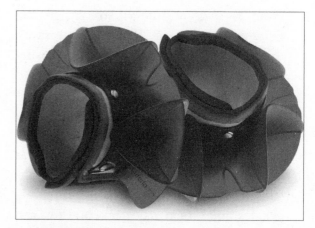

Speedo Hydro Kickboxers.

a swim after my shallow-water run. An upper-body workout like swimming is a great complement to running.

And who knows? With enough water running, maybe you'll become a triathlete. Then you definitely won't have the urge to run every day.

DEEP OR SHALLOW?

The effectiveness of shallow versus deep water has been examined in many studies over the years. A 1991 study conducted at Wheaton College with nine cross-country runners found that neither one could match the VO_2 max levels of treadmill running, but shallow-water running elicited 90.3% of the VO_2 max versus 73.5% for deep water. A 1999 study of 15 runners at Liverpool John Mores University in England found shallow best by 83.7% to 75.3%.

But a world record or two may throw a monkey wrench in the equation.

Kiplagat exclusively uses deep-water running with a floatation belt, which has no foot-strike impact at all and allows her to concentrate on form. With approximately 90% of body weight supported by the water, deep water is an excellent venue to increase effective stride range of motion and running mechanics, promote active recovery from running and other athletic movements, and increase and/or maintain cardiovascular fitness. AQx shoes and the various ankle resistance devices shift more of the muscular demand to the large muscles of the leg instead of the smaller, weaker muscles of the upper body.

Others like shallow water running precisely because it does retain impact (a 50% reduction in body weight with the water line at waist level, according to Kilgore), allowing for more of a realistic push-off off the bottom of the bottom and dynamic effects that can't be found in deep-water training—power training, speed, agility, and dynamic flexibility. I personally favor chest- or shoulder-deep running because its ground contact seems to better simulate real running and allow a focus on both a vertical arm swing and butt-kick heel lift. Done with the full-body resistance offered by the hand and ankle resistance devices, it really drills in the soft-running form described in Section 1. I throw in Sprint 8 ultra-intervals and get a superb high-performance running workout.

WATER WORKOUT DRILLS

For the injured runner, Phase IV's Bob Forster uses a progression from deep- to shallow-water running that tracks the healing process. The athlete starts off with no impact in deep water. "Be sure to use a running motion, not bicycling," he says. As the injury heals, move to chest-deep shallow water with belt flotation, so you have feet on the ground but are supported. The final stage is standard shallow-water running in waist-deep water.

If you are not injured, Forster promotes mixing up deep and shallow workouts. Intervals, fartlek, whatever you do on land, you can do in the pool. A study on water running by former 800-meter runner Tim Quinn, Ph.D., and colleagues at the University of New Hampshire concluded that for runners to maintain fitness during water running it is necessary to include intervals, tempo, and/or fartlek training.

For shallow water, Forster recommends alternating running-in-place and leap-and-bound drills, doing sets of 25 each.

One of his favorites for deep water is "Deep-water walking," in which you imitate a wooden soldier, keeping arms and legs straight. "This creates a lot of resistance because it gives you a lot more surface area," he says. "But beware: It can blow out your hip flexor if you go too hard too long." For lateral strengthening in deep water, you can use a variety of adduction and abduction exercises.

Bottom line: Whatever you do on land, you can do more safely in the pool. Use shallow-water running as cross-training or as a full-bore replacement for a regular running workout if you are uninjured, deep if you are. Use AQx shoes (there are no competitors as of 2008). To multiply the effect, strap on the Speedo devices. But at first, do the workouts after your workday is over. Because believe me, you will have no trouble falling asleep that night.

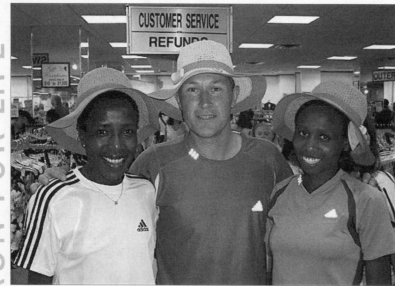

The final water-running tip: Wear a hat for sun protection. That's Lornah (left); coach-husband Pieter; and niece Hilda Kibet, 2007 New York Half-Marathon winner, shopping at Macy's.

Photo courtesy of noted running journalist Toby Tanser, author of several books including the new *More Fire: How to Run the Kenyan Way*

NEXT: AQUA POWER TRAINING

A famous NFL trainer thinks water plyometrics is the next big thing

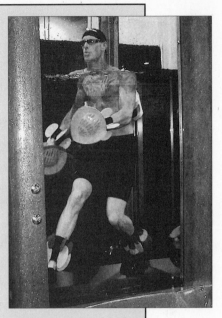

In the shallow end of a pool in Santa Margarita, California, former Stanford running back and Oakland Raiders draftee J. R. Lemon gasps for breath as he works out with aquatic dumbbells that look like wiffle balls with fins. Wearing matching widgets on his ankles, he does hip rotations, hip extensions, hamstring kickbacks, low-ab twists, and various upper-body exercises, all while thrashing his hands and feet back and forth so fast it bubbles the water like a spa. "Faster, faster," yells his coach from the deck. Then, grabbing a thick elastic band tied to the pool ladder, Lemon leans back, loads his calves and quads, and explodes rearward before the taut band flings him back.

Aqualogix water resistance workout

When the 40-minute workout ends, Lemon drapes himself over the coping, exhausted. "In the water, the harder you push, the harder it resists, yet I feel great—not beat-up like with weights," he says. "You definitely can't push this hard in the gym—you'll get hurt. It's definitely helping my first step get faster. Just like Marv said it would."

That would be Marv Marinovich, the burly poolside coach barking out orders to Lemon. As with running, he says water resistance can improve weight-room-style strength and power for any athlete. The former Raiders lineman and strength trainer, long known for an unconventional program that avoids conventional weight lifting, is pioneering a new genre: Water Plyometrics.

Plyometrics are rapid-fire, stop-start, explosive exercises that work on the principle that stretching a muscle right before you contract it fires more bundles of muscles at once than if you just started from a stopped position. Plyometrics enhance performance because they build power, which Marinovich describes as "strength-speed"—how quickly you can apply your force. The result is instant speed when you need it—to hit a tennis ball, to change direction to avoid a tackle, to swerve away from an open car door when you're on your bike, to catch yourself when you trip.

175

Marinovich believes that conventional weight lifting is incompatible with plyometrics. "Weights stress your connective tissue, weaken joints, generally detract from fitness, and make you too slow," he says, "three times too slow." He claims that the feet of a player running at full speed contact the ground for just 0.2 of a second, while it takes 0.6 of a second to change direction with weights.

The need for plyometric power and speed turned Marinovich into an instant aqua-convert in the summer of 2006 when he saw perforated water dumbbells from Aqualogix. "I have seen nothing that facilitates my training methods like this, that lets you do real-world movements with resistance in every direction." Aqualogix inventor Tad Stout calls it "Omni-directional resistance," which means that aqua-bells and fins provide resistance every which way as they are dragged through the water—side to side, front to back, and in all rotational movements. Unlike regular weights, they work both agonist and antagonist muscles at once, providing resistance to, say, a bicep curl as well as the returning triceps push-down.

Drag resistance, introduced with Huntington Beach–based Hydro-Tone baffled water-weights in the 1980s, offers a significant benefit vis-à-vis regular weights and land-based plyometrics: it's virtually injury-proof.

A 2004 study in the *Journal of Strength and Conditioning* found that aquatic plyometrics provided the same performance enhancement benefits as land plyometrics with significantly less muscle soreness.

Being able to train harder, without injury risk, has yielded positive results for Marinovich clients like Troy Polamalu, the longhaired, All-Pro safety who led the Pittsburgh Steelers' Super Bowl win in 2006. "I love this," he told me one day after a water workout that summer. "It's an extremely tough, high-intensity workout, but not so taxing on your joints. That's the most important factor—you can fire up the nervous system without getting injured." Impressed, he committed to a twice-a-week off-season schedule.

As the word about water gets out, innovations that might have once seemed goofy are becoming cutting-edge.

Tim di Francesco, a physical therapist/trainer in Swampscott, Massachusetts, says he got good results when he set up a hoop over his office's aqua-treadmill for his basketball player clients. "People are getting the message," he says. "The water is becoming the new gym."

CHAPTER 15

ULTRA MOUNTAIN MOMMA

Monster bike climbs + swimming = ultrarunning bliss?
A wild woman says "yes."

Cycling is often used as non-impact cross-training for runners, which makes it great for injury rehab and a run-to-100 program, but the knock on it is that it is not specific enough to maintain runners' running fitness and speed. Thomas S. Miller, Ph.D., a Salt Lake City–based coach and author of *Programmed to Run*, says it is—if you do two things: 1. Follow your run with a bike ride, because it aids recovery; and 2. Do standing bike hill intervals. Miller says if you stand up as you bike uphill and crank like hell for at least 30 seconds, you can replicate a runner's position with a lot more torque. He says it's the ultimate runner's interval. Find his plan at the sidebar at the end of this chapter.

But first, meet a runner who's never met Miller, yet unwittingly became a guinea pig for his plan. She even added a twist that makes you run even faster: a swim. Here's the story of how a "reverse triathlon" a day turned a part-time shoe clerk pushing 40 into one of the hottest women on the trails:

"Go faster, Mommy!"

Those three words, uttered repeatedly in 2002 by 2-year-old Sierra Barton as she rode shotgun in a jogging stroller on an Orange County dirt trail, were taken to heart by her mother, Michelle. "I was afraid *not* to push it faster—or else she would start to cry," said the auburn-haired mom from Laguna Niguel, California. Soon, the erstwhile

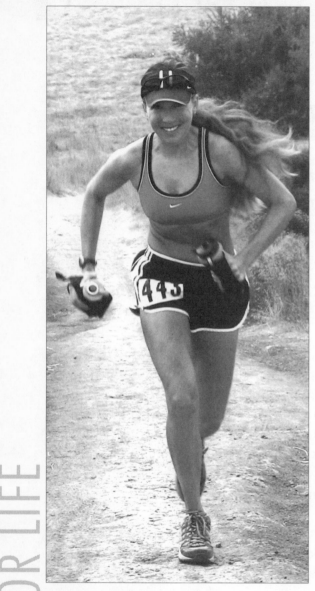

Ultrarunner Michelle Barton.

and the wins—all flying by at a furious pace that's still picking up speed.

In 2007, Barton set 12 course records at ultraruns all over the state, often beating the men. She suddenly vaulted to eleventh on the *Running Times* list of world's best ultrarunners. She won first place in the mixed category at the inaugural TransRockies Run, a 5-day, 113-mile mountain footrace in Colorado.

Pretty good for someone who only runs six miles a day, was virtually unknown until '07, and almost never ran at all until she was 32 years old.

Barton, 38, a part-time shoe store clerk, was always athletic while growing up, but seemed to do everything but run. She biked from Seattle to Vancouver at age 12 with her father, accomplished inventor-engineer, Doug Malewicki, who built the rocket-bike with which Evel Knievel tried (and failed) to fly over Idaho's Snake River. They went on long hikes together every time she stayed over his house after his divorce from her mother, and backpacked through Yosemite, often with a friend in tow, every summer from age 5 to 10. She played guitar and danced at Dana Hills High. After graduating from the Musicians Institute of Technology in Los Angeles as a virtuoso guitarist, she traveled the world, joined two rock bands, then taught dance and funk classes, where she stood out as, in her words, "a white, Polish girl with the rhythm of a black girl."

nonrunner was running so fast and far that she literally wore the tires bald on the stroller. And soon after that, in storybook fashion, came the marathons, the ultras,

In early 2000, Michelle had a child she named after the towering mountain range she'd come to love, Sierra. A couple months later, her father brought her the running stroller that changed her life.

"From all those backpacking trips, the outdoors was in my blood," she said. "I started pushing the stroller uphill on the local trails, taking Sierra on gnarly stuff. She loved it, and soon, I was running. To this day, people in the neighborhood still remember me pushing that stroller!"

When Sierra outgrew her wheels, Barton remained on the trail, running an hour a day, 2 hours a day, then more. She couldn't get enough. And she was getting pretty good.

By the time she and Sierra moved back into with her mom after Barton's own divorce 4 years ago, she was running 3 hours every day, 130 miles a week, and starting to place well in ultrarunning races.

"If you run trails, you eventually do ultras," Barton says. An ultra race, usually off-road, is defined as anything longer than a marathon. She ran her first one in 2003 at the San Juan Trail 50k, finished in the top ten, and was hooked.

After several wins in short races and high placings in ultras, Barton scored her first ultra win in 2004 at the Lake Hodges 50k, followed with an age-group win at Bishop High Sierra 50-miler and a second at the Saddleback Mountain Marathon.

Barton realized she was clearly good at this. But she didn't have a clue how much better she could be until she caught a break—literally.

On December 12, 2004, Barton broke her ankle on a 22-mile trail run. "I broke my fibula right in half," she says. "And I knew why: It was because I was always running, running, running—training like a madman. I'd knew I'd been feeling blah, getting stale, no faster, aches and pains all the time. I was always tired and hungry. Something had to change."

A TRIATHLON A DAY

After she healed up in 2005, it took Barton about a year to figure out what she had to change. She DNF'ed with stomach issues at mile 70 of Western States 100 in June. But by the time she won a San Diego 12-hour race in November, doing 69 miles around Sea World, she had it figured out.

"The broken ankle taught me that I had to cut back on the miles," said Barton. "No more 100-plus miles a week. And there was only one way to do that and stay in shape: I had to cross-train."

Cross-training isn't easy to do without a bike. "I had to borrow a mountain bike from my mom's coworker," she said. And as she began riding more and more up the steep Alison Woods trails in back of her house, she noticed something odd happening with her running: She was going up the hills faster.

RUN FOR LIFE

179

"I always used to get passed on the climbs," she said. "But the biking really was helping me kick butt going up [while running]."

Soon, to further reduce the running stress on her bones, flush out her leg muscles, and work her core, arms, and shoulders, Barton added another element to the experiment: She replaced an hour of running with an hour of swimming. Her former workout of 3 hours (18-20 miles) of running was now replaced by 1 hour (6 miles) of running, 90 minutes or more of biking, and an hour of swimming.

The nearly 4-hour-a-day regimen is made doable by her light hours at work and convenient living arrangement with her mother. Barton runs at 5:30 A.M., gets 8-year-old Sierra off to school, mountain bikes at 8 A.M. (concentrating on hill repeats), works at Fleet Feet Sports from 10 to 1, swims for an hour, then picks up Sierra at 2:25. She often bikes another 45 minutes in the afternoon, and is in bed by 9 P.M.

Bottom line: Barton roughly does an Olympic-distance triathlon every day. And lo and behold, on just six daily miles of running, she found that her running races were getting faster and faster.

The first proof came in February '06, when Barton beat the men at the Orange Curtain 100k in Cerritos. More came in August with a first place in 5:04

STANDING BIKE INTERVALS
How to raise running speed by pounding uphill on pedals

Dr. Tom Miller, Ph.D., a 65-year-old Salt Lake City running coach, college instructor, and running-book author, believes that bike intervals done while standing up on the hills and pedaling all-out make for some of the best training a runner can do. "Standing out of the saddle replicates the motion of running but at a higher resistance that stimulates higher contractive muscles in the quads," he says. "I prefer it to running speed work. And the chances of injury are nil."

Miller's study, done for his doctoral dissertation in exercise physiology, found that runners' 10k times shrunk by 10% over ten weeks after a series of intense, 30-to-60-second all-out bike hill climbs over 18 minutes. As proof, Miller, himself a runner since 1965 and triathlete since 2003, pointed to, "my star student: 85-year-old John Cahill. At 78, he ran a 3:30 marathon." See Cahill's *Run for Life* interview following Chapter 23.

at the Bulldog 50k in the Santa Monica Mountains, and in November at the Javelina Jundred 100-mile trail race in Arizona. There, she finished first female and fourth overall in 19:42. That was four hours ahead of the runner-up female.

In 2007, Barton exploded into the top ranks of world-class ultrarunners, breaking female course records 12 times.

It started in February, when she beat everyone—men included—at the Twin Peaks 50k, in 4:26. The course had 6,500 feet of climbing up Orange County's Mojeska and Santiago Peaks.

That was just a warm-up for a phenomenal 4-week, May–June streak of records that left the running cognoscenti buzzing: wins at the Wild Wild West 50k in Lone Pine, with 5,500 feet of climbing (time: 4:41); the brutal Pacific Crest 50 Miler in San Diego (6,500 feet of climbing in 8:44); the High Sierra 50k, which tops out at 9,000 feet (5:03); and the Shadow of the Giants 50k in Yosemite (3,100 feet of climbing in 5:22).

In September, Barton won the co-ed division of the inaugural 5-day Trans-Rockies run stage race with her partner, celebrated ultrarunning journalist Adam Chase. They pocketed a cool $3,500 for their effort, making her a bona fide professional athlete.

Here's the 18-minute workout (not including cooldown), which can be done or a hill or on a stationary bike.

- Warm up for 10 minutes
- Gear up to as much resistance as you can handle at 70 to 90 rpm
- Do 30 seconds all-out while standing climbing/60 seconds easy recovery
- 30 all-out/60, easy recovery
- 30 all-out/60, easy recovery
- 45 all-out/60, easy recovery
- 60 all-out/60, easy recovery

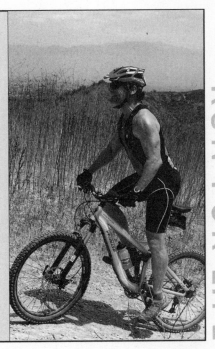

RUN FOR LIFE

"I was good before, but nothing like this," she said. "It's the cross-training."

Ironically, to Barton's wonder, a lot of runners won't do cross-training. "They think it takes away from their running training," she says. "But I'm beating them by doing a triathlon every day."

Barton hasn't beaten them yet at her dream race, the Western States 100. In 2005, she DNFed at the "Boston Marathon of Ultras," as it is known, when she threw up and her pacer quit at mile 70—four hours ahead of the cutoff. In 2008, primed for a top finish, the race was snowed out and cancelled.

"I love that trail, and have gone to the training camp every year," she says. "To win it would be a dream come true. . . ."

Win or lose, she'll certainly be greeted at the end by two of her big-gest fans, serious runners themselves. Her dad Doug, spurred by his daughter's success, finished his first ultra on March 28, 2004, on his 65th birthday. At 69, he and his 64-year-old partner Steve Harvey took 51st of 64 teams at the 2008 TransRockies Run. Now he's one of the nation's best senior runners. His granddaughter Sierra, whose demands for more stroller speed 6 years ago started this whole thing, also caught the running bug in a big way.

"One day we hiked 13 miles—and she didn't complain once," says Barton proudly. "Pretty good for an 8-year-old. And she recently got an award for being the top runner at her school."

Sierra's following in her mom's footsteps. In fact, given Barton's success, you might say that everyone is.

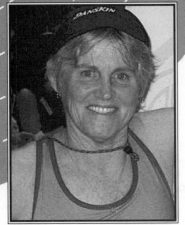

SALLY EDWARDS

The Relentless Pioneer

No word describes Sally Edwards as a runner, an ultrarunner, a businesswoman, a triathlete, an event organizer, and a sports educator better than "pioneer." Born in 1947, she grew up a tomboy in a world of limited sports opportunities for women, and helped to lead the way for women's athletics. As an athlete she's done 100 marathons (including 10 in one year), won the Western States 100 in 1980, done 16 Ironmans and finished in the Top 5 of the Hawaii Ironman five times, including second in 1981. She's also won the 100-mile Iditashoe Snowshoe Race, the Race Across America Relay division, and participated in adventure races around the world, such as the Eco-Challenge. She's been as prolific as a businesswoman, having founded 6 companies, including Fleet Feet Sports in 1976—one of the first athletic-shoe retailers—plus the triathlon-specific Fleet Feet Triathlete, Yuba snowshoes, and Heart Zones, which markets heart-rate training programs. On top of that, she's also written 22 books about triathlon and heart-rate training, and is the national spokesperson for the Danskin series of women-only sprint triathlons. A Triathlon Hall of Fame inductee in 1999, Edwards sat down for her *Run for Life* interview on November 6, 2007.

Although I'm only 60, I grew up in a world not so different from 100 years ago. We had to wear dresses to school. We couldn't play a lot of activities on the playground because of the dress requirements. We wore these stupid shoes. There were really no athletic shoes at all to wear to participate in sports for women. All the shoes were for men.

I grew up in a little town of 1,000 people, Loomis, California, 30 miles northeast of Sacramento. My dad, a World War II naval hero, a pilot, retired there when I was 13. Before that we moved every couple of years. Our last duty assignment was Athens, Greece. The traveling was great. Before Greece, we were stationed in Nebraska, we had horses and cows and chickens—great for a city kid. We also lived in Fairfax, Virginia, and Coronado Island, San Diego Bay. I was the youngest of four kids born in five years. It was post–World War II, and Marge just kept having babies after babies.

I was always athletic, and all I ever wanted to do was play sports. I had to be good to keep up with my three older siblings. In basketball season, we played basketball. In the other seasons, the other sports. But as for girls' sports, there just weren't any opportunities—this is pre–Title IX. There were no sports in high school and very few in college.

I was labeled a "tomboy." A tomboy was a negative term at that point. It was the precursor of "athlete." It always bothers you when you are labeled as something different. Yeah, it bothered me.

But I said screw it, I'm doing my thing. I played sports. And none of the other girls did.

There were social stigmas. There were apparel inadequacies, the lack of opportunities in teams, coaches, budgets, and resources. And you had to realize—boys didn't like the girls who were tomboys. They wanted to go out with the cheerleaders. So you had to play two different roles: You had to cheer the boys, so I was a cheerleader, and take whatever athletic opportunities there were in high school and college.

It was weird. I was gifted with a lot of athletic talent, but there was no place to go with it. So, you're kind of raised as a fighter—three older brothers, a system that is against you …. But luckily my parents were really supportive, they encouraged me. They didn't tell me I had to be like all the other girls. When I was on a team, they'd come watch the game. In the summertime, we played summer league softball, slow-pitch. It was really fun—I'm 14 or 15 years old, I was the shortstop, and had a uniform! Girls today would laugh at that and say, what do you mean? Back then, all the resources went to boys.

There was AAU swimming. For most of that, you had to belong to a swimming pool or country club, and we lived out in the country, so we didn't have that. There were girls' gymnastics clubs, because that was an Olympic sport.

At least college had teams. At U.C. Berkeley, we had a volleyball team, a tennis team, a swimming team, a basketball team. I liked basketball. We had six women on a side—three on each side of a centerline. We had a five-game season. We played teams nearby, like San Francisco State, San Jose State, U.C. Davis; all were within a radius of 100 miles at most. We had no real travel budget. Of course, we didn't play in the big gymnasium. We played in the women's gymnasium, which didn't have any bleachers or anything. There were no spectators. The women's athletic department was practically non-existent. It was appalling.

We didn't have a women's track-and-field team; I would have gone out for it.

THE RUNNING TEST

When I was at Berkeley in 1967 or '68, a guy named Dr. Ken Cooper came to talk about his new book he'd just written, Aerobics. He was on a national lecture tour to talk about the benefits of aerobic training. He was in Air Force uniform, and he had just done all this testing on Air Force cadets. He was speaking to the graduate school of physical education.

I listened to him and I decided, "I'm going to take his little 12-minute Aerobics Points test." It was the very first cardiovascular fitness test—all quantified with a bunch of research. I found it personally challenging rather than having any sort of application. He said, "go out and do this for 12 minutes and see what you score." That's what started me running. I went out and did the 12-minute run-walk test and scored the top of what you can score. I thought, "Well, that's good—I thought I was pretty fit."

I'd been jogging—and when we jogged, I mean just one or two miles. Nobody ran then or lifted weights or did base conditioning. You did your sport. If you were a basketball player, you played basketball.

Then the boyfriend challenged me. "I can outrun you in a mile." And I said, "I don't think so, but let's try it." He led the first lap. I caught him on the third and won. He was humiliated. He got in better shape, and I never beat him again. But this is when I started officially jogging.

I graduated in 1970, and volunteered to go to Vietnam for a year. I joined the American Red Cross as a volunteer. It was like all things: it was wonderful and it was absolutely horrible. I hadn't quite finished writing my master's thesis, so I had to finish that in Vietnam. So I went from protesting the war at U.C. Berkeley with a sign to getting on a C5-A [cargo plane] in Fairfield, California, where the troops were being transported and flown to Saigon, and putting on a little blue Red Cross worker's outfit and being paid almost nothing. Our job was troop morale, so we traveled around with officers and would visit the enlisted troops in forward firebases and we'd put on these little recreational programs.

And it was really bad, really tough. We'd see body bags, and deal with depression and lots of those issues.

It changed me tremendously—had a huge impact. I was there in Vietnam in 1970 and '71. We had 500,000 American troops fighting there. The big protest movement in the United States continued, and troop morale was really low. We announced a withdrawal while I was there. So everyone knew that we had lost the war and were going to come home, and there were tons of drugs. I mean, the drug problem in America is so closely attached to the Vietnam War and the use and abuse of drugs there.

I ran while I was in Vietnam. Since Dr. Cooper did say the more the better, I jogged for 30 minutes. There wasn't anyone else out there jogging. The only safe place to run was on the military base. I always took a guy with me so I wouldn't get harassed—because I tried running by myself at first in Vietnam and I got harassed a lot. I'd wear shorts and a T-shirt and pair of running shoes and I'd go run. And the guys—there weren't many white American women who were there, and there were none running. Sometimes, the soldiers would know what my schedule was and would come out of their barracks, and they had a chair and would sit there watching us run 1-mile loops. I can remember we'd run 4, 5 miles a day. That's what I got up to by 1970.

I took a year off after Vietnam and traveled around the world with my boyfriend. We went everywhere—Japan, Trans-Siberian Railroad across Russia, Eurail Pass down to Spain, over into North Africa. My boyfriend got out of Vietnam and met me in Spain. I didn't run at all on the trip.

FLEET FEET

I came back August 30, 1972, with $300, without a job or a place to live. We got a house, and in five days, I got a job teaching at an intermediate school in Sacramento. Seventh and eighth graders weren't my ideal, so in '74 I took my master's degree in exercise science and a secondary teaching credential, and got a job teaching at Monterey Peninsula College (junior college), coaching intercollegiate athletics.

I was running 5ks and 10ks myself, but I didn't coach running; I coached women's volleyball, women's basketball, women's softball, and men's volleyball. I was the only woman on the staff with nine men, and they gave me all the things they didn't want to coach.

I was competing all the time. I ran the Bay to Breakers Race in San Francisco when I first got back to California. It was pretty big. There were probably 5,000, 10,000 people there. It was the biggest race in the state. The only race, I think.

There were very few women out there. It was 80% male and 20% female probably, maybe 90:10. Women played tennis, but they didn't run.

There were other big, famous races going on—like the Boston Marathon. But they weren't around me. We didn't have a marathon in Sacramento. When I was teaching, I ran the Lakes at the Pines 10-mile race. It was the furthest I ever ran, and I really liked it. There were 100 people in the race, and 10 women. And I won. I said, "If I can run 10 miles, then I can probably run a marathon."

I won most of my races, because there was no competition.

I lasted at the college for two years. Teaching wasn't my calling. At the same time, my boyfriend broke up with me after almost ten years together, and I was up to running 10 miles and really liking it.

So I went to my best friend in high school, Elizabeth Jansen, and said, "You know, we have to go to sporting goods stores to buy shoes. Let's start a shoe store." There weren't any athletic shoe stores. If you wanted athletic shoes, you can't find them, the stores don't have a good selection, and you don't have experts to fit you correctly or who were athletes who know anything about sports. Elizabeth was teaching elementary school and said, "I don't want to teach school, either. Let's do it."

She was a serious tennis player. Tennis was really popular in the late 1970s. So I like to run, she likes to play tennis. We came up with the name "Fleet Feet Sports," and we opened the first retail athletic footwear store in California.

We thought, we don't have much money, so if we lose it all, we can just go back to teaching.

In our initial 2-page business plan we wanted to get involved in the community and sponsor running events. Fleet Feet started some of the very first running events in Sacramento. Later we started the first triathlons in Sacramento.

Fleet Feet was founded in 1976. We started hosting the St. Patrick's Day 5k, the California International Marathon, and the American River 50 Miler, the first ultramarathon in Sacramento. There was a Western States 100 miler; I ran it in '79.

The store wasn't an immediate success. Running wasn't popular right away. It started to grow. Running was so small compared to what is going on today. There were no coaches, no teams, no support. At first, there were no shoes for women. Nike was one of the first companies to come out and make a running shoe for women. I know because we sold it at Fleet Feet in 1977 or '78. The Lady Cortez was the name of it. White with nylon uppers, as opposed to Adidas, which was all leather.

When we opened the store, we started a community class on "How to Run." It was a 6-week class put on by the Learning Exchange, which was a community education program. The new boyfriend and I taught them. They were extremely popular. We'd get 30 and 40 people to take a running class. It was huge.

In fact, he found his new girlfriend through that and married her.

People didn't know how to run, what to do. We had community events and we'd host speakers like Joan Uloyt, a medical doctor and marathoner in San Francisco, who had just written a book called Women's Running. Brian Maxwell was our Adidas sales rep; he then went on to found PowerBar. Runners would get jobs in the running shoe companies, and Brian was a runner from Berkeley.

Running was a tiny, little world, and we knew everybody.

We started to sponsor some of the first trips—the first group outings to go to running events. I went from 10 miles to 13 to running marathons. After I started running marathons, I started running lots of marathons. So Fleet Feet would host trips to, like, Avenue of the Giants Marathon, the Boston Marathon, and we had a little travel business, where we'd rent buses, go to travel agents to organize travel.

To this day, we have a running club in Sacramento that we helped sponsor: The Buffalo Chips. We didn't have a lot of money, but everybody kind of worked together to make it happen.

It was really, really hard work. Yes, satisfying. And we didn't make much money at first. The whole thing was a circle. The number of runners was low. A decade later, the same thing happened with triathlon.

We could not have made it on running shoes alone. So we sold football and soccer cleats. We became successful after I franchised it in 1979. We weren't the only chain; there was Phidippedes, The Athletes Foot, and others later.

I didn't know I'd love business. I found that I truly love it. I've started a half-dozen businesses now. A couple didn't make it. I had a triathlon business that went broke, Try Triathlon, which made the very first triathlon apparel an all-in-one tri-suit.

UPPING THE PACE ATHLETICALLY AND COMMERCIALLY

As the boom picked up, I won a bunch of marathons and started running 50-milers. I did my first Western States 100 with a friend in 26 hours in 1979—she was slow and didn't finish. Then I won it in 1980 in 22 hours and 15 minutes and did it a third time in 1981—came in second even though I dropped my time to 20 hours.

I had no idea running could be like it is now. But I thought triathlon would. I just got an e-mail saying that there are now 100,000 registered triathletes, that it surpassed swimming and running and cycling.

I did my first triathlon in 1978, the Davis Triathlon that Vern Scott, Dave's dad, started. It was a run-bike-swim in that order. Then I did the Lodi Triathlon, and I won it. So then I decided to do the Ironman in 1980. There were 120 people, 30 women.

I didn't read about it in Sports Illustrated, like many did. When you're in the athletic shoe business and a lot of events are going on, you hear about them. People said, "Hey, you ran the Western States, well, you ought to do the Ironman." So I went to Hawaii in 1981 and finished 2nd. I did the next five Ironmans, finishing 3rd twice and 5th twice. So I was five times in the top five. I was actually a professional athlete, because I raced on contract with Nike and Specialized then.

After that first Ironman in 1981, I wrote my first of 22 books: Triathlon: A Triple Fitness Sport. I self-published it in 1982. It was the first book written on the sport of triathlon. Everyone laughed at me. They told me, "Sally, nobody's going to buy this book. Nobody does triathlons."

Then we kicked off the first triathlon retail stores in America: Fleet Feet Triathlete. We still had Fleet Feet Sports. We started Try Triathlon, an apparel and event company. We started putting on triathlons. By the time I sold the company in 2003, there were 5, but they weren't very successful. It was really hard to figure out the formula to make a triathlon store work.

But that's okay. Part of it is I'm ahead of the curve, ahead of the wave. I'm out there pioneering—this is a classic scenario in my life. It happened with retail stores, with books, I opened a snowshoe business, then heart-rate monitors. I like being on that side of the curve. I'd rather be on that side of the curve than the side where the cash cow happens.

MAKING SENSE OF HEART-RATE TRAINING

I bought my first Polar heart-rate monitor in the early 1980s and absolutely fell in love with it. By 1984, I used it to train for the Olympic Trials in the Marathon. They took the 200 fastest women in America; I ran a 2:50 marathon, which qualified me, so I went off to Olympia, Washington, with Joan Benoit and the gang. I wasn't one of the top three at the trails. I was 20 minutes behind Joan. But I wasn't disappointed; I was 35, never in contention. The event was a celebration of the emancipation of women— the first marathon. After all, we'd been warned that our breasts would get droopy and ovaries would fall off. It was a huge celebration. And I was sponsored by Nike the whole time. ABC telecast the whole thing. They wouldn't do that today.

I tried to qualify for the 1988 Olympic marathon. I missed by one minute. It was disappointing. A couple trials would have been great, but the quality of the women has risen.

Anyhow, I just thought a heart-rate monitor was the coolest tool in the world. "Everybody's going to want a heart-rate monitor. This is so cool," I said. And I was absolutely wrong.

No one knew what to do with it. I loved knowing my heart rate, but the other runners didn't seem to like it. So I tried to make it understandable.

The basic concept is to train in zones. The methodology you use is called "heart zones training," which I created based on time in zone and training load. Either you use your maximum heart rate or your threshold—find those out and choose one way or the other. There are three different kinds of threshold: lactic threshold, anaerobic threshold, and ventilatory threshold (shifts in ventilation—that point that you can no longer talk while you're running). They are all so close together that in our system we just call them, "Threshold." For consumers it makes it much easier to understand that threshold is a crossover point between aerobic and non-aerobic. It's easier to measure ventilatory threshold than to measure oxygen with a mask or lactate by drawing blood. But all those thresholds are within a hair's width of each other, so it doesn't really matter how you measure a threshold—it matters that you do measure a threshold.

So now you get an anchor point—a threshold—and now you've got your zones. So the strategy: On different days you train in different zones to get different benefits.

Say your threshold is 150 beats per minute. We set up 5 heart rate zones based on that threshold—from easy to all-out.

The higher the zone, the less time you have to train in it. So if you want to train less, you train a shorter time in a higher zone. You can spend a lot of time in a low zone and not burn very many calories and not get much of a training effect. Or you can move it up a zone or two, and then get a whole lot of aerobic benefit and train half the time.

It is real logical, but most runners don't understand the concept. What you're doing is getting yourself something called "load." There are different kinds of loads—there's emotional loads, metabolic loads, and there's training loads, cardiovascular loads. You give yourself a due quantity of load on your body and then you measure—you either get fit, you get positive training effect or a negative training adaptation. So, if you want to get positive, you give yourself the right amount, and give yourself more and more and more, and you get fitter and fitter and fitter. And this is how you get fit. Very, very simple to get cardiovascular fitness by using a heart-rate monitor.

The way we set it up is that you get points for time in zone. It's simple math anyone can do. Example of a 30-minute workout:

- 5 minutes in Zone 2 = 10 points
- 20 minutes in Zone 3 = 60 points
- 5 minutes in Zone 4 = 20 points

When you add all that up, you get a number for your workout—a number that you can compare to those of other days' workouts.

One minute in Zone 3, you get 3 points. One minute in Zone 4, you get four points. In the case of the above example, you got 90 points (10 + 60 + 20). Over time, as you get fitter, you'll do more points per workout.

It's easier than counting calories. It's an exercise prescription methodology that measures how much exercise you just got. It's the only way to quantify cardiovascular training: Time in zone multiplied by the number of the zone. Easy. No calculator needed.

It gives you a framework for using your heart-rate monitor. You say, "Today I did a workout of 100 points. Tomorrow, I want to take it up a zone, add 10 minutes—it's worth 180 points." Thirty minutes in Zone 3 is worth 90 points. 40 minutes in Zone 3 is worth 120 points.

If you do an hour, which is what I recommended people do, you do a lot of Zone 3 and Zone 4 time, which are your best zones, because they are high enough intensity to stimulate a cardiovascular improvement in oxygen consumption. Walking doesn't really do it—it's too low-intensity. That's why a walk-run is a good idea. Because the running part gives you enough intensity to get improvement.

If you are using Threshold, then your threshold is 100%.

- Zone 3 is 70–80% of threshold
- Zone 4 is 80–90% of threshold
- Zone 5 is 90–100% of threshold

So 40 years after I met Dr. Cooper, I've put together my own test. Cooper was, and continues to be, such a good role model as an exercise scientist and applied physiologist. And that's ultimately where I am now in my career: I'm an applied exercise physiologist. And I'm working now on what's called power-based training, which uses Power Meters, using a threshold system with metabolic charts, which measure metabolism and metabolic responses. And we're using HRMs for using zone-free methodology.

You absolutely need an hour a day to work out. You need stretching, strength training, and cardiovascular. And it takes an hour to do those things. Most of that hour will be aerobic.

FOOD AND ANTIOXIDANTS

I am not worried about oxidation and anti-oxidants. I don't think there's enough support for that theory. My reading of the research does not indicate free radicals are as curious a thing as Cooper has alleged they are. Cooper hasn't convinced me of it

Besides, the problem isn't overtraining, it's undertraining. Oxidation is a factor. But a bigger, more significant factor is non-oxidation. If you don't move, it's worse for your health than if you do move. Yes, if you move you have this release of free radicals that can mutate into all kinds of other problems. Yes, that's bad. But a worse scenario is inactivity, a sedentary lifestyle, and the disease that I call sedentaryism. Sedentaryism is the root cause of the obesity epidemic. Not the food we're eating, not the ratio of carbohydrates to protein—carbs are bad this year, and protein is bad that year, there's too much coffee—it's a very complicated issue.

The root of it is when you stop moving, all … things … change. Your metabolism, your emotions, your muscle mass, your mood and outlook, your brain functions all change. If we can get the human body to start moving, we start a cascade of change. And that's what we need—to get America active. And not worry about free radicals. (laughs)

What it all boils down to is lack of activity. Activity is more important than food, although food is really important. In fact, I took the Heart Zones framework and applied it to what we call "Food Zones." Taking foods and making them into the five different zones from "healthy foods" to "moderately accessible foods" to "practically lethal foods." We even created a Food Zones chart.

The one question people always ask is, "Sally, I don't know what to eat." And I always say, "Eat the healthiest possible food you can, so you're in the Blue Zone." Not-quite-healthy is green zone, yellow is worse, orange is bad, and red is toxic.

I put chocolate ice cream in a separate category. But it's really in the orange zone—straight sugar, not good nutrients.

You can categorize anything in a "zone" format. Now we've got power zones for power meters (laughs). We even put emotions on a zone system—productive zone, safe zone, et cetera. In context, am I out-of-control emotionally, to where I've lost all rational thought and I'm going to flip someone off on the freeway, or am I calm and peaceful, meditative? Am I Zone 1 or Zone 5?

BEWARE RUNNER'S BACK

I have a serious disc disease. In other words, I wore out my back.

In 1997, I had done the Race Across America, an adventure race in China, and then a month later I thought I could do the Ironman. I was pretty beat up and didn't realize it. I took 4th that year in the 45–49 age group. The next year, I specifically trained for the Ironman and I lost by five minutes; I took 2nd. And then my back started to hurt.

It got worse and worse and I went to see a surgeon. He showed me the X-rays. I had no disc in my L5 S1 (lumbar 5, sacral 1), which is the last disc in your back, the bottom one. He said, "Not so many people exercise so much that they wear out their back. That's really unusual."

Actually, this particular joint has brought a lot of runners down. It's a huge problem for runners because that's where all the compression happens. One way to avoid it is not to run on asphalt. Pay attention to your technique. Run in higher zones for less time. Cross-train more.

You get this, and you're stuck. Get a heavy dosage of steroidal anti-something medication. Pretty much I haven't been able to race because I can't train hard. I can train. I run twice a week now, but not at high intensity. So my speed is poor. If I go for more than an hour, my back just kills me—so I don't. I'd rather run the rest of my life if I have to run slow, than not be able to run at all.

Ironically, having to run slow has helped other women. I did triathlon through the mid-nineties, did the first Eco-Challenge, got into adventure racing, then got involved with the Danskin women's triathlon series.

The president of Danskin called me and said "I want to do this. Will you be the spokesperson?" At first, I was not convinced that women's triathlons could be successful. And

189

then, after our first race, I decided it could. We had 2 races the first year and 5 the next, 6 the next, and now we're up to 8. After Year 3, I got a torn Achilles tendon doing another event, so I volunteered to finish last. That worked well, so for the last 15 years, I've finished every event last. It's the best place in the race, of course. The woman with me has the toughest time of all.

For me, the Danskin series has grown into one of the two crown jewels of the sport, along with the Ironman. This event has substantially changed 20,000 women's lives. And when you change a woman's life, you change her family, because she is quite often the head of the household. Other women's series have not had the endurance of the Danskin.

I attribute to Danskin the reason that almost 50% of the field in all triathlons is now women, excluding the Ironman.

I never got married. Never wanted to. I never wanted to have kids. I came from a culture of Berkeley in the sixties. It was free love. It was follow your heart. And it was do good things for society and volunteer your time; that's why I went to Vietnam. I wanted to do volunteer work.

I have no regrets. So I ran a business, wrote books, and raced professionally. It's been a great life so far.

RUN MOTIVATED

Staying motivated is easy when you're a young stud or studette reeling off new PRs every month. But many runners over 40, 50, 60, or 70 need to find new motivation when times start to slip and friends drop out. This section gives you six case studies to draw ideas from. You might try pushing the envelope at a crazy, far-out race, such as the legendary Badwater Ultramarathon. You might develop a rivalry with another runner you occasionally cross paths with and spend years and years trying every imaginable training method and oddball performance product—like a hyperbaric chamber—to beat him or her. Consider joining a club, and better yet, start a club for age 65+ runners, like a group did in New England. You could pick a grand goal that'll keep you going for years, like running 50 states or 100 marathons, or use running as an excuse to take a vacation to an exotic locale you've dreamed of for decades—like Tahiti. And there are even ways to use running to help you give back to the community in some way, helping lead blind runners or teaching kids to run, which will teach them—and you—lessons about life.

CHAPTER 16

MOTIVATION CASE STUDY #1:

PUSH THE ENVELOPE

*The 135-mile Badwater Ultramarathon was
out of my league. So I signed up.*

"**W**hy don't you cool off in the pool for a couple minutes?"

On the evening of July 11, 2005, that seemed like a good suggestion after 12 hours of jogging and walking through the blistering 120-degree heat of Death Valley, California. So I heeded the words of my brother Marc, my crew chief, and jumped into the deep end with a big cannonball splash—and gasped!

The pool water was a tepid 80 degrees—but to me felt as frigid as the Arctic Ocean. An ice-watery shockwave literally knocked the wind out of me. My body shook and shuddered so violently that I could barely breathe. "I'm f-f-freezing!" I yelped to the delight of amused bathers, who thought my cries were a joke. But I felt like I was going down on the Titanic, my veins freezing up like Leonardo DiCaprio grasping for flotsam. When my teeth-clattering shivers and all-body shakes didn't abate after a warm-water shower and laying on the deck for 10 minutes, Marc carried me over to the medical team in a room across the parking lot, where I eventually fell asleep under several layers of blankets as my confused body tried to reconstruct a damaged internal thermometer that had transformed bathwater into a sea of icebergs.

The doctors were alarmed but not surprised. I'd lost 8 pounds in 12 hours. A blood test determined I was dehydrated and quite low on sodium, which will bring on chills and eventually cause hypothermic seizures. "Bottom line: weird things happen when you subject your body to this abuse," said Dr. Lisa Stranc-Bliss, who did it herself the year before me. "That's why this is no normal race. This is Badwater."

The Badwater Ultramarathon is unlike any other ultramarathon. First of all, as race director Chris Kostman puts it, "It's 35 miles longer and 35 degrees hotter" than the 25 other 100-mile footraces in the U.S. Traveling 135 miles with 13,000 feet of elevation gain, Badwater is held in one of the harshest sports arenas on the planet—Death Valley—and at the most forbidding time of the year, mid-July, when temps regularly rise to 120 or 130 degrees. From the banks of the brackish saltwater pond called Badwater, at 280 feet below sea level the lowest point in the Western Hemisphere, the race route climbs over the Inyo and Panamint Mountains, into the Owens Valley, then up to the 8,360-foot portal of Mt. Whitney.

The Badwater route was mapped on August 3, 1977, by Al Arnold of Walnut Creek, California, who had noticed that Whitney's 14,496-foot peak, the highest point in the continental U.S., was a mere 146 miles from the hemisphere's low point. Attempting to become the first man to connect them by foot-power, the then-49-year-old started at Badwater in 135-degree heat, the world's highest recorded temperature that year. He told me that the air scalded his lungs like a blow dryer; the rubber soles on his tennis shoes began melting; sweat dried before it

could cool his skin. Still, Arnold ran. And after 84 hours, he had given birth to what would soon become the world's most grueling endurance event.

"I did it to prove it could be done—like Roger Bannister breaking the 4-minute mile," reflected the founding father, now in his ninth decade and unable to run anymore due to a bum knee. "Now, I just sit back amazed at the world-class names who do it."

Some of the best runners in the world have done Badwater—but most haven't. "Badwater's a different planet," says Ann Trason, the 12-time winner of the Western States 100. "At Badwater, I felt like I was in *Star Trek* 9—and I wanted to be beamed out." Trason, by the way, merely crewed the race for a friend; she had no desire to run it.

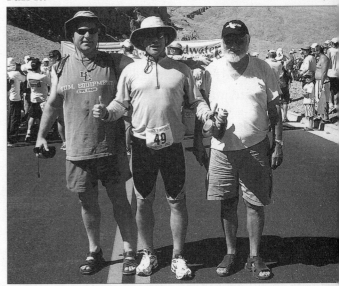

2005 Badwater Ultramarathon. Team Wallack at the 10 A.M., 110-degree start.

For years, neither did Scott Jurek, the closest thing ultrarunning had to a rock star. The long hair; the tall, thin Mick Jagger body; the 7 straight wins at Western States, including the record of 15 hours and 36 minutes.

"Badwater didn't attract the biggest names in the sport because we have no interest in pounding pavement for 135 miles," said the Seattle resident, who was 31 at the time of the 2005 race. "Besides that, it falls two weeks after Western States; I couldn't be at 100 percent." But Jurek's reservations faded when he started seeing all the media interest in Badwater over the previous year, such as the *60 Minutes* story about the 2004 race featuring Pam Reed and Dean Karnazes, and the many magazines saying it was the world's toughest race. "And I was looking for something different," he said.

That made Jurek sound a lot like most of the 80 other runners who joined him that July 11 at the 28th annual Badwater. There was 2-time women's winner and occasional David Letterman guest Reed, who became the first person to run 300 straight miles earlier in the year. There was Canada's Monica Scholz, who beat Reed in 2004 and was the latest women to win the coveted Death Valley Cup for completing Badwater and its sister cycling event, the Furnace Creek 508, in one year. There were the usual large contingents of French, German, and English runners. And of course, on hand were long-

time regulars like 9-time finisher Scott Weber, 52, of Mount Shasta, California, and 10-time finisher Jack Deness of Great Britain, 70, the oldest competitor.

And then there was me, the poser. Standing onstage at the prerace meeting the day before the event, I listened as racers with huge 50-mile and 100-mile race résumés were introduced. Not only do I prefer 10ks and had never run beyond a mere 26-mile marathon, but a strained abdominal muscle in March had left me unable to do anything but bike, swim, and elliptical until early June. So with 30 days to go, I began my running.

Over the previous months, I actually had called up race director Kostman several times to bail out of the event, but he told me to wait, "You are the Second-Fittest Man. You'll be okay."

It was our little joke. In my race résumé I explained that I'd completed the World Fitness Championship in the previous fall; this was a crazy event that included a 10-mile run, 10-mile power walk, 10-mile elliptical, 2-mile swim, 20-mile row, 100-mile bike, and lifting 300,000 pounds of upper-body weights. Instead of dozens of competitors showing up, as expected, only three did. Since one of them couldn't swim, it more or less guaranteed me second place.

I finished the WFC, held at the YMCA in Plano, Texas, in 21:59:02, three hours behind Rob Powell, who holds the Guinness Book of Worlds Records title of the

World's Fittest Man. So I was now officially the World's Second Fittest Man—and still am today, since the contest disbanded after that.

Of course, this hardly qualified me to run Badwater. But Kostman, an iconoclast who'd once set a number of cycling records in events no one had ever thought of before, was fascinated.

"Everyone else here is an ultrarunner," he said. "You are ultra crazy. You're in."

A Harvard University research team, which fitted me with a heart-rate monitor and GPS unit the morning of the race as part of a volunteer study of exercising in heat, weren't impressed. They craned their necks in disbelief when I told them that my maximum run-walk that year had been 20.5 miles two weeks before Badwater. "Are you insane?" one blurted.

But I honestly wasn't worried. In fact, I was aiming to finish under 48 hours—half of Al Arnold's original time—in order to win the coveted Badwater Belt Buckle. After all, I reasoned with a fool's confidence, I completed the 1995 Eco-Challenge—which included a 100-mile hike with a heavy backpack—on two weeks' training, and ran the 1999 Boston Marathon under four hours after literally training a week for it (see Chapter 1). Neither finish was pretty, and this one wouldn't be, either. But a finish is a finish. My base fitness—quite high with a resting heart rate in the low 40s from intervals, weights, and cross-training—always gets me through.

And realistically, I wouldn't be running, as would Scott Jurek, who despite winning Western States just two weeks earlier was out to blow the doors off his first Badwater. He'd set his sights on the record of 25 hours and 9 minutes established by Russia's Anatoli Kruglikov in 2000. He had to average about 5½ miles per hour to do that. I, on the other hand, only had to go a bit under 3 mph to make 135 miles in 48 hours—literally, a walk. Walking is easy on your body—running isn't. Heck, I can walk 4.5 mph on a treadmill at 8% grade for hours. Only 3 mph? Piece of cake!

THE HEAT IS ON

July 11, 10 A.M. I'm soaked already, and I haven't moved a millimeter. Why I'm in the 10 o'clock wave with the elite runners I do not know. But I promise not to let it affect my game plan of walking every step.

Then I see Scott Jurek. "I did my homework," he explains. He wears a special Brooks-designed hat with an "ice pocket" to keep his head cool. He has an ice bandanna around his neck to cool off his main arteries. He is the only one wearing full-length white pants, which keep you cool and insulated when the temperature—110 and rising—is higher than 98.6. His two support vehicles hold eight people who will continually spray him with cold water and have an ice bath ready when he overheats.

In fact, everyone has two vehicles. I have Marc and my father Norm, 76, in a van with 2 ice chests. And Dad, normally as regular as the morning newspaper, has been complaining of being constipated since we arrived in Death Valley two days before. We were the last ones to arrive at the start line because he'd been stuck, unsuccessfully, in the bathroom.

When the gun sounds everyone takes off *running*. No one's walking! "It won't look good on film," a cameraman yells. So I run. My heart rate rockets to 160. After a mile, I start walking. My heart rate is 140—20 beats higher than it is when I walk the same pace back home. I am passed by 63-year-old Art Webb, who's done this 7 times. He and I begin a cat-and-mouse game where I run the downhills, pass him, and he jogs past me as I walk. It's fun. Then I remember that I am not trained for 135 miles, that I'm wearing out my legs. By mile 25 I can't run the downhills, anyway; they hurt too much.

By mid-afternoon, heading west with the sun ricocheting up from the blacktop and microwaving my face, my pace is steady—but my nerves are not. I am alone. No sign of life, human, animal, insect, tree. Among the missing: My 2-man crew.

"I'm a lot more worried about him than you," Marc had told me 30 minutes earlier. "Dad is scared. He's so constipated that he feels like he's going to rupture,

like an interplanetary predator is going to burst out of his belly like in the movie *Alien*. He feels like he's got a battleship in there. He's been moaning and crying for the last four hours. I've never seen him in pain like this."

He handed me two water bottles, then raced away to drop Dad at Stovepipe Wells, 15 miles up the road, where a medical team could look after him. He promised to be back in 30 minutes, max, and had arranged for the crew of Badwater rookie Rob Harsh to supply me with liquids.

But it never happened. In two minutes, the crew dropped back to let Rob rest. Stupidly, I didn't join them. I was feeling too good to stop.

So as the temperature crept into the 120s, I was now alone, rationing my one bottle of Gatorade and the other of water, both of which are morphing from warm to hot. As I feel my engine winding down, my feet aching, my mind as empty as the stark desert around me, I look for shade. Of course, there is none. I look at my watch. Forty minutes. I'm cooking alive, and he's late.

A car pulls up. I don't know who it is and they don't say, but they see I have no crew. "Listen, this is illegal and dangerous—you can be kicked out for this," says the driver. I tell him about my dad's constipation and that my brother ought to be back in seconds. He hands me a gallon jug of water. (Thank God, I was down to fumes.) I fill up my bottles, and he drives off.

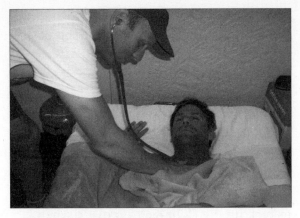

Electrolyte deficiency after 11 hours.

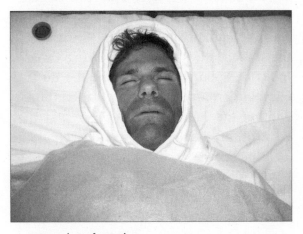

Frozen asleep after 14 hours.

When my brother returns, alone, 60 minutes after he left, he says, "You look broiled." I am. It's been 8½ hours non-stop, 32 miles. I grab some potato chips and a turkey sandwich. I lay down in the van for an hour, feet up on a cooler, my toes and every muscle in my legs aching, and fall asleep thoroughly depressed. "This is hopeless, there's 100 miles to go," I tell Marc. "This is the stupidest thing I've ever done."

But after an hour of rest, something unexpected happens: I'm rejuvenated, my feet and body feel great! It's just 10 miles to Stovepipe—2½ hours. As the sun dips toward the horizon, I hammer past the Devil's Corn Field in full 4.5-miles per hour stride, and don't begin to fatigue until the last hour. Finally, we see the tiny lights of the three-building town of Stovepipe Wells.

All I'm dreaming about is jumping in that pool.

DEATH AND RESURRECTION

My eyes slowly open at 1 A.M. To the right, I see my dad sprawled out on a cot. To the left, my brother is laying faceup, eyes shutting. I close my eyes and go back to sleep, when it hits me: I've been off the road for three solid hours. I have 93 miles to go! And I am the Second Fittest Man!

In 20 minutes we bolt off on the 16-mile assault up 4,956-foot Towne Pass.

A big help from that point was the 12 Endurolyte electrolyte replacement capsules Dr. Bliss told me to take per hour. (We'd misread the instructions and only been taking one—contributing to the sodium deficit.) My salts restored and body rested, I attacked the ascent at full speed in the cool night air. It was beautiful out there, just us, alone, the headlights from behind me pointing the

197

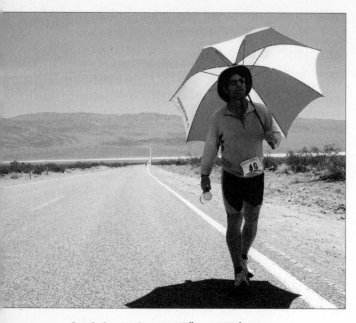
Day 2: Crossing Panamint Valley at 125 degrees

way, throwing my shadow ahead like a ghostly monster. The black velvet night is splattered with millions of stars

Sunrise broke before 6 A.M. as we reached the 4,000 FEET ELEVATION sign and passed Jack Denness, the legendary septugenarian. *How do these old guys do it?* I think to myself as I sped up while passing him. The final 1,000-foot climb up to Towne Pass was a pleasure compared to the steep, 9% descent, which is harder and much slower to walk than it is to run. Every eccentric contraction pulverized my quads. That slowed my arrival at the scalding 8-mile-long Panamint Valley below.

When I arrived at Panamint Springs Resort checkpoint at mile 72.3, it should have been a call for celebration. We had just 62.7 miles to go! That meant I had 21 hours remaining to "Buckle"—to make the 48-hour time limit—an average of a mere 3 miles per hour!

But there was a problem: I was despondent. Desperate for shade, I had opened up a huge red-and-white umbrella as I crossed. It did help a lot psychologically. But I emerged from the valley so wasted and hurting that I couldn't move once I stopped at Panamint. I literally had to pick up my right leg to move it when I sat in a chair, as if it were a piece of wood. The soles of my feet felt were so blistered it was like walking on hot coals. Worse was the math: If I was barely walking three miles per hour now, how would I do it climbing 3,000 feet up the Panamints and another 4,000 up Mt. Whitney?

One of the doctors who'd seen me freezing in the medical room the night before stopped and pulled out the race program, detailed the course profile, and cautioned against it. "It's all hills the next 13 miles," he said. "You've achieved enough." On top of that, we were out of ice, and there was none in town.

"There's no hope," I told Marc and Dad, then laid down on a bench and fell asleep for an hour.

As usual, the perspective suddenly changed when I awakened. First, Marc told me that another crew had just given him some valuable tips. Number 1: Keep an ice-cold towel around your runner's neck. Chilling all the neck veins—among the largest in the body—helps chill the

198

whole body. Number 2: Keep the runner's water bottles filled with ice at all times; it encourages the runner to drink more and keeps his core body cooler. Number 3: Splash the runner in the face every few minutes with ice water. The face is like the radiator of car—if it's hot, the rest of the body feels bad.

Next, out of nowhere, an elderly waitress handed Dad a large bag of ice. "I thought there was no ice," I said. He smiled. "I made her a dollar ring (a ring he constructs from a dollar through an origami-like series of folds). Women always swoon over that ring." Not more than a minute later, a Badwater van pulled up. "We've got ice!" they shouted.

The doctor saw us talking and shook his head. "Not worth it," he said.

An image of Kostman popped into my head. "Dude, screw him," he says. "You're the Second Fittest Man."

Flying uphill at 4.5 miles per hour, I tore through the Panamints. Properly educated, Marc had morphed into a one-man Indianapolis pit crew, bolting in and out of the van every five minutes to ice down my shoulders and bottles, never letting me out of his sight. I mainlined ice water and Enduralite capsules and spritzed my face endlessly. For the first time all race, we were functioning as a unit, like a single, integrated organism.

I went 7 miles in 90 minutes. My feet were crying, but I refused to recognize their pain. The Buckle beckoned.

Then my right heel exploded.

It literally went off like a bomb. A blister under the thick heel callus ruptured. I staggered like a car with a blown tire, hobbled over to the van, and ripped my shoe off for the first time in 30 hours. Oh my God, it was ugly. Blisters everywhere—like tumors! And my heel was on fire. I had no idea how to deal with this. All I knew is that touching the heel brought red-hot pain and that I needed a sandal—anything without a heel backing.

"It's over, guys," I said.

"What about this?" said Marc. From the back of the van he tossed over a pair of Nike Frees, ultralight shoes new on the market then that I'd tested months ago and thrown into a junk box. They had no structural material on the back of the heels to speak of, just a thin membrane and a sandal-like strap.

And it worked!

I tore through the rest of the Panamints, made up more time, and emerged on the long, gradual descent of the Owens Valley. At mile 90 we posed for a picture at the "Leaving Death Valley" sign and gazed west at 35 easy miles into Lone Pine before the final 15-mile, 4,500-foot push up the flank of Mt. Whitney. The impossible had become probable. We'd completed two-thirds of the course in 32 hours. Marc and Dad could smell the Buckle.

Victory seemed a given. My leg muscles were fried, but no worries—they've been

RUN FOR LIFE

much worse at other events and always seemed to recover with short rest breaks.

But then there were my feet … my wimpy bike/swim/10k feet. The last couple miles took my breath away. I was slowing precipitously. My soles were hamburger, every step raw terror, like smashing against hot coals, and getting worse. Just standing made me grimace.

I ran 200 yards, and stopped. I walked 30 yards, and stopped. I waved over Marc and Dad. "The pain is too much," I told them.

My race was over.

I couldn't fake it anymore. I couldn't fake tough feet. I had the soul, but didn't have the soles. Years of 30-minute runs don't armor them for ultrarunning—or even ultrawalking. For this, you need months and years of training with three, four, five hours of foot strikes. The torturous chain of blisters metastasizing across my unhardened feet was proof. If I could only resole them …

Days later, when I told Scott Jurek, who set a new Badwater record of 24 hours and 36 minutes, that I didn't finish, I could hear the disappointment, even the disrespect, in his voice. But I don't feel that way.

I consider Badwater 2005 one of my greatest life experiences. Shackled with ignorance, error, and undertrained body parts, my brother, my dad, and I learned on the fly, jelled as a team, and by the end, completely changed our tune. From "I would never do this idiotic thing again," our rallying cry became, "We'll be back."

And we will. After all, I was only 49 at the time. Just a kid, really, compared to someone like Jack Deness, who retired after finishing his 11th Badwater in 57:52:12. So I've got at least a couple more decades to get in shape for the next one.

CHAPTER 17

MOTIVATION CASE STUDY #2:

GET A RIVAL

How a fast-swimming nurse made a doctor a better runner

At 6-foot-6, 225 pounds, Dr. Samir Shahin, a general practitioner from Manhattan Beach, California, stood out at any race he went to. He stood out above the crowd in his 60 marathons, including the day he and 30 others ran the San Diego Rock 'n' Roll Marathon dressed as Elvis. "We each had names; I was called 'Tall Elvis'—of course," he said. It was the same thing at triathlons, of which he's done dozens, including four Ironmans. Even in the 200-plus pound "Clydesdale" category, his head would poke out of the corral on the beach like a lone submarine telescope.

That is, until the 1997 Hermosa Beach Sprint triathlon, when the then 39-year-old lined up next to the year-younger Martin Spencer, a 6-foot-7, 250-pound registered nurse from Santa Barbara by way of Manchester, England.

"We bade each other good morning, and then I took off," said Spencer. "The sprint events favored me. He's a good cyclist and remarkably good runner, which I can't do well. After a fracture in my 20s, a podiatrist told me that I was too big to run. But my swimming background gave me a real and psychological edge." The Englishman built a huge lead on the swim. Shahin, a 4-plus-hour marathoner with a PR of 3:45, inexorably closed the gap as the race went on. But there wasn't enough time in the short race. Spencer took 3rd, Shahin 4th.

It continued like that for a couple years—Spencer 2nd, Shahin 3rd. Spencer 4th, Shahin 5th. They were always among the Top 5 in the Clydesdales, which often would account 20 or 30 people out of a field of 600 triathletes. It ate at the doctor.

"Despite all the races I've done—including a marathon a month one year—I don't think of myself as being a hardcore athlete," says Shahin, who coauthored the book *50 Trail Runs in* *Southern California* and is the inventor of SportSlick, the lubrication gel. "But being beaten by Marty again and again changed me. I wouldn't miss a workout—thinking 'I've done 99% of the work, but that guy beat me by 5 seconds and took away my third place.' So I'd push it to 100%."

"I read every article on training. I did track work; I could debate every side on nutritional issues," says Shahin. "I did the normal carbo-loading, then went to a diet of high-protein powder made of egg whites and dried milk, a can or two of tuna fish, topped off with honey."

His running seemed to get faster. In 2000, at a buffet at the Luxor Hotel the night before the Las Vegas Marathon, he ate roast beef, fish, fried chicken, and one piece each of cherry, apple, and peach pie. "I ate so much that I could barely walk," he said. "And guess what happened? I broke my 5k, 10k, and half marathon records during the marathon, running 7-minute miles."

There seemed to be no limit to what he'd try to beat his rival. "This would make normal people laugh, but I even tried a hyperbaric chamber," he says. Super-saturated with oxygen, hyperbaric chambers were originally developed to help burn victims and diabetics. Diseased tissue that doesn't get enough oxygen heals better this way. As a physician, Shahin had access to it for free.

"My conclusion: There is no benefit to normal people," he says. "But it's relaxing—1½ hours breathing 100%

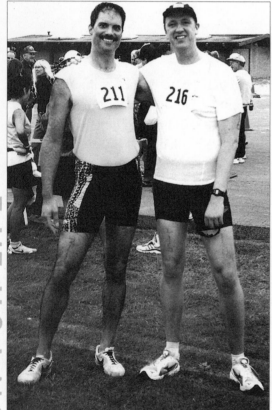

Big rivals Samir Shahin (6-foot-6) and Martin Spencer (6-foot-7).

oxygen with no phone calls. I felt good. And psychologically, I was ready for him."

Finally, in the Catalina Island Triathlon in 2001, Shahin beat Spencer. And for the next two years, the two Clydesdales traded places.

"It was good motivation for me to get better—especially on the bike," says Spencer. "We competed probably 10 times—five times at Hermosa. We used to call it "our event." Even when I moved to Monterey, I came down to compete against him."

He'll never forget one of their last races, the Catalina Sprint, which he lost. "It was a long, hard sprint race: ½-mile swim, 9-mile bike, 5k run," says Spencer. "There were three ascents on the bike. He had the advantage there and was fresher on the run. There's some footage of me hobbling after the bike transition."

The supersized rivals became friends. "He came to my wedding," said Spencer. That was 2003. It was the last time they saw one another.

Spencer moved away with his wife. Seattle was too far from L.A. to sustain the rivalry. But neither has forgotten it.

"Looking back, our competition did make it so exciting," says Spencer. "The anticipation for months and months, motivating you to train harder..." He doesn't do triathlons anymore due to a foot injury.

Shahin doesn't race triathlons much anymore, either. "I miss the passion of having a rival," says Shahin. "The competition makes you enjoy life. With it, you want to learn everything you can to get better. It was fun knowing that I *had* to go out and exercise. But when he left, I lost some motivation. It even may have hurt my running."

But it hasn't stopped him. Five years later, still furiously thinking of a new way to motivate himself, Shahin's thinking about shooting for what he calls, "The world's most expensive T-shirt: the 50–50 club." As in 50 marathons in 50 states.

John Strand, whom you'll read about next, knows a little about that.

CHAPTER 18

MOTIVATION CASE STUDY #3:

SHOOT FOR BIG NUMBERS

How John Strand became the 100-Marathon Man

D r. John Strand is a slow starter, but he gets up to speed fast. The physician from Yorba Linda, California, 70 when I met him in early 2005, was a 39-year-old aerospace engineer when he decided to move his wife and two children to Guadalajara, Mexico, to study medicine. Then, at age 53, as a confirmed middle-aged couch potato with a thriving geriatrics practice, he suddenly took up running and got swept up in marathon mania. Soon, Strand was chasing races around the U.S. and Europe and even Antarctica—and chasing history, too. That's what led him to do 42 marathons in four years starting in 2002. And it's what led him to Pacific Coast Highway on the foggy, overcast morning of February 6, 2005. If he could finish Huntington Beach's Pacific Shoreline Marathon, he would gain membership in one of the most historic, exclusive, rarified fraternities in the sport of running: The 100-Marathon Club.

At the time, about 180 people in the world had run 100 marathons in their lifetimes. But Strand's achievement would actually be more impressive than that. He had already run a marathon in all 50 states of the U.S.—a feat accomplished by only 210 people (as I write this in 2008). In 1995, at age 62, he became the 5th person in the world to run a marathon on all 7 continents. By '05, 118 people had done that. But add all of them together—assuming he would finish the Pacific Shoreline Marathon—and Strand would become one of just 11 people in history to have completed the exalted "triple crown" of marathoning: 100 total marathons, 7 continents, and all 50 states.

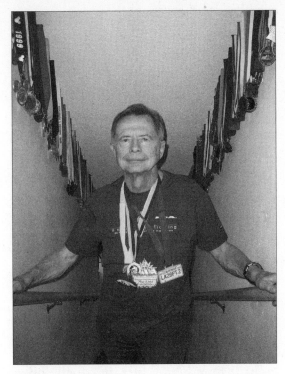

Strand's stairway of fame.

Eleven people on a planet of 6 billion is not a high percentage. "It's roughly 2 times 10 to the negative 9th power," says Strand, in the pleasant, matter-of-fact, faintly ironic manner of an otherwise-conservative man amused by his predilection for doing the far-out. "But if you add 'cancer survivor' to the mix, I could be the only one in the world," he adds, referring to his successful 1997 prostate cancer surgery.

THE 53-YEAR-OLD ROOKIE

Strand didn't start running until 1988, when he was 53. "It never struck me to run or exercise, even though I know that it was good for your health," he says. "But I started running to kill time, then found I enjoyed it." It happened when he found himself driving his then-15-year-old son Eric to weekend running races, then sitting around bored for hours through the event and the awards ceremony. "It dawned on me: By the time Eric got his award, I figured I could run a 5k," he said. He started walking, then jogging.

Years of inactivity left a mark. "No matter how slow I ran, I'd get winded," he said. "Took me a month to run 5k without walking. Soon I was entering 5ks. And I'd often say to myself, 'How did I get myself into this?'"

Strand stopped questioning himself the day that the marathon bug bit. "One fine day, in a moment of insanity after I finished a 5k, I did the 10k immediately following it," he said. "Just like that, I was hooked—it was like crack cocaine. The first one is free. The next one, you negotiate prices." As Strand already proved in his late-blooming medical career, once he gets started, he commits. Within months, he was training for the 1989 Los Angeles Marathon. Soon, he was doing several marathons a year all over the world. He did the Moscow marathon in 1992, just after the fall of communism. He did Germany and England and Korea. He did the 100th Boston Marathon in 1996. The year before, he was one of five people to do the first Antarctica Marathon, making him one of five people to do a marathon on every continent.

His motivation? "It's the thrill of reaching a pinnacle," Strand says. But to the unbiased observer, it may be more than that: "completion-mania." After finishing the first Disneyland Marathon in Anaheim in 1995, he thought, *wouldn't it be nice to have a matching finisher's medal from Disney World Marathon in Florida?* When he picked that one up in 1999, it set off a whole new series of goals.

As it turned out, Florida was the eighth state in which Strand had run a marathon. "So, from that point, I made it my new goal to do all 50 states," he says.

For the next 4 years, Strand kept a pace most runners would consider insane, if not impossible: nearly a marathon a month.

Some of those he really had to dig for, like the Delaware Marathon, which is only held sporadically and once

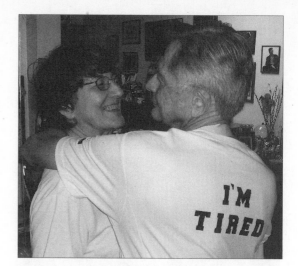

cancelled on him. He collected his 50th state marathon at Columbia, Missouri, on Labor Day, September 1, 2003. Then he slowed down a bit.

You see, the 50-state accomplishment only inspired him to reach for another monumental goal. After all, by then Strand had racked up a total of 90 marathons. If he did 10 marathons in the next 15 months—a piece of cake!—he could attain his 100th in his Orange County homeland at Pacific Shoreline.

A TORTOISE, NOT A HARE

How does Strand's body handle a marathon a month or every three weeks? Most people, like Bob Gamez, manager of the Snail's Pace running shoe store in Brea—Strand runs with him every Saturday morning—are astounded. "Dr. Strand's recovery rate is rare. Few people can recover month to month," he says. "Maybe it's because he's thin and

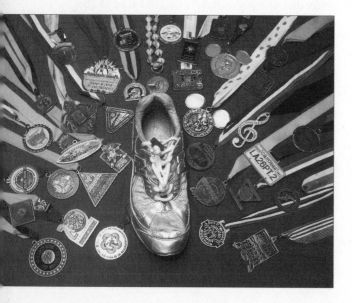

light—5-foot-6 or so, cross-trains with cycling, and didn't start running until he was in his 'golden years.' He didn't put his body through the pounding early. You don't see a lot of people over 60 running. Mostly, though, he can keep it going because he doesn't run fast enough to get hurt."

Strand, who trains 22 miles a non-race week, would not disagree. "Have fun, don't get hurt. No need to go fast; someone's always done it better than you," he says. "I don't peak—I just maintain. I run my marathons nice and slow—between five to six hours, up from 4½ in my early years. My goal is to finish before sunset. Out of courtesy to our foreign visitors, long ago I decided to let the Kenyans take first place."

There are usually 180 to 190 runners in Strand's age-group at the L.A. Marathon. He finishes in the top 20%, an hour or an hour-15 back of the winners. Strand set his PR of 4:04:56 at the Valley of the Flowers Marathon in Lompoc, California in 1991. His slowest time of 8:54:20 was recorded at the Laramie, Wyoming, Marathon in 2001. Apparently, high elevation—8,642 feet above sea level at Laramie—bothered the sea-level dweller more than the cold. (He ran a 6:28:26 in subzero temps in Antarctica on February 5, 1995.)

Strand is most proud of having have finished every marathon that he's started, which is why the 2004 Phoenix Rock 'n'

Roll stands out. "I didn't think I would finish that one," he says. Hit with a viral infection and nausea the day before the race, he didn't eat and slept 16 hours. "Most people carbo-load before a marathon; I fasted. Do not try this at home," he says. "I started the marathon carrying my trusty cell phone, so I could abort when things got too tough. But, at 10 miles I started to feel good, and so I did finish—standing up."

Marathon globetrotting can be an expensive, time-consuming hobby. Describing himself as "frugal," Strand guesses he's spent about $500 on every domestic race he can't drive to, about $25,000 total, plus another $25,000 attending 14 foreign races. His schedule—often flying into a city on Saturday and flying out Sunday—doesn't leave time for conventional sightseeing, but that doesn't bother him. "I figured anything worth seeing is on the marathon course," he says. So like any good tourist, he brings a camera. His album includes shots of Berlin's Brandenburg Gate, London's Tower Bridge and Parliament building, and Moscow's Red Square—although he shot the latter the day after the marathon, which didn't pass by Russia's most famous tourist attraction. He has a shot of himself running on the Great Wall of China taken a day after the Beijing Marathon, 180 miles away.

Future plans include a marathon in every country in the Caribbean. "But

Puerto Rico may be a problem," he says. "It only has one marathon, and it has a cutoff of 3½ hours because it's an Olympic tryout. Speed isn't my thing."

There are some places, however, that he will not go. "If I get the 100th," he said the day before the inevitable, "I'd like to get back into [cycling] centuries again once I can reduce my workload. (He sold his practice in 2003, but was still working it fulltime.) No ultramarathons for me. No Badwater 135. Death Valley in 110 degrees? People my age can die from that."

THE BIG DAY

On February 6, 2005, Dr. Strand arose at typical marathon wake-up time: 4 A.M. Like always, he fixed one bowl of oatmeal, with no butter or sugar. He drank one glass of milk and a glass of orange juice, and topped it off with one slice of wheat toast spread with peanut butter. At 5 A.M., he grabbed his fanny pack, threw in his cell phone and a Hershey bar, and hopped in the car with his wife Dorothy, 65, a fellow runner. If all goes as planned, Huntington Beach's Pacific Shoreline Marathon would be her 36th marathon finish—and his 100th.

Physically, Strand was ready, having tuned up with a 21-mile run 3 weeks earlier. Yet, when the gun went off at 7 A.M., he found himself with an unusual "slightly nervous state of mind."

"It was cool, cloudy, and kinda threatening," he recalled. Yet it wasn't the weather that bothered him. It was the expectations.

"Normally, no one knows or cares about what I'm doing," he says. "But today, everyone seems to—the race promoters, the police, and my two running clubs: Snail's Pace and the 642 Group." He runs with the former on Saturdays and meets the latter near Villa Park High School every Sunday at 6:42 A.M. Both feted Strand's 100th at a party the day before.

Strand settled into his 12-minute-per-mile groove early. "Everything was going smoothly as expected," he said. Then came a minor crisis at the 13-mile turnaround point at Bolsa Chica Beach: the can of Pepsi he'd stashed in a bush had been stolen. Strand religiously gulps sports drinks at every aid station and sucks down two chocolate GUs per race, but eagerly looks forward to the cola's sugar jolt.

Composing himself, Strand resumed his normal routine of talking to other runners and looking for photo ops. Soon, he handed his camera to a spectator and posed with the pier in the background. A small burst of exhilaration came at mile 16 with the discovery that his next secreted can of Pepsi remained unmolested. Spirit soaring, he slowly, luxuriously drank in the bubbly, caffeinated sugar water over the next ¾ mile.

By mile 24, Strand was on cruise control. "I really didn't have anything left in terms of emotions," he said. Then came the last mile. A dozen of his Snail's Pace buddies—most of whom had already finished the half marathon—suddenly appeared around him. Then at the half-mile mark, he looked to his left side and noticed his son Eric. He looked to the right and saw his younger son Bill. With Dorothy running alongside him stride for stride, the whole Strand family was running together.

"I don't do a whole lot of crying—I'm not sentimental," Strand says, "but I was flabbergasted to see my sons … although at that point, I didn't have much moisture left in my body to cry."

He crossed the line in a time of 5:28:42 with a police escort. The entire Strand clan—including his daughter-in-law and two grandkids—collapsed in joy around the 100-Marathon Man.

WHAT'S NEXT?

When I caught up with Strand again, he was 74, retired half-time, and up to 112 marathons with no signs of slowing down. In fact, he was speeding up.

Perfectly content with his standard 4.5-mph pace and his multi-generation pals in a new running club he helped start, the California Cruisers, he was forced out of his comfort zone in 2008 by the biggest challenge of his running career: The hilly Big Sur Marathon.

The two-mile climb didn't bother him. But the six-hour time limit did. He hadn't run under that since Pacific Shoreline.

"That meant I had to do some hefty training—on hills," he said. He ended up doing two 27-mile training runs on a hilly nearby loop. And when Big Sur ended, he'd officially finished not by a minute or two, but by a stunning 34 minutes—in 5:26. That was good for a 4th place medal in the 70–74 age-group.

"I was elated!" he said, with rare emotion. "It shows you that you can improve at any age if you train properly. Train just to finish, then do 20 miles. To train for speed, you have to do the whole thing. And you have to do hills."

So what's next for the new, high-performance Dr. Strand—200 marathons, 100 countries, a sub-5? "Just one goal right now," he says. "Look for a marathon in interesting places. A marathon is more or less an excuse to go somewhere you've never been before."

Like, for instance, Tahiti. Check out the next story.…

RUN FOR LIFE

CHAPTER 19

MOTIVATION CASE STUDY #4:

TAKE A RUNNING VACATION

Head for the exotic, 150-strong Tahiti Marathan

Crystal-clear turquoise lagoons. Lush volcanic mountains. Romantic over-water bungalows. Technicolor coral-reef necklaces that surround islands in aqua-blue bathtubs of calm, clear water. And don't forget the buffed, bare-chested outrigger paddlers and the bodacious, bare-breasted brown-skinned bathing beauties (on the ubiquitous postcards, that is). On 118 South Pacific islands about 2,500 miles due south of Hawaii, the spellbinding pleasures of French Polynesia—commonly referred to by the name of its biggest isle, Tahiti—have dazzled Westerners from the time of Captain Cook's visit in 1775. Yet for American travelers who are serious about fitness—both physical and fiscal—Paradise Found has a major image problem:

"It's too far away," they complain. "It's too hot. And it's only for jelled-out honeymooners." The only physical activity on Tahiti, so goes the thinking, involves power shopping for black pearls.

Tell that to the 150 hardy, world-traveler runners—call them globetrotters—who came here in 2002 to do the Tahiti Nui Marathon before anyone else heard about it.

Picture Hawaii with 3% of the tourists, no Kentucky Fried Chickens, all the coconuts, and a 7½-hour flight from L.A. instead of 5. Throw in 250,000 laid-back descendants of the intrepid sailors who paddle-canoed all the way to Hawaii 1,000 years ago. Take a 12-mile, half-hour ferry ride from the airport to the spectacular isle of Moorea, a white-sand-fringed volcanic crater wrapped in a shimmering blue lagoon and shaped

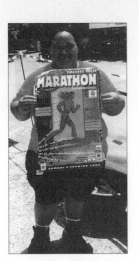

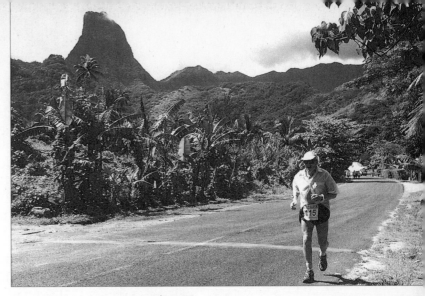

Aussie Ken Matchett, 80

like a three-toed sloth. Then line up at the only marathon in the world that starts in the dark at 5 A.M. The reason? As the sun joins the runners on their journey on the coastal road that encompasses two of the island's "toes," they will be broiled like marinated mahi-mahi.

Tahiti's average summer temperature of 79 degrees is misleading. "The humidity is so high here that it feels like you're running in a sauna," says Wolfgang Pinnow, a 71-year-old TV repairman from Rodgau, Germany. With his thick mane of grey hair, he looks 60. He's done 32 marathons since he started running at age 35, including a PR of 3:16 at 53. He trains every day, including an hour of yoga, and can still peel off a 50-minute 10k. "But this heat will hurt," he says. "I hope it rains."

So does Gordon Ludt, 64, a Canadian who works as a freelance translator for Fuji in Japan. He's used to competing in cool-weather events, like an 84-kilometer ultramarathon in the Arctic Circle and the Antarctica Marathon, the latter having made him one of the first 25 people to run a marathon on every continent. "If there's a special marathon somewhere," he says, "I'm there."

Ken Matchett came to Tahiti with a similar philosophy. The great-grandfather of six from Melbourne, Australia has spent the last 25 years running in 122 marathons all around the world—Rome, Copenhagen, London, Boston, Vienna, you name it. It's done him good, too—he's 80, but looks 70. I tell him 65, and he smiles toothily. "I get that all the time," he says with pride. His skin is smooth and pink, punctuated by a splatter of brown age spots. He combs his white hair over the deforested portion of his head like Rudy Giuliani before he ran for president. The voice is boisterous, confident, authentically Aussie. The legs look like steel rods.

RUN FOR LIFE

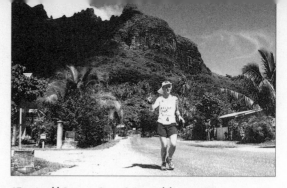
67-year-old German Gerta Gruenwedel

Still, the heat was on his mind. The night before the race, as Matchett talked about how he started running at age 57, averaged 6 marathons a year, and scored a PR of 3:40 at age 68, his forehead glistened with sweat like it was a piece of deeply varnished beech wood. "I'm slowing down the last few years, but I've never not finished," said the former university math/science lecturer and pro bike racer. "I finished the sweltering Fiji Marathon. I'm good for 5 hours. Maybe more here …"

In the darkness the next morning, Matchett lined up next to the man most Tahitians were rooting for: 2-time winner George Richmond of Papeete, a 37-year-old deliveryman for Tahiti Premium Water. The father of three started running a decade ago. Since then, he's become a hero in Tahiti, trailed by a handful of kids whenever he trains, like Muhammad Ali in his Rumble in the Jungle in Zaire. His best time came on a cool day in 2001, 2 hours, 36 minutes, when he finished third.

At 5 A.M., when the gun sounded, the cool air was already beginning to percolate. By 6 A.M. as the sun poked up to reveal towering silhouettes of the lush volcanic mountains all around, the temperature was 73 degrees. The hoped-for rain would not appear from the cloudless sky. Soon, the mercury climbed to 90; it feels like 115 in the humidity. Some runners go by in Arab headdresses.

By 6:30 A.M., leader Thierry Lacroix, a 32-year-old college physical-education instructor from Rennes, France, begins to wilt. This is his fifth marathon and his third Tahiti Nui. He finished 2nd here last year to Yamone Fumio, a Japanese half marathoner, who, on a bet, jumped into the marathon at the last second, set the course record of 2:32:53, puked at the finish, and vowed never to return. Lacroix, who loves coming to Tahiti during the cold French winter, had trained to set a new record. But the heat and an "exploding knee," as he put it, began to wear him down. By mile 18, it had become "zis big," he said, cupping his hands around it like a cantaloupe.

That's when George Richmond blew by. He didn't look back, finishing in 2:37:50—not his best, but nearly seven minutes up on the hobbled Lacroix. "It was a gift, but I'll take it just the same," he said in French through a translator, between bites of coconut and pineapple. "After all, how often can a guy like me take first in a marathon? It'll be at least a couple years before the Kenyans make it to Tahiti."

Due to the heat, no PRs were set this day. Wolfgang Pinnow, the German TV repairman, came in at 4:57, 20 minutes

FUNKY RACES IN FAR-OUT PLACES

Of course, if you want to spice up your running life with an extraordinary race, you don't have to go to paradise. Do a running vacation at 12,000 feet in the Himalayas. Run naked in San Francisco, or through pig poop in England, or do Phidippides' original three-day 270-mile route in Greece. *New York Times* adventure writer and syndicated columnist Stephen Regenold, my teammate at the 2006 Primal Quest, a 400-mile, 8-day adventure race through Utah, and principal of the popular GearJunkie.com website, put together a great piece about the "World's Weirdest Footraces." In it you'll read about:

- **Animal activism** at the Boom Days Pack Burro Race in Leadville, Colorado, where you pull a burro or donkey on a rope through a mountainous, 22-mile-long course.

- **Bare-naked running** at the Bare to Breakers in San Francisco, which runs the same day as Bay to Breakers, and the Kaniksu Ranch Bare Buns Fun Run in Spokane, Washington.

- **High-altitude adventure** at the Nepal Trek and Trail Run—6 days of hiking plus a half marathon.

- **British masochism** at the Tough Guy race, 8 miles of mud, manure, water, fire, ice, and electric charges.

- **Greek tragedy** at the Spartathlon, which traces Phidippides' route from Athens to Sparta to Marathon.

For more races, go to http://thegearjunkie.com/the-worlds-weirdest-footraces.

slower than his previous worst. And octogenarian Aussie Ken Matchette? He almost melted away altogether.

Matchett's sartorial strategy—wear a safari hat and an ordinary collared, button-down white business shirt to vent the heat and ward off the sun—made him

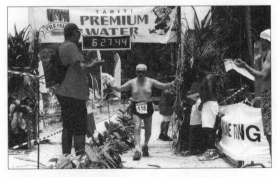

Matchett finishing with a PW.

the best-dressed runner. But that's all. Planning to outwit the heat by running 1k and walking 200 yards, he ended up walking all of it after the 9-mile mark—except for brief bursts of speed when he saw me aiming my camera at him and on the downhills. That saved his strength for a final 5-mph burst across the finish line, by then in the process of being dismantled.

Matchett's time was 6:27:43. "It was grueling. I don't think I'll do a marathon again in such heat. But there's still something to celebrate tonight: a PW!" he said, taking the arm of his 50-year-old female companion. In case you don't speak Australian, that's "Personal Worst."

CHAPTER 20

MOTIVATION CASE STUDY #5:

RUN WITH A PURPOSE

*Generations of kids become marathoners
because of Students Run L.A.*

"I'll see you at the finish line, okay?" said Manuel Garcia to Jennifer Caudillo at the start of the 1993 Los Angeles Marathon.

Manuel was 16, Jennifer 15. Students at Francisco Bravo Medical Magnet High School in East Los Angeles, they met on the track team. Then they trained together in the SRLA program—Students Run Los Angeles, a fitness and mentoring program that has trained thousands of schoolkids to run the L.A. Marathon over the years. Friendly for months, they'd just recently been out on one date.

"It was hard to tell her good-bye, but she was a slower runner than me," said Manuel. When the gun sounded, he immediately left Jennifer behind and raced off with a bunch of his buddies. It was his first L.A. Marathon, her third.

One by one, Manuel's friends dropped off the pace until he was running alone. Halfway through the marathon, though, his pace slowed precipitously as fatigue set in. His stride shortened, his breathing labored. Soon, things were looking grim and finishing this beast was no longer a sure thing.

As he stumbled past the mile-16 marker, Manuel glanced to his left and got a surprise: Jennifer!

The experienced marathon veteran was fresh and upbeat; she'd learned to pace herself, to avoid the rookie mistake of going out too hard. But instead of passing her friend, waving good-bye, and saying, "see you at the finish line," she slowed down.

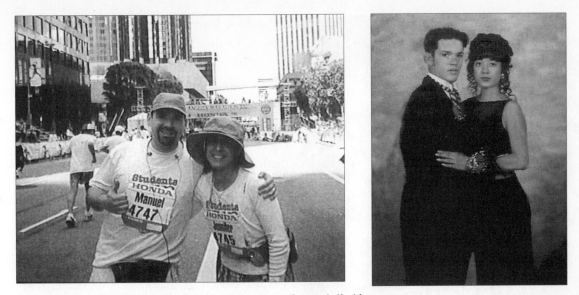

Going the distance: Manuel and Jennifer have been running mates for over half a lifetime.

"Come on, Manuel, you can do it!" she said, running next to him.

Jennifer did not leave Manuel's side for the last ten miles, fueling him with words of encouragement the entire way.

"I gained so much respect for her—how she kept her pace, how she helped me out," said Manuel. "We crossed the finish line together."

And they haven't been apart since. It's been 15 years. The last three, married.

Manuel and Jennifer, now 32 and 31, have had the run of their lives. They were first in their families to go to college— her, UC Santa Cruz, him, San Diego State. Both have Master's degrees and now are teachers in the L.A. Unified School District. Both are as fit as ever; she's done the marathon 6 times, him 4.

They say they owe it all to SRLA.

"SRLA and the marathon helped bring us together and get us to where we are today," says Jennifer. "It teaches you to plan. The training gives you the time to think and relax, to think about your goals.

That's exactly what Harry Shabazian, an East L.A. continuation high school teacher, had in mind in 1989 when he founded SRLA. Feeling "transformed" after he finished his first L.A. Marathon in 1986, he challenged his students—all misfits, troublemakers, and underachievers—to let him train them. Not only did all of his 18 student runners finish the race, but most went on to finish high school, college, and find good jobs at much higher rates than their non-marathoning peers. The teacher-led

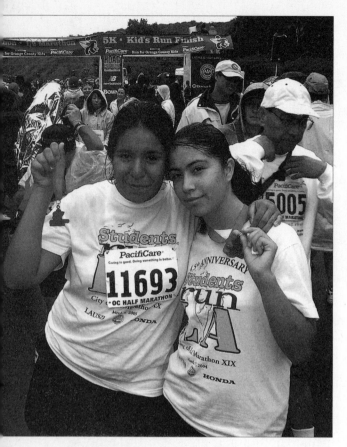

Patricia Garcia and Yurico Rodriguez of Students Run L.A. finished the OC Half Marathon.

SRLA training program trained 3,300 kids last year at L.A.–area schools, leading them over 200 miles from September through March, and paying entry fees and transportation to a number of preliminary races and the marathon itself. Ninety percent of them finished the 26.2-mile course. All are running in a positive direction.

Not surprisingly, Manuel and Jennifer have been SRLA coaches for the last three years. They train 15 student runners at Belvedere Middle School in East L.A., where Manuel teaches 6th grade math, science, and art. They lead 5- to 6-mile runs after school on Monday, Wednesday, and Friday, and long runs on the weekend.

"I tell my fourth graders my story and they are fascinated," says Jennifer, who teaches math, science, and history at several central L.A. schools. "A lot of them are first-generation. Their parents don't have the education, and the kids wouldn't think of going to college or running a marathon. But running teaches values, opens up other pathways. You realize that you do have the power to continue and succeed."

"After all, when things get tough, I'll think, 'how did I feel at mile 22 or 23?'"

Probably better than Manuel did that day 15 years ago. Which brings us to another thing that running can teach you about: relationships.

"Find something you have in common," says Jennifer. "Something healthy that you can share for a long time. It might last a lifetime."

For more information about Students Run L.A., go to www.srlastudents.com.

CHAPTER 21

MOTIVATION CASE STUDY #6:

JOIN THE OLE' BOYS (AND GIRLS) CLUB

Old folks roam with the New England 65-Plus Runners Club

This club proudly discriminates. At the New England 65-Plus Runners Club, young whippersnappers under age 64½ need not apply.

Formed by eight runners in 1991 to encourage race directors to include older age-group categories (it worked—a decade ago, races in New England had none beyond age 50+, but now 95% have 80+ divisions), NE 65+ now has over 600 members from six states, with a satellite in Florida. About 25% are women. Eight are over 80. Fifteen did the 2007 Boston Marathon, ranging from youngster Phil Pierce, 65, of Falmouth, Maine at 3:52:40 to 86-year-old Phil O'Connell of Plymouth, Massachusetts at 8:55:00. The club's average age is 72. The oldest is 96.

"I like it because I feel so young around these guys," says club president Fred Zuleger, 70, a veteran of 30 marathons, including 10 Bostons, with a PR of 3:01 at age 51. "It's social. And inspiring. It gets you out of the house. At this age, most of your friends are running friends. The rest are either dead or have moved. The club keeps people running."

The membership roster includes doctors, lawyers, businesspeople, and blue-collar workers. "Generally, we have people well-off enough to have time off to engage in sports," says former club president Bob Hall, 80, of Sudbury, Massachusetts, a semi-retired neuroscientist who specializes in cochlear implants for hearing stimulation.

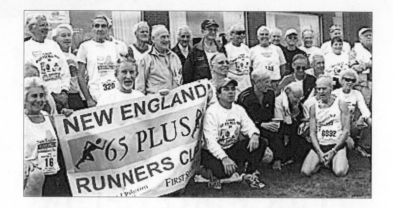

When I note that his voice sounds remarkably vital and young, he was pleased. "All my friends are the same way," he says.

As the number of older runners has risen, NE65+ has served as a crucial lobby group. "If I go to races and they only have a 60+ age-group, I try to convince the director to put in a 70+ category," says Zuleger.

When he started running, there were no age-groups over 50. "There was just 50+," he says. "It wasn't fair—you couldn't compete against the younger guys. But when I was turning 70, I was looking forward to it, because I was going to be in a new division."

Competition is as important to a 70-year-old as it is to a 30-year-old, but the math can be cruel. "You have three good years that end with 0, 1, and 2," says Zuleger. "After that, you're losing speed even though you're putting in the same effort. Psychologically, it can get you down."

Hall knows the feeling. He began running at age 53 when he had to run his daughter's dog for her when she left for college, and has been a top age-grouper in New England for almost three decades. He nearly always medals in everything from 5ks to marathons and has set 5 course records, including a 2:01 half marathon. "But I'm slowing down and I don't like it. I've always been at the head of the pack, and now I'm at the middle. I've been losing half a minute to a minute a mile since 75," he laments.

Of course, there are some club members who seem immune to the ravages of time. Bill Spencer, 71, ran a 5k in 20:14 at age 69. Four-time Hawaii Ironman finisher Bill Riley, 71, the club's acknowledged best runner, is number one in the country in the 70–74 age-group and still can pull off a 1:30 half marathon. "He beats people in their 60s," Hall marvels. But he's humbled by the legendary 115-pound Ed Whitlock of Toronto, now 74, who runs 90 miles

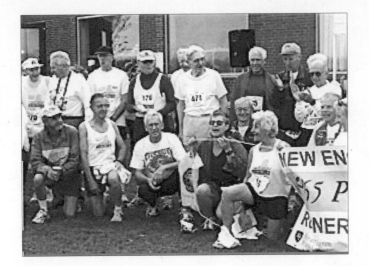

a week and is the only person over 70 to have run a sub-3 marathon (2:56).

Surprisingly, club members rarely discuss anti-aging strategies. Hall plays tennis and does calisthenics, but like most members does not lift weights. He wants to bike more, but fell on the bike on a downhill at 30–40 mph and got a big gash.

Lifetime membership in the New England 65-plus Runners Club is $35, with no annual dues. There are no meetings since members are scattered across the Northeast; the 600 members meet by chance at races and get their results published in a quarterly newsletter. The club has a Hall of Fame and inducted four people this year, all of whom hold world or national records.

More important is the example they may be setting for other older runners. "The social aspect at this age is so important that I wouldn't be surprised to see 55-plus clubs popping up soon all over the country," said Hall. "Oops. Senior moment. 65."

For information on the 65-plus New England Runners Club, go to www. NE65plus.org.

RUN FOR LIFE

INTERVIEW 7

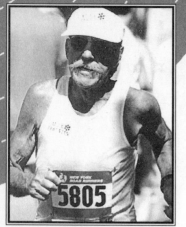

JOHN D. CAHILL

The Fastest Old Ponytailed Dude Of All Time

RUN FOR LIFE

Like many top masters runners, John David Patrick Cahill, 83 at the time of his *Run for Life* interview on January 16, 2008, came to the sport later in life. But it isn't the just pure talent—a 3:04 marathon at 65, a 3:05 marathon at age 72, and his being named 2000 USA Track & Field age 75–79 Runner of the Year—that make this lawyer-turned-resort hotelier stand out. It isn't even the salt-and-pepper ponytail that bobs halfway down his back. It's his world-class joie de vivre.

"He's a character," says USA Track and Field media director Ryan Lampa. "He loves life, and has an energy that's contagious. Some of the dirtiest jokes I've heard have come from John. And some of the funniest memories...."

Like the time in the mid-nineties when Cahill, wearing a beret and a mischievous smile, picked Lampa up in Salt Lake City driving a black Porsche. He took Lampa to his property in Alta, then handed him the keys to his "extra car"—a Jaguar—and said to drive it back to Salt Lake. That Sunday night he met Lampa in town on foot. He'd run all the way from Alta—25 miles.

Cahill is a high achiever. When his brain was rattled by a severe concussion in a car accident a few years ago, doctors thought he'd never be the same again, given his age. It took 4 or 5 months of speech therapy to bring his speaking voice back. Today, he's learning to speak Italian.

In fact, the interview below was conducted from the airport while Cahill was waiting for a flight to Sicily, where he planned to stay for three months. He'd just finished the Rock 'n' Roll Phoenix Half Marathon the previous Sunday and had plans to run the Marrakech Half Marathon in Morocco and the Agrigento, Sicily, half-marathon in the next month.

"That will be three half marathons on three different continents," he said. "Cool, huh?" When the task was completed, he promptly returned home in April and ran the Salt Lake City Half Marathon in 2:09:56.

Running's been very good to me. It saved my life, got me on the right track. I owe a lot to running.

I suppose you could say I was always athletic. Born and raised in Shawnee, Kansas, I played high school basketball, but I knew I was really too little to play in college at Notre Dame. So when I saw a sign out on the bulletin board, TRYOUTS FOR CROSS-COUNTRY, I went out there, even though I didn't know what the hell cross-country was. I don't know how far we ran, but I'll tell you, when I finished, I felt like shit. But that same night, I was surprised to see a sign up there that said TRYOUTS FOR THE FRESHMAN BASKETBALL TEAM. In those days, freshmen could not play varsity ball. So I went out for the freshman team, and I made it.

And I always wondered, if I hadn't made that freshman basketball team at Notre Dame, I'd have probably kept running. I often wondered how good I would have been—how fast. I'm sure I would have been a good college runner given what I know now. It just took 45 years to find out.

I went to law school at Marquette University in Milwaukee and stayed there practicing law for about 29 years, raised a family, divorced. Was married for 27 or 28 years, and I've been divorced 28 or -9. To a wonderful woman; of course, we're better friends now than we ever were when we were married. Nine kids. Well, I was a Catholic in the fifties, and what the hell do you think? Who ever plans to have nine kids? Nobody!

Then I went to Salt Lake City and got into the hotel business. I'm not retired. I bitch at my general managers, and I bitch at my financial people. We own four hotels at the moment, me and my children—the Alta Peruvian Lodge in Alta, the Park City Peaks Hotel, the Tyrolean Lodge in Ketchum Idaho, and the El Pueblo Lodge in Taos, New Mexico—all associated with ski areas.

I skied and played a lot of racquetball in my middle years. And screwed every chance I got.

Running came into the picture when I was driving down to Cuerna Vaca, Mexico in the late winter of 1985–86; I was 62 years old. It was a weeklong solo trip and I was in no rush. I remember going to some athletic store and buying a pair of running shoes for $30—God, I wish I still had 'em, I remember they were red and white. And the

first night I drove down to the Arizona-Utah border, Kenab, Utah, I got up the next day and ran—probably about half a mile.

I did it because I was a little overweight. I weighed about 165—I'm 5-foot-8½—and I'm about 140 now. Nobody told me to run. I wanted to lose weight. That first half-mile run was terrible. I said, "This sucks big-time!" The next day I drove to a town just north of the border, and I ran around the parking lot some more. Anyway, I ran every day on the weeklong drive down and every day for the three months that I was in Cuerna Vaca. By the end, I was running an hour, maybe an hour-15 a day, no idea what my pace was. Maybe seven miles per hour.

When I came back from Mexico, I got on the scale and, by God, I weighed 148 pounds. And I thought that's pretty cool. So I kept running around Salt Lake and then I entered a race, the Desert News 10k on July the 24th, Pioneer Day, 1986. And I ran 46 minutes and change—and I liked it.

It was kind of eye opening when I first saw my times. I don't know where I placed in my age-group; I didn't even check. I don't think I even knew about things like that then. But I found out that for an old fart of 63, I was pretty good.

I started reading these books about the average speeds for people 65 years old, and I thought, "Jesus Christ, I'm 10 minutes better than that." I did a couple more 10ks. Then I started winning everything.

A year later, running actually saved my life. I was running in Acapulco, I had this strange feeling over my left breast. It happened several times. And when I got back to Salt Lake City, I went to see my doctor and he said, well, I'll send you to see a cardiologist. The cardiologist suggested I go see a funeral director.

In June or July of 1987, I had an angioplasty. I didn't run for a year—the doctor told me not to, because my arteries were healing. I swam a lot. Those were the days before stents. But mine worked very well. So I started running again in 1988, after a year off. I ran my first marathon, the St. George Marathon, in October of 1989 when I was 65½. I ran 3:04:49. Not bad for an old guy.

I was first in my age-group. I lowered the age-group record by 42 minutes. I had the record for 10 or 15 years. Eventually, my age-group record was lowered by a guy who did it in 2:55.

Then in 1990, I started traveling around to all these races. I went to Peachtree two or three times, others four or five times. If there was a big race around, I went. I had a list of the 25 biggest races in the country, and I was going to run every one of them. Usually 10ks to marathons. My 5ks will be high 26s, low 27s. My 10ks will be 54.

I've done around 35 marathons total, including 11 St. Georges, New York eight times, Boston twice, Honolulu, Los Angeles, Moscow, Rome, Berlin one time each. I did the first Antarctica marathon. The 3:04:49 is still my PR, but my best marathon came at age 72 when I ran a 3:05:49—just a minute slower 7 years later.

The one I disliked the most was Antarctica—wet shoes for 26 miles. I think the most exciting marathon in America is New York City. Of my 8 times there, I've won my age-group 5. It's a tougher course, goes through Central Park, of course tons of spectators. And Boston doesn't interest me. It's an easy course. It's way hyped more than it should be, in my opinion. Of course, the other thing that pissed me off about Boston is that the first time I ran it, the age-group stopped at 60. I wrote them a letter and said, "How about changing it?"—and they said, "No." They are too hidebound. They changed it since then. I think the top age-group now is maybe 70 or 75. They haven't kept up with the times.

Last year, I did no marathons—because of the training. The training is the brutal part of any marathon and gets more brutal when you're old. But I did 12 half marathons in 2007—with a best of 1:57, just under 9 minutes a mile.

GOOD RACES AND GOOD FORM

You just don't see that many racers over 80. I ran the half marathon at Phoenix last Sunday, and there were 4 people in the age-group. Three 80-year-olds and me. And in New York, they will have maybe 4 or 5. I'm handsomer than any of them, of course. Most of the times, though, I'm the only one.

Most of 'em have died. Most of the living probably have health problems. And I notice the aging in myself: a certain amount of laziness. For example, I used to get out and run 7 days a week, rain or shine. Now, I get up and it's 15 degrees outside, and I'll say "screw it" and go get a newspaper. So I don't have the passion I used to have. Lack of passion and laziness: It's easier to sit on your ass than it is to get out there and run.

One way I stay motivated is by doing a lot of races. I think it's great training. Some people do tempo runs. I do races. I think it's kind of the same thing. Those races keep me motivated, you bet. I've always loved to race. Interesting: getting a medal used to be important. Now, it's like "ehhhh—what do I do with them? Should I throw 'em away or let my kids throw 'em away after I die?" I have them in a room with trophies and all kinds of shit. It don't mean anything to anyone but me.

I rarely lose. To the best of my knowledge, there's only one guy who is faster than I am. I thought, "you shouldn't be ashamed of that." (Laughs.) His name is John Keston of Sunrise, Oregon. He's about 6 months younger than me, and he's the only one in this country who I knew could beat me anywhere, any day, at any distance. We've only run in the same race 3 times, maybe 4. And he's kicked my ass every time.

It's not hard to take. There's worse things than being number two, you know.

When I was a kid of 70, I'd train up to 70 or 75 miles a week. Now a big week for me is 20 or 25, so I think that that might have had something to do with it. And by the way, when I was running that much, I mean regularly 50 miles a week, every week, and a race every Saturday. I'd run 42 to 45 races a year. And this past year, at age 83, I ran 32 races, including 12 half marathons. I love to race. It's my reward for busting my ass.

As you train, find out what works for you, and do it. Adopt your own training. Don't read that horseshit in Runner's World. Do what works for you. If hills work for you, do 'em. I hate hills, so I rarely do them. If speed workouts work for you, do them.

Here's some speed work for you: At the Alta Peruvian Lodge, we started a "Downhill Dash and Bar-B-Q Bash." It's an 8k downhill. When I was 69 or 70, I ran it in 30 minutes and change. So it's fast. The record on the course is 21 minutes. We get 150 runners.

A running career is going to last for 10, 15, 20, 30 years. You can develop your own program. And if you enjoy running with other people, do it. I don't. I much prefer to run by myself. The only person I run with is a dear friend of mine, my coach, Dr. Tom Miller, who is 65 years of age. I met him in 1989 when I was 65 myself, two or three months before my first marathon. God gave me physical talent, but Tom taught me the technique and mental skills to fully utilize that talent.

The main thing Tom did was shorten my stride length, which increased my turnover rate. And it's all turnover rate, as you know. That increased my speed.

Tom's a nut case for running form—how runners move their arms and move their legs. He studies the Kenyans, and has a series of photos of Jim Ryun, the great miler, pasted on his wall. If Ryun ran with today's nutrition, today's track, I bet this guy would have run 3:40 something.... Anyway, Tom took a TV camera out to the track and taped me. Then we went over the tape, he showed me how I was landing on my heel. He said, "you gotta land flat or forward; you gotta shorten your stride length." A miracle. Until I met him, I thought the way to run fast was to increase your stride length. You know, I was a rookie; I didn't know shit. Then I found out it's all turnover.

Heel-striking—I'm glad I got over that as early as I did, thanks to Tom. It saved my knees. My oldest boy is 57. He's been running since 21. His knees are worn out, but he still runs.

I think I did help motivate my kids. They were adults when I started running. The youngest son, now 42, was excellent; he ran at SMU. My daughter Kathy runs; she's good, got some of my genes. Mike, 47, is very good; he ran at Southwest Texas State, did New York in 2:28 his first time, and did a half marathon last weekend in 78 minutes.

My knees and hips have been fine all these years. I had a problem with my right knee for a while, and I took glucosamine. Either it worked or the knee healed by itself.

I used to have a lot of muscular problems, hamstrings and stuff like that. But when you slow up—start running 9- or 10-minute miles—you don't have those problems anymore.

LONGEVITY TIPS: BIKE, SWIM, WEIGHTS, PASTA

I do one triathlon a year. And I regularly bike and swim to stay in shape for that one triathlon. I do intermittent weights—no regular program, even though I know that's good for you.

I eat pasta 7 nights a week. I love pasta. When I go out to dinner, I eat pasta. I don't know what's wrong with me. If I cook at home, I will cook pasta every time. And a huge salad, and a little chicken or beef or fish, too. A wise athlete finds out what works for him. I have a daughter who says carbohydrates make her fat. Well … fine. But I process them extremely well. That's a buncha horseshit about that anti-carbohydrate diet. Wait two years, and it'll be carbohydrate diets are hot. I watch my intake. Huge plate of pasta and a huge salad. I rarely eat bread and butter, never have salad dressing.

Because I have serious cardiovascular disease, I have to watch what I do. I take an anti-cholesterol pill, Vytorin, which has fallen into disrepute all of the sudden, and Zetia, which yesterday also got knocked. [A study released in early 2008 said the drugs failed to improve heart disease despite reducing several key risk factors.] You know, I think people expect too much out of their drugs. For example, it never occurred to me, and it still doesn't, that an anti-cholesterol drug is supposed to prevent a heart attack. It's NOT supposed to prevent a heart attack. It's supposed to lower your cholesterol.

The medications work for me—you bet your life they have. I take a blood-pressure pill; I suffer from high blood pressure. I take fish oil, because my cardiologist tells me to. I take vitamin B complex, vitamin E, calcium, the One-A-Day brand. Shit, I'm a pill lover (laughs.) I don't know if they're any good or whether it's psychological, but what the hell.

I'll take Viagra, if I ever get a chance to use it.

HIS PLANS FOR AGE 100

That's easy: Trying to get laid.

And If I'm physically able, I will run. Yeah, I think you can run to 100 if you're healthy. I'll let you know in 17 years. Unless I become disabled, I will run to the bitter end.

The older you get, by the way, it doesn't seem so bitter. (laughs) Everybody else is dead, you know. All your friends, everyone you know. You reach the point where you think, well, I've lived long enough. And the world doesn't owe me anything. I'd like to live another 20 years, but if I die tomorrow, I've had a wonderful life. I've been healthy. I've been lucky financially. I've been a very lucky guy.

I run with a singlet that says, 83 AND STILL RUNNING, and I get tons of comments in a big race. I'll bet I had a hundred people say something to me in this Phoenix Rock 'n' Roll Half Marathon last Sunday. Like, "you're my idol, I hope I can do this at your age." And I tell them the key to success and running longevity is the following: Lots of illegal drugs, lots of booze, lots of cigarettes, and all the sex you can get.

Actually, I only have a glass of wine now and then, don't smoke, and I don't screw anymore, dammit. But I look good. Weight 146, 5-8 and a half. For some reason I have a limited amount of gray hair, I don't know why, except that my mother didn't get it until her 90s. That's why I can pass for 79. The good news is that Mother lived to be 101—and I got her genes.

You know, there was a 92-year-old East Indian who broke the marathon record for 90+ [Fauja Singh of Great Britain, who ran 5:10:01 at Toronto in September 2003]. And I want to break that record. If I'm healthy I think I could do that.

RUN REPAIRED

In April of 2008, I drove over to Torrance Memorial Hospital in Torrance, California, I put on a light-blue dressing gown, a hair net, and shoe covers, then watched a knee replacement operation. I gawked in awe as Dr. Stuart Gold, a highly respected surgeon in the Los Angeles area, led a five-person team that peeled open the right knee of James T. Bisson, a 6-foot-5, 250-pound plumber who'd worn out both knees crawling on floors for 30 years. Gold did his left knee two years earlier. Bisson was so happy with it that he came back for the right.

I got very intimate with Bisson, even though I never talked to him. I saw a surgeon's assistant pull a "fat pad" out of his knee area and slice his quadriceps muscle open like raw sirloin. I watched Gold grab an electric saw and, like a good carpenter, slice off the two beautiful round condyles at the end of his femur—like it was a giant steak bone. Next to go was the end of Bisson's tibia. I shut my eyes as his blood splattered all over me, and brushed away bits of his bones as they were sanded and planed. Gold then drilled holes for an alignment device, and began stacking and gluing down the various parts of the new artificial knee. The new "bones" of the Journey BCS Bi-Cruciate Stabilized Knee System, made by Smith and Nephew, were covered not in something resembling the original white cartilage, but in "Black Oxinium," a new high-tech metallic compound. In 90 minutes, Bisson was sewed up and rolled out of the operating room, and Gold and his team were ready for operation number two.

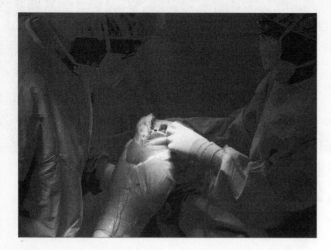

(see Chapter 23), there is an unspecified risk to consider: The release of millions of microscopic bits of metallic and plastic particles inside your body (see sidebar). So, the best advice is clear: fix your form and take care of what you have. In 20 years, bionic parts will be a lot more effective and safe.

For now, when injuries do happen, the best strategy is to minimize the damage by dealing with them promptly. Don't risk wearing anything out. The bionic body parts are amazing things. But give me a choice between cobalt-chrome and old-fashioned cartilage, I'll stick with nature every time.

"Wanna stay for that one?" he asked.

"No, I've seen enough," I said. I got plenty of notes and photos. I also got scared.

Seeing a human sliced open like a carcass in a slaughterhouse is sobering. It makes you want to take care of what you have. After all, a lot could go wrong. For one thing, what if Gold had sneezed? For another thing, as good as the new knees are, recovery is painful, and durability for hard-core athletic use is unknown. "I'm ecstatic over my new left knee," said Jim Banach, 55, a Los Angeles. S.W.A.T. Team cop, 20 months after his February 2007 operation. "It's as good as new; I run 3 to 5 miles a day on it. But I'm hesitant about jumping from high places on it and won't run a marathon. I try to only run on a treadmill so I don't wear it out."

Although knees are fast improving and hip resurfacing has restored some ultrarunners to their full-striding glory

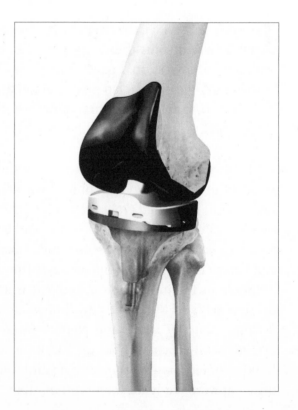

CHAPTER 22

QUICK FIXES FOR RUNNING'S "BIG 6" INJURIES

A *Run for Life* runner isn't supposed to get IT band syndrome, Achilles Tendonitis, Runner's Knee, tendonitis and chrondomalacia, shin splints, plantar fasciitis, and hamstring strains. Theoretically, if you build a strong, balanced body, running form, and workout program, you won't get injured bad enough to have to pay a physical therapist like Bob Forster to repair you. But we're all human, subject to overtraining and biomechanical inefficiencies. "If you have pain in the same place for two workouts in a row or over the course of a week or two, consider yourself injured," says Forster. "For every two days you train in pain, it will take two to get better." Below are the six most common runners' injuries and—besides swimming, cycling and other logical cross-training options—what you can do yourself to rehab them.

1. IT BAND SYNDROME

What it is / Symptoms: Iliotibial (IT) Band Syndrome, one of the leading causes of lateral knee pain in runners, includes extreme pain on the outside of the knee, pelvis, or hip, while running, squatting, and doing knee-bending exercises. The pain, often worse while walking or running downhill, is caused by the continual rubbing of the IT Band (the thick sheath of tissue on the outer thigh running from the outside of the pelvis, over the hip, down to the knee, attached to the tibia) against and over the lateral femoral epicondyle (the outside hump of the end of the thigh bone). The IT is crucial to stabilizing the knee during running, shifting from behind the femur to the front during the gait cycle.

Causes: Tight muscles in lower extremity and pelvis; structural or functional leg length inequalities (a short or long leg); excessive foot pronation from poor shoe choices or faulty running mechanics.

Treatment: Fix incorrect running mechanics and keep the IT and outer thigh muscles loose with stretches, deep tissue massage, foam rollers, and The Stick. Also, stretch the glutes, strengthen the hip abductors (especially the gluteus medius), which control ITB tightness, and strengthen the quads to lessen the load on the IT bands.

2. ACHILLES TENDONITIS

What it is/Symptoms: Dull or sharp pain above the back of the heel due to inflammation of the Achilles—the tendon that connects the two major calf muscles, the soleus and the gastrocs—to the heel bone. Over time, it gets covered with scar tissue and, in extreme cases, can tear or rupture.

Causes: Running too far, too fast, or too steep on tight, fatigued, or untrained calves, which transfer the burden to the Achilles. Natural overpronators are at highest risk.

Treatment: Stop running and avoid weight-bearing activities until the pain disappears; be patient—it could be weeks.

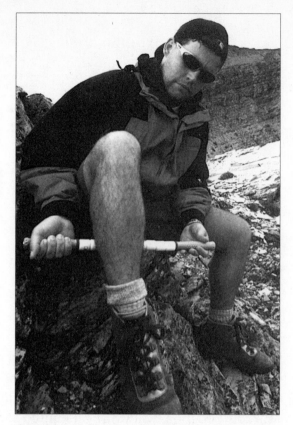

The Stick

Stretch and massage the both the gastroc and soleus (see Chapter 12, stretches #3 and 4), gently at first, then more rigorously and frequently. Use The Stick (see photo). Don't run until heel raise and jumping are pain-free.

3. RUNNER'S KNEE

What it is / Symptoms: Any pain in the kneecap. The two most common forms of runner's knee are patellar tendonitis, a tendon strain, and something much worse and permanent: chondromalacia, a fraying and deterioration of the cartilage that coats the end of the femur and the backside of the kneecap.

Causes: Overtraining, poor biomechanics, overpronation, and tight, imbalanced leg muscles. In chondro, the culprit is "lateral tracking," in which the V-shaped backside of the kneecap no longer rides in the center of the groove in the end of the femur, but high on the groove's lateral side, scraping off cartilage in the process. It will not grow back.

Treatment: For tendonitis, rest and cross-train until pain disappears. For chrondro, cut your loses by stretching the IT bands and outer part of the quadriceps, the vastus lateralis (VL) to loosen their lateral pull on the kneecap. At the same time, strengthen the inner part of the quad, the vastus medialis oblique (VMO). This will realign the kneecap back into the groove between the two condyles (humps) of the femur. Do pool running until pain disappears. For overpronation, try motion control shoes.

4. SHIN SPLINTS

What it is / Symptoms: Razor-sharp pain on the inside of the shin bone from knee to ankle, technically called Medial Tibial Stress Syndrome (MTSS), caused by any of a half a dozen problems. The most common is trauma to tendons and muscles where they attach to the front of tibia. While trying to stabilize the foot, ankle, and lower leg, the muscles exert great force at this point, often causing strains and microtears.

Causes: The sudden shock of hard running after a long layoff, a too-big increase in mileage, tight Achilles and calves, excessive forward lean, worn-out shoes, sudden change in running venue from soft to hard surfaces; lack of warm-up and stretching.

Treatment: Stretch the calves three times daily and before and after activity. Warm up the area before running; ice it after cooldown. Cut back to half your current mileage and stop all hills and speed work. Water-run. "Do not wait," says Forster. "This injury can lead to stress factures in your tibia, which will keep you off your feet for a longer time."

5. PLANTAR FASCIITIS

What it is / Symptoms: Pain in the bottom of the heel due to inflammation of the plantar fascia—a thick, tough, fibrous band of connective tissue that runs along the bottom of the foot in a fanlike manner from heel to the base of each toe. During running and walking, it acts to stabilize the metatarsal joints (the joints associated with the long bones of the foot) during impact with the ground, acts as a shock absorber for the entire leg, and helps to lift the longitudinal arch of the foot to prepare it for the takeoff phase of the gait cycle. The fascia is thinnest near the heel, which is why the pain occurs there.

229

Causes: Inflexible calves, especially the tibialis posterior (a muscle located underneath the soleus and gastrocnemius that connects from the arch of the foot up to the back of the knee) that limits the tibia's ability to move forward at the ankle joint. This lifts the heel early and increases the tension in the plantar fascia. Also, a sudden increase in hill training or general volume, and large weight gain or pregnancy.

Treatment: Stretching or deep massage to relax calf muscles to allow less stressful bending at the ankle. Putting about a small lift under your heel will reduce the ankle bend a bit. Strengthening the fascia with toe-grasping drills and barefoot running will help, too.

6. HAMSTRING STRAIN AND ISCHIOGLUTEAL BURSITIS

What it is / Symptoms: These are two similar conditions caused by biomechanical imbalances. Both can cause persistent or growing pain and tenderness in the back of the thigh during and after workouts; loss of flexibility and pain when stretching; bruising; and pain during sitting. It is caused by a sudden tear (you may hear a "popping" or "snapping") or accumulated microtrauma (from overuse) in the hamstring group, the three large rear-thigh muscles that extend from the pelvis at the "sit bones" (the ischium) to the top of lower leg bone (tibia), below the knee. These "two-joint" muscles are very active in running and biking. Ischiogluteal Bursitis refers to inflammation of a fluid-filled sack (bursa) that lies between the sit bone (ischium) and the butt's huge gluteus maximus.

Causes: All causes are biomechanical and may be exacerbated by: overuse (too much work with too little recovery); leg length discrepancy; tight glutes, hamstrings, hip flexor, and quadriceps; poor running mechanics; improper bike fit.

Treatment: Rest from all painful activities; cross-training if it produces no pain; cross-fiber massage to break up the scar tissue that makes the muscle unable to contract in that area, causing weakness, pain, and frequent reinjury, restrengthening the muscle; stretch associated muscles but avoid directly stretching the injured muscle before scar tissue is resolved, as the scar tightens with aggressive stretching. Physical therapists like Forster use ultrasound, electric stimulation, and icing to fight inflammation and swelling.

CHAPTER 23

BIONIC BODY PARTS

A resurfaced chrome hip that you can do an ultramarathon on—and set a PR on—is now available. But is there a hidden downside?

By December 2007, Scott Tinley's hip hurt so bad that the 49-year-old, two-time Hawaii Ironman champion walked with a noticeable limp, had a hard time bending over to tie his shoes, and hadn't run in five years.

The previous summer, after dragging her right leg sideways "like a crab" and having it repeatedly buckle beneath her at the world championships in Scotland, 40-year-old Robyn Benincasa got an X-ray and some bad news. "You've got end-stage osteoarthritis in your hip—no cartilage, bone on bone," the doctor told the adventure-racing superstar. "Unless you like running in extreme pain, your athletic career is over."

In January 2007, 51-year-old Beverly Hills trainer-to-the-stars Gary Kobat, a world-class age-group duathlete who's run 51 marathons, frantically tried massage, chiropractic, Rolfing, and body work to relieve the excruciating hip pain that had ended his running. "Your only option for a normal life is a total hip replacement," said a surgeon, a spinning-class client who offered to do it for free. But Kobat turned down the gift because it wouldn't leave him "normal" as he defined it. A replacement traditionally lasts only 10 years and is recommended for low-activity people over age 60. That's because it is not strong enough to handle athletic activity like long-distance running.

No more running. That thought is chilling to the millions who've made megamile fitness part of their lives and livelihoods over the last couple of decades.

"I thought: What if I'll never be what I was again?" said Benincasa, a former child gymnastics star and 1998 National Judo champion who'd run up to 70 miles per week

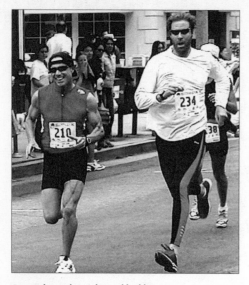

Gary Kobat with new hip and buddy Will Ferrell.

for two decades, completing hundreds of running and adventure races and nine Ironmans, including four World Championships in Hawaii.

"What if I can't do a 10k? What if I can't hike to Macchu Picchu? Oh my God!" she says she screamed to herself. "This is the end of my athletic career!"

But that was then. In March 2008, Benincasa ran a marathon, Kobat was doing four 1-mile track repeats at a 5:45 pace, and Tinley was surfing and planning to run by July. The reason: A new medical procedure and technology largely unknown in the U.S. that promised to rewrite the rules of athletic longevity: Hip resurfacing.

HOW IT WORKS

Hip resurfacing is a procedure that literally resurfaces the worn-out ball-and-socket structure of the hip with steel. The operation cuts a 6-inch gash in your buttock and installs a finely honed cobalt-chromium steel cap and cup that slide smoothly on one another, assisted by synovial fluid that leaks in from the surrounding bones.

In a damaged hip, the slick, lubricated hyaline cartilage that once coated the rounded head (the ball) of the femur (the thighbone) and the cuplike acetabulum (the socket) of the pelvis has deteriorated, leaving the bone-on-bone surfaces painfully grinding on each other and reducing range of motion.

"A 45-year-old person with bone on bone is miserable—he's disabled, but not ready to sit down yet," says Dr. John A. Rogerson, who has done about 300 of the surgeries at Meriter Hospital in Madison, Wisconsin, since the FDA approved it in May 2006, including Tinley's in December. He expects to do thousands more, because bad hips are showing up earlier today.

"In the past, arthritic hips didn't appear until later in life," he says. "But now there's a whole new demographic: those who have been extremely active through their 20s, 30s, and 40s."

Reasons for the deterioration can be osteoarthritis, caused in people 45 and up by a combination of overuse and imbalances; rheumatoid arthritis, an immune-system foul-up in which the body attacks its own cartilage; and trauma from a fall or accident, which may lead to avascular necrosis, the weakening and eventual collapse of bones due to lack of blood supply.

The latter happened to Floyd Landis, the drug-deposed ex-winner of the 2006 Tour de France. He had a hip-resurfacing operation in late 2006, and took 2nd place nine months later in the Leadville 100 mountain-bike race.

Hip resurfacing has been performed on 60,000 people over the last decade in Europe with no reported wear-related failures. Its apparent ability to restore hobbled athletes to their old selves is a big contrast to the clunkier total hip replacement, now annually done on over 200,000 Americans, most over age 60. A total hip replacement involves complete removal of damaged parts of the patient's hip joint and replacement with a prosthesis. The head of the femur is sawed off and replaced by a metal ball and arm held in place by a long spike hammered deep into the shaft of the femur. The surgeon then scoops out excess cartilage and bone from the socket part of the joint and fits a new socket. While pain-free mobility is restored, gait and skeletal stress is altered and vigorous activity, like running marathons, is not encouraged. Two years ago, California governor Arnold Schwarzenegger broke his artificial hip skiing.

Resurfacing, on the other hand, preserves virtually all of the femur, precisely shaving a few centimeters off the surface before capping. "It's a trickier, more difficult operation," says Dr. Rogerson,

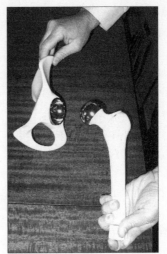
Resurfaced hip joint, exploded view.

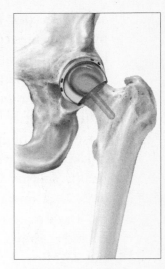
Completed hip resurfacing.

who like most uses the Birmingham Hip Resurfacing (BHR) technique and device pioneered and patented a decade ago by Dr. Derek McMinn in Birmingham, England. (BHR is now owned by Memphis-based Smith and Nephew. A similar device is made by Stryker, of Kalamazoo, Michigan.) The procedure takes 90 minutes or so, twice that needed for a hip replacement. The socket cupping is similar to that of a total hip replacement, although it uses more durable cobalt-chromium instead of plastic. The resurfaced femur head is much larger than a total hip's smaller-diameter total-hip hardware, and therefore less prone to dislocating.

Of course, the higher quality of life comes at a price—$30,000 or more in the U.S. for a hip resurfacing, roughly double that of a total hip replacement. Over-

RUN FOR LIFE

seas is cheaper: £11,995 in England (see mcminncentre.co.uk) and half that in India by McMinn-trained doctors. Until two years ago, Americans had to go overseas for the operation. Resurfacing, invented in the seventies, got a bad rap when the plastic parts of the early devices wore out quickly. The lingering apprehension about quality delayed U.S. approval, even after durable, all-metal parts arrived.

The big question: How fast can you get up and running after the operation? From the McMinn Centre Web site: "1 year after operation. At around 11 months, you may start jogging on a treadmill with good quality running shoes or trainers. Do this for a couple of months before you start running outdoors or participating in high-impact sporting activities like squash, cricket, football, etc."

To many, waiting a whole year to run after hip resurfacing seems too conservative. To Corey Foulk, the poster boy for this operation, even a month was too much.

THE PIED PIPER

Foulk, a 49-year-old Hawaii architect and lawyer who writes environmental impact statements for luxury resorts, earned his hip resurfacing with a megamile résumé that's off the charts. He has finished the UltraMan (a triple Ironman distance) 15 times. He's done 50 ultramarathons, 50-plus marathons, and has 41 Ironman finishes. He ran 40 miles in a typical week and totaled 66,560 lifetime miles.

"I never considered not doing this forever," Foulk said. But 9 years ago, he broke his hip in a bike accident. A few years later, the pain began. Like Landis, he had avascular necrosis—part of his hip was dying. "At the 2001 Ironman South Africa, I had a great bike," he said. "But I couldn't run a step."

His hip was a mess. X-rays showed pieces of bone all over the place. "If you were older, we'd do a hip replacement this week," the doctors said. "But you're too young and active. Wait 5 years for the technology to get better. Until then, take pain drugs."

So Foulk did—and kept doing Ultramans. He switched from running to deep-water running. He put in a wood floor, tried inversion therapy, crystal therapy, acupuncture, and took glucosamine, put lifts in his shoes to even out his leg length. And his hip got worse.

Finally, Foulk heard about hip resurfacing from Drew Dixon, a 50-something triathlete who'd had the operation done in Belgium and finished an Ironman 3 years later. Quickly, he settled on a McMinn-trained doctor in India who offered an $11,000 package deal that included a luxury hospital suite and a beachfront recuperation villa.

RUN FOR LIFE

The pampering worked wonders. Six days after the operation, to the horror of his doctor, Foulk ran a 5k on a treadmill. He ran a marathon on his 3-month anniversary, did Ironman Germany in month seven, and a 24-hour run soon after.

Since his operation on December 21, 2005, he's done five Ironmans and three Ultramans, finishing 11th out of 35 at the world championships. "All with a fake hip!" he chuckles. "I am bionic."

Being one of the first hardcore athletes in the U.S. to have the operation, Foulk wasn't sure what to expect. At his last race before flying to India, he said good-bye to the race director, competitors, and even the aid-station volunteers he'd seen over the years, thinking he might never see them again.

"But now I have a bar code and a warrantee," he says. "The doctors are worried that I'm pushing it, but the engineers tell me that it won't ever wear out."

Whole again, Foulk started spreading the word. By way of *Competitor* editor Bob Babbitt, he was connected to Tinley, Benincasa, Kobat, and even Landis, who switched to a hip resurfacing instead of a planned total hip.

Foulk turned a half-century in 2008. "The 50s are the gravy," he says. "You're still fit, you've made the money, got it all figured out. I got a second chance, and I'm not going to waste it."

LAB RATS ONCE AGAIN

Years and years of megamiles pound, tear, and pulverize the hidden structures that make us move with a fluid grace we only think about when it's gone. The baby boomers, the first overtrained generation, thought they were hammering the road to endless health, only to find themselves staring at an X-ray of a gimpy, arthritic joint better suited to a battered ex-NFL lineman.

"The crazy endurance stuff didn't happen until our generation," says Benincasa. "I always laughed at people who said 'Wait till you're 40 and all your joints are worn out.'"

The laughter stopped for a while. But it's back now every time she goes for a run—or sets off the metal detector at the airport.

"We knew we were lab rats, erring on the side of excessive miles," said Tinley, who guesses he's run, biked, and swam "to the moon and halfway back."

"I always knew I was doing too much. I always knew I could get by on two-thirds of the mileage I was doing." The warning signs were there. In 1997, when a lab test showed that he wasn't producing cortisol, a doctor told him he needed to take 2 years off. So he took off a month.

Although he was already surfing 11 weeks after the operation—against doctors' orders—Tinley was toeing the

line on takir
running," he said. "Not
And then, no 40 miles a we

He looked forward to a
present on his 50th birthday
2008. "I'll have a life back," he say

METAL, METAL, EVER
Metallic hips leak millions of micros

As hip resurfacing racks up thousands of
baby boomer athletes transformed back into ultramara
we should all know about: Pollution.

Internal pollution. A study in the 2007 issue of the *Lancet* medical journal
cobalt-chrome hip replacements and hip surfacings, implanted in 300,000 people in the last 10 years, spit off microscopic shards of metal and plastic that get into the bloodstream, the brain, and every cell. That's not good. Metals are known to produce complex biological actions with immunological, mutagenic, and toxic effects, which is why there are laws preventing exposure to them in industrial use. Still, the *Lancet* couldn't find a smoking gun of folks who'd died or were diseased from the cobalt chrome. Same with the March 2008 *Journal of Bone and Joint Surgery*, which found that the number of chromosomal aberrations in the metal-on-metal group was 31 times greater than in normal people. Thirty-one! It called that "statistically significant" — and added that "there was good evidence for an association between cobalt chrome-on-cobalt chrome and increased genotoxicity in patients. Metal ions in solution or in particulate form have been shown to cause delayed type IV T-cell hypersensitivity, dose-dependent cell necrosis and mutagenic changes." But the conclusion was the same: Yes, mutagenic changes are documented, but so what? Their implications are thus far unclear.

The *Lancet* concluded that the changes in patients' demographics and the materials used for the articulation will increasingly result in younger patients being exposed to higher amounts of metal ions and particles for extended periods. Since both particle-mediated and metal-related diseases could have long gestation periods, they may be the first people to exhibit signs of any ill effects.

Will you be running a sub-40 10k with a resurfaced hip at age 50, but be hammering the highway to Alzheimer's or cancer at 70? There is no answer to this question yet. Your best bet: Improve your form and posture now to reduce damage and avoid the issue altogether.

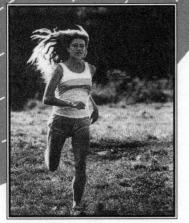

BOBBI GIBB

The First Woman To Run The Boston Marathon

When Roberta "Bobbi" Gibb ran the Boston marathon in 1966 at age 23, she not only became the first woman to start and complete the event, she also changed history. By shattering the stereotype that females couldn't run long distances, Gibb hoped to stir up change—and succeeded. Six years later, women were legalized at Boston; other marathons followed, as did the Olympics in 1984. That makes the Cambridge, Massachusetts–born daughter of an MIT professor a true hero of the women's rights movement.

Unfortunately, she's mostly an unsung hero.

Gibb's name is virtually unknown to runners and to women. Oprah Winfrey, that other famed marathoner, hasn't invited her on her show. Despite a *Sports Illustrated* article about Gibb and some TV appearances, her landmark achievement was soon forgotten by a short-attention-span media that didn't check the facts. That's why, when you ask most people today who was the first woman to run the Boston Marathon, 99% will say "Kathy Switzer," who read the SI article about Gibb and finished an hour behind her in the next year's race (1967). Switzer grabbed headlines when the race director unsuccessfully tried to toss her out. Over time, she proclaimed that *she* was the first woman to run Boston. Forty years later, even after Gibb has been officially feted several times by the Boston Marathon itself, inducted into its Hall of Fame, and run it on her 20th, 30th and 35th anniversaries, the misinformation persists. Most people today believe Switzer was the first female marathoner, and don't know Gibb.

So for the record, here's Bobbi Gibb's amazing story, told in a *Run for Life* interview conducted on January 22 and 23, 2008, when she was 65 and still happily running an hour a day. It's a story of a woman of intellect and purpose who simply loves to run and wanted to give women the opportunity to experience the same joy.

I was always running. When I was a toddler, my mother just couldn't keep me still. I was into everything. From the earliest times, from two or three, I can remember running under the chestnut tree, seeing the rays of sunlight come randomly through, how the world seemed beautiful, with all the patterns going by.

When we moved to Winchester, Massachusetts, when I was 10, all we did was run around. We didn't have a TV in those days; we'd play cowboys and Indians and horse. My mother basically threw us out of the house and said, go play! And we were out there, in December in the wind and the snow, through March. We climbed trees, played softball and capture the flag, and ran all over the neighborhood. When my cousins would chase after me, my uncle would say, "look at her—she floats when she runs." I'd run by myself along the river. When my best friend Debbie Usher's dad saw me down there, he used to say that I looked like a gazelle or a wild animal or something. I felt like I was a bird flying. I found in running a sense of peace and joy and love.

In high school I played field hockey, one of the few sports for girls. I'd run on my own up in the woods with the neighborhood dogs at the Winchester Fells reservation, a huge piece of deeply wooded Indian land about 5 miles across. It was beautiful up there. There were hemlock trees, and ledges, and streams and lakes. To me, it was like a holy place, sacred ground.

When I went to college at Tufts, I kept running. It was a very inner-directed thing—I felt close to the creative being of the universe or something. Eventually, I met a guy who ran cross-country, Will. The only way I got to see him was to run along after him. Pretty soon, I could keep up with him. And we went all over greater Boston together on foot.

Oh gosh, we could run an hour or more. One of the longest runs we took was from Boston to Blue Hill. He lived in Canton, and we ran down to Blue Hill, south of Boston. I'm sure we covered 7, 8, 9 miles. And then I used to run from my home in Winchester to the Museum School of Fine Arts in Boston—about 8 miles. I ran along the Mystic River, over the hill in Medford, and followed the Charles River down into Boston. I'd actually commute on foot; it would take me about an hour. I'd spend all day there. Sometimes I'd run back at night, or take the subway and bus back.

I was doing something that was waaay far outside the social norm for a woman. And it wasn't just the running. In those days, it wasn't very common for a girl to study physics, math, Spanish, and philosophy at the Tufts School of Special Studies, and sculpture at the museum.

But my family was determined to raise my brother and me equally. So within the family there wasn't gender discrimination. I'm very thankful to my parents for that. It wasn't until I got out in the real world—I was shocked (she laughs) to find out in those days that women were barred from the professions. In the sixties, it was very difficult to get into law school and medical school. As a women, you were expected to pretty much get married right out of college—if you were lucky enough to go to college. You might work as a secretary or a nurse or a telephone operator. But that was about it if you were a woman—unless you took a blue-collar job or worked on an assembly line.

Here I grew up in this highly intellectual environment, and suddenly I was faced with the horrible realization that it was stacked—you couldn't even get a credit card in your own name if you were a woman—you couldn't get a mortgage for a house. Really the only chance that women had of surviving pretty much was getting married. And the husband was expected to provide for the wife and the children. That was the deal.

I did get married. I actually married my track friend, Will. But it didn't last. That's how I got to California. But before that, in 1964, I first saw the Boston Marathon and truly fell in love.

TRAINING TO THE PACIFIC AND BACK

Although I grew up in the Boston area, I'd never heard of the marathon. When I was 21, Debbie's father told me about it, and I went out there with my dad to Wellesley (mile 13). We watched the runners go by. I instantly fell in love with it. It was just totally irrational. I fell in love because I recognized these runners felt the same thing that I felt when I ran—that bond with the earth, the unity of the physical and the spiritual, which gave me such a sense of peace and wholeness and health.

I knew I had to do it.

I didn't say, "Oh there are no women here; I must make a statement." I just saw these people running—and felt that's what I was supposed to do. I never questioned it.

I didn't tell my dad this. I kept it a secret, because I knew they'd think I was nuts. Only several friends knew.

I didn't know how to train. I was actually running in nurse's shoes. Of course, they didn't make women's running gear. I thought, "I'll just start running farther and farther." So that's what I did. I didn't know if I'd have a heart attack or if my body could do it. Twenty-six miles! So I'd just go out every single day. Some days I could run far, and some days I couldn't. But I just gradually built up.

Then in the summer of 1964, my parents were on sabbatical in England—which is how I got away with this:

I took the family Volkswagen van and Moot, my Malamute puppy, and started off on a spiritual journey across the country.

It wasn't that I was wild or anything. I wanted to see the country. People think I must have been a hippy or flower child, But it wasn't so. I never did drugs. I hate that, would have never put that stuff into my body. I don't even drink coffee.

Every day, I would run in a different place. I just loved the land. I was in love with the earth and this country, America. In the day, I'd run. At night, I'd camp. I was a good camper—been going to camp for many years. Knew how to take care of myself in the woods, how to build a lean-to. I had a sleeping roll, and every night I'd sleep out under the stars. I'd eat in cafes and truck stops and meet all kinds of interesting people.

I went out across Massachusetts across the Berkshires, then across New York, parts of Pennsylvania, West Virginia, then to Ohio and Indianapolis, where my aunt and uncle lived. In Kansas I met a woman farmer who had a paralyzed son. I stayed there a week or so painting fences. Back in Pittsburgh, my engine had seized up, and I had to put a new one in. So I had to earn some money by painting. Then I went on out across Nebraska and

Colorado, to Denver. I could run all day across the Plains. It blew my mind.

At night, I'd sleep out, and I'd hear the grass blowing in the wind and see the stars. To me, it was the most beautiful thing, so miraculous.

I stayed in Wyoming for a while. My old friend Debbie Usher was out there, married, with a kid, living in a trailer park. Then I went on across Utah into Nevada—never saw so many stars. I really got a sense of position in the universe, on this blue earth, and how beautiful it all is. It was like a spiritual revelation.

In California, I ran in the Sierras. I saw the Pacific Ocean for the first time as I crossed the Golden Gate Bridge. I plunged into the ocean at Stinson Beach with my puppy Mooty, camped out and made a campfire right there and slept in the sand. A bunch of kids with a guitar came over. We all sang songs. Then they curled up in their blankets and went to sleep around the fire, too.

The next day, I headed back across the country.

That's the way I trained for the Boston Marathon. I would see a mountain peak way off in the distance—a pale blue peak. And I'd spend all day getting to the top of that peak and back, maybe 30 or 40 miles at a stretch. I was in incredible shape—like a wild animal.

Actually, the VW van didn't make it back to Boston. Near the end of summer, driving back with three guys from NYU who answered an ad I ran, we had an accident—rolled down an embankment. I ended up selling the car for junk and taking the train with Moot. My parents were glad I was home safely. I have to give my father credit. He did not say one word about the microbus; he never said anything. He loved that bus; had it all fixed up with a camper and a table inside.

In September, I was back in Museum School full-time studying sculpture. I was going to run the marathon in April '65, but sprained both my ankles. So I had to wait a whole year, and during the year I kept training. In September '65 I went up to the Woodstock 100-miler horseback race; I ran 65 miles of that. And then I knew that I was ready for Boston.

So now my problem was that I had to hold my conditioning from September until the next April. Then Will turned up during Christmas vacation and asked me to marry him. It surprised me because we had never had a romantic relationship. It was a friendship. I said "sure." I went out to San Diego—he was in the navy. I stayed there and trained while he went back out to sea. The Vietnam War was raging.

THE SOCIAL STATEMENT

In February of 1966, I wrote for my application to run the Boston Marathon and got a letter back from the Boston Athletic Association. Will Cloney, the race director, said that women were not allowed to run the marathon, and furthermore, are physiologically not able to run it. In those days, the AAU didn't allow women to run more than 800 meters—half a mile. That was the longest women's sanctioned race. The Boston Marathon was a men's division event.

At that point, I could have said, "well, too bad, I guess I won't run."

But I said to myself, "All the more reason to run."

I realized right then that my run was going to be a social statement. Because it wasn't just that the guys at the marathon didn't think that women couldn't run—but that women thought they couldn't run marathons, either. Or course women didn't train to run long distances. If you were in sports, they told you that you couldn't run more than 800 meters because you might hurt yourself, you might die, you might hurt your reproductive organs. But having been outside the world of sports, I didn't know that. If I had been in sports, ironically, I never would have run the marathon.

It was at that point that I realized I was running for a lot more than just my own personal challenge. I was actually running to change the way people thought about women. I realized if I could overturn this prejudice about women, it would call into question every other prejudice about women. All those restrictions that said "you can't be a doctor, you can't be a lawyer, you have to be a secretary and a wife and mother." Being a wife and mother is wonderful, but what about all your other gifts? That really kind of irritated me as I began to see how restricted my life was going to be as a woman,

At first, I was really outraged. It didn't matter that I could run 30 miles at a stretch. It only mattered that "you're a woman, therefore you're not allowed to do this." And then I chuckled to myself. "Oh, I have a small way here, a little wedge. This'll really give people something to think about. This is going to change some attitudes." And I knew that once I did that, they'd change the rules. And that'll throw into question other misbeliefs. And it'll open up the question of what people were capable of—men, too. They were in these rigid roles, too.

So from San Diego, I took the Greyhound bus back to Boston. Three days curled up in a ball. I arrived at my parents' house the day before the race and broke the news to them. And my father thought I was nuts. He was really angry, convinced I was going to hurt myself. But I convinced my mother to drive me out to Hopkinton, the beginning of the race.

She dropped me there an hour before the race. Then she had to go do something with my dad—they had a sailboat race to go to. She didn't say anything when she left, but I remember the expression on her face. It was a look of concern, like "Will you be all right?" But it was also a look of pride, like, "I know you can do it."

She had been frustrated for her whole life. She's a very intelligent, gifted woman. She had not ever been able to do anything but be a housewife. So she understood when I said that this was going to open things up for women, that this was going to set women free. It'll help. It'll be like a wedge, a pivotal point.

So she understood. But she was also worried. She and I both knew that sometime when you do something so far outside the social norm that people can get angry and hostile. I also knew that I had to do it in a very upbeat way, that I couldn't make it as though it were a negative thing. I wanted to inspire people to run, for one thing, and inspire the officials to open it up to women without having to make it into a confrontational thing.

So now I was confronted with this double bind: "How can you prove that you can do something if you're not allowed to do it?"

In those days, the men started in a pen that was roped off. There's no way that I could get into the pen; they would see me, and see that I was a woman. There were between 400 and 450 men. Running wasn't at all the big thing it is now. The Boston Marathon was the only marathon I knew of. I kind of trotted around the downtown area to warm up. I was wearing my brother's Bermuda shorts. And I had a blue, hooded sweatshirt on to cover my hair, because I knew that if they saw me they'd throw me out. I thought maybe I'd be arrested. I knew it was important that I not be stopped. I had reddish-brownish blond hair pulled back in a ponytail.

So I was running around downtown trying to figure out how I was going to get into the race without being seen. There are people all along the sidewalks and police barricades. So I found some bushes in a little hollow as near to the beginning of the race as you could get. For the hour until race time, I went up behind some buildings, and I ran up and down 2 or 3 miles. I was still a little stiff from that 4 days in the bus. As the start time got close, I got back into my hiding place in the bushes.

Then the gun went off, I let about half the pack go by. Of course, the front-runners start really fast; I wanted to stay out of their way. The rest of the pack, of course, started very slowly. I was able to slip into the middle of the pack.

Very quickly, the guys around me realized that I was a woman, studying my anatomy from the rear. "Are you a girl?" they asked. I turned around and laughed. They asked me if I was going to go the whole way. "Yeah, if I can," I said. "I'm trying to." I said I was hot in my sweatshirt and wanted to take it off, but I was afraid to because if they saw I was a girl they'd throw me out. And the men said, "We won't let them throw you out. It's a free road."

The men were great. They loved the fact that I was running. It was not a male-versus-female thing. They were very protective and encouraging. I ran along with a group. I talked the whole way with Alton Chamberlain from Connecticut.

For most of the race I was on a sub-3-hour pace, Of course, the press saw that a women was running, that was a big story. They started phoning it on ahead. And soon my position was being broadcast on the radio, where I was: "There's a woman in the race!" When I got to Wellesley College, the women knew I was coming from listening to the radio and were waiting for me. Diana Chapman Walls, the president of Wellesley, later wrote an article about what it was like. When they saw me, they let out an enormous scream. They were crying, jumping in the air, laughing, and screaming. One women standing on the side with a bunch kids, she was yelling, "Ave Maria, Ave Maria ..."

It was a great thing—everybody cheering and screaming. I'd thought maybe they'll throw tomatoes or the police would arrest me and that the spectators might boo and hiss or the officials would throw me out. You never know how people are going to react; I was doing something that had never been done.

I ran on and on. I got to Heartbreak Hill. You know, I had been running up and down mountains out in California. But Heartbreak Hill! I thought I was at the top, but no. I ran a few hundred more yards, and then it started going up again. I thought, "surely this is the top," and then no, no. I kept going up. And finally reached the top. That wasn't so bad.

But coming down the other side, with all the descent, my legs started to bother me probably about a mile or two from the finish. Of course, I hadn't drunk any water or eaten anything the whole way. Because I thought if you drank water while exercising, you get cramps. That's what they told us in high school. The whole thing—no water, no electrolytes, no oranges. And my feet were bleeding with blisters; I was wearing new running shoes—boy's size-6 shoes I had bought in San Diego before I left on the bus. My first pair of running shoes. I hadn't broken them in. And I wasn't used to running on hard pavement like that; I'd done all of my running on dirt.

So a couple miles from the finish, my pace really dropped off. And I was just tiptoeing along, literally tiptoeing. I could see my time was really spinning out. And

RUN FOR LIFE

I was really disappointed; I felt like a total failure. And I wondered if anyone was going to be at the finish when I got there. But I still kept going because I knew that I had to finish—because there was a big weight of responsibility on me. If I failed to finish I was going to set women's running back 20, 30 years. They'd say, "See? This is why we don't let women run these long distances. Look what happened to her." So, I had to finish. And I had to finish well.

My time was spinning out. Finally, I got to Boylston Street. Lo and behold, the crowds were still there. The bleachers were filled, people were screaming, and the press trucks were rolling. As I ran down that last stretch, I picked up my pace a little. I finished in a time of 3 hours, 21 minutes, and 40 seconds.

That was ahead of about two-thirds of the pack. Even though I thought it was not one of my better runs, it turned out to be pretty good. And the governor of Massachusetts came down—he heard I was running. He also lived in Winchester, my hometown—Governor Volpe. He came down and shook my hand.

When I got home, the entire street was wall-to-wall lined with cars. I thought somebody was having a party until I realized that the entire press was at my house. Asking my parents questions about their daughter.

It was front-page headlines, and it went all over the world by wire. I mean, my parents' friends from Malaysia sent them articles on this. It was all over Japan. Of course, the Japanese had finished 1-2-3-4. It was in all the Japanese papers.

It was unbelievable that a woman had run a marathon. Even after I ran it, some people didn't believe it. That's how deeply ingrained the prejudice was. But hundreds of thousands of people saw that a woman could run a marathon.

Nobody tried to stop me. Everybody was friendly and happy and upbeat. It was very positive. Because I think part of it was, when I run it's a way of expressing my love of life and love of people. And I think that kind of came across that I was a loving and positive person and it was a neat thing. I found running so healing, mentally and spiritually and emotionally healing, that I felt if everybody could run

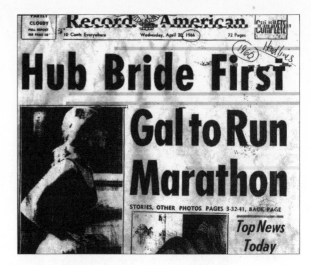

and could feel like this and could heal themselves with it this way—even if they are not doing top times—just getting out and breathing the air and setting one foot out after the other on the earth; it's so basic, it's so fundamental. I just wanted to inspire people to find in running the same thing that I did.

In fact, women would call me up after the race and say (in a high-pitched voice), "Oh, I just ran around the block for the first time. I'm so proud of myself." It's like, for women being able to run from Point X to Point Y was the first step in their sense of autonomy.

I was on To Tell the Truth. I went down to New York City; there were three of us sitting there, and the panel had to guess which one was the real woman who ran the Boston Marathon. And I won something like $65, which would be like $650 now. But I gave it to the Tufts Medical Center as a donation. Because in those days if you wanted to retain an amateur status you couldn't take any money. So I was thinking, maybe someday I'll run the Olympic marathon, someday I'll be in the Olympics, and I don't want to ruin my potential amateur status by taking any money whatsoever.

Of course, Sports Illustrated ran an article on me. And then, there was an article in the Record American newspaper that said ROBERTA GETS OFFICIAL SUPPORT. The April 21st issue. In there was a spokesperson from the Amateur Athletics Association, which was going to push for a rule change to allow women to run marathons. So that was exactly what I wanted! I knew that would happen once that they knew that a woman could run, and run well. So they on their own initiative were going to allow women to run. And that was in '66.

Another big article was entitled, GAME GIRL IN MAN'S GAME. It called my run a "feat."

That feat really stunned the world. People don't really understand it now—it was just as though you'd flown to the moon or something. It was so unbelievable that a woman could run the Boston Marathon. It didn't fit into people's stereotypes. A woman baked cookies; she didn't run marathons.

OUTRUNNING UNBELIEVERS AT HOME

When I got back to San Diego, I still ran into unbelievers. I had a friend named Bill Gookin, who was part of San Diego Track and Field. I had met him running around Balboa Park. In fact, if you read Hal Higdon's book on the Boston Marathon, published around 1996, you'll see one of Bill's anecdotes about meetings with me. Anyway, his brother Ed still couldn't believe a woman could run a marathon. So Bill and a couple of his buddies and Ed invited me to go for a little run from Del Mar out to Black Mountain. In those days, it was all open pastures, sagebrush, wild lilacs, dirt roads, and cattle grazing. We started out from Del Mar; they went on ahead. After half an hour, I caught up with them. Then we started to climb up the mountain. Bill and I went scampering up the mountain. Climbing boulder to boulder, looking out for rattlesnakes—you had to be careful then—we got to the top, looking back at the Pacific, shimmering in the sun, so peaceful. It took over an hour, closer to an hour and a half, to get to the top.

Then Bill and I came back down. We passed Ed and his friends, still struggling to get up the mountain, and Bill and I ran all the way back to Del Mar. We were waiting for them, cooling our heels when they got back. Bill still calls

that the day Ed became a believer. "Oh man, she ran 20 miles to the top of Black Mountain and back. And she did it a lot faster than I did," Ed said, and he became one of my staunchest supporters. Bill and I have stayed friends to this day.

People had to see it to believe it. Remember, only 100,000 people actually saw the marathon. Women wanted to believe it, but even they couldn't. Remember, it wasn't like there were thousands of women runners out there, clamoring to run marathons, and the mean, bad old men weren't allowing them to run. Lot of times, I tell women this and they don't want to hear it. Women coaches wouldn't let their girls run more than 800 meters. It wasn't like women knew they were being repressed. They didn't know they could do this, either. So when I did it, it was like a bolt of lightning—an enlightenment. "Wow, I didn't know we could do this! We can do this!" they said. And that really triggered women starting to get out there and run.

That's exactly what I hoped would happen. There is such a thing as quietly leading by example. Not trying to force people to do anything. Not selling a product. Just revealing the truth. Revealing that the truth really has an effect on changing how people think. And once you do it, then the world is open, because people's false beliefs keep them locked into their old patterns.

NOT ALONE IN 1967 AND 1968

I still had to finish my undergraduate degree. In fall of 1966, I came back and enrolled in the University of California at La Jolla, now UC San Diego. It was just opening. I was in the second graduating class. I loved biology. A number of my friends back in Boston were at Harvard Medical School, and I liked the idea of going into medicine. I took pre-med courses with a major in philosophy and minor in math, figuring I'd go on and be a doctor. It was a really tough course. We probably had more Nobel Laureates here per student than anywhere—Linus Pauling, Harold Urey, Maria Goeppert Mayer, the physicist. I found a place where I could flourish. I painted a mural on a 300-foot water tower here. People loved it.

RUN FOR LIFE

On this campus, and I think California in general, I always get the feeling that people not only accept you for who you are, but they love it when you do things that express who you are. You say, "Oh, I want to make a film." They go, "Great! Make a film." You say, "I want to write." They go, "Great, write a book." There's no sense of, "you can't do it." It's a can-do, upbeat feeling.

I did very well in school. But I also kept running. I couldn't train the way I did before, but I still ran. I'd run on the beach.

So the next year, 1967, I went back to run the marathon again for two reasons: One, I wanted that experience again. And two, there were still people who couldn't believe that a woman could do it. I thought I'm gonna go back and run this thing however many times it takes until everybody admits, knows, and realizes that a woman can run.

So in 1967, the press knew I was coming. They were calling my parents for days ahead of the race. "Is she coming, when is she coming?" This time I flew back, but I ended up getting the flu. So there was this period of time when I didn't know if I was going to run or not. The press would call the house, and my mom would say, "She's sick, she doesn't know if she is going to run . . ."

Finally, I realized that I had to run whether I was sick or not. I had to do it, because there were still a lot of Doubting Thomases out there—like Ed. So my mom drove me out to Hopkinton again. This time, I didn't have to hide in the bushes. I stood outside the pen, out of the way of the lead runners. I waited, the gun went off, I slipped into the middle of the pack. Again, I didn't want to interfere with the men, I wanted to run with them, the sense of camaraderie. Again the importance was to demonstrate that a woman could run the marathon and run it well. And until I did this, all the petitioning in the world wasn't going to change the rules. On the other hand, you could yell and scream and say it was unfair, but the fact of the matter is that there weren't any women marathoners. It wasn't like women were saying, "we want to do the marathon."

But there was another women there when I started, and I didn't know it until that night.

That was one of several differences about that year.

One was that the men were not friendly anymore. I couldn't figure it out. One man tried to push me off the course.... Now, the spectators were still cheering. When I went by Wellesley, the women screamed and yelled. And the press was following me, taking notes, asking if I was running the whole race. I'd answer "yes indeed"—even though at one point in the race, I couldn't breathe, my lungs were so congested. I actually laid down on somebody's lawn for about 10 minutes. The press found out, called my father on the phone, and were about to call the ambulance when suddenly, whatever it was, the spasm released, and I sprung up off the lawn to their astonishment and ran off.

Then I ran all the way. That year, it was rainy and cool. A spectator near the end ran alongside of me with an umbrella. A photo of that was in one of the papers later. So the crowd was very supportive. Then I got all the way to Boston, and the racers were very antagonistic. I couldn't figure out what the difference was; they'd been so supportive the year before. I got to Boston and there were half a dozen men standing with arms linked on the finish line; they wouldn't get me go across the finish line.

I said, "What on earth is going on?"

I just went around them and crossed the line. In 3:27:17—which included the ten minutes lying on that lawn, and waiting at the start until half the pack left.

When I got home and read the evening paper, I realized what happened at the finish line: They mistook me for another woman who also did the race. There were pictures in the paper of Jock Semple, one of the race directors, trying to rip off her number. She was dressed in a sweatshirt. I guess there were 3 or 4 men around her who were blocking Jock from getting her number. There were pictures of me—that year I was wearing black leotards and a paisley-print blouse—and there were pictures of her. And the headline read, BOUNCING BABES RUN MARATHON.

Well, it turned out that this girl Kathy Switzer, who finished an hour behind me in 4:20, had gotten a number illegally. And it enraged the race officials. I didn't have a number. I had written the organization the first year asking for one, and didn't even ask the second year.

The marathon was a men's division event. And no woman could run a men's event any more than a man could run in a women's division event. The reason that the men had been so unfriendly is that if an unsanctioned runner runs in the race, it can lose its accreditation. So Kathy put them at risk. Jock Semple claimed it was subterfuge—that she'd tricked them into giving her a number. To get one, I'd have had to lie on the application form about my name or use another name. Kathy just used her initials, K V Switzer, so they didn't know. She also had to falsify her medical records.

I wouldn't do that. Besides, what's the point? All Kathy did was enrage the officials and make them say, "If this is what women's participation means, we don't want it." After this, all consideration of opening the marathon that had begun the year before closed down completely.

Kathy set the cause back about five years. She made the officials dig in their heels. Now, they were never going to open it if they could help it.

It was not until 1972 that the AAU rules changes and marathon had an official women's division race. In fact Nina Kuscsik, who had already run it three times by then, was the first official women's winner that year (in 3:10:26) and the first official women's marathon finisher anywhere. There has been a lot of disinformation in the press about who was the first official finisher. She was.

The important point that has been lost here is not that I could get an illegal number, but that a woman could run, and run well. The next thing that had to happen is that women had to get inspired to take up long-distance training. Until there was a critical mass of well-trained women running marathons ...

I never saw Kathy in the race. We've since met. I don't know whether to get into this or not. I didn't run into her again until the late seventies, claiming to be the first woman to run the Boston Marathon. I usually don't talk about it—A. Because it's so painful for me, and B. Because I don't want to sound...

A lot of people still think that she was the first to run Boston because she is still saying that. I will talk about that later.

I actually ran again the next year, '68. I went back to the University of California. I had my final math exams. I was really studying hard. I'd gone from art school to abstract algebra and calculus. When I came back and ran the 1968 Boston, I had not trained. I was occasionally running on the beach.

I didn't know how I'd be received. The situation the previous year was so hostile, so I was almost hiding shyly before the race. But this time, the men were all funny and cheery, just like the crowd. It was like a cloud had gone over the race the year before, and now it had lifted. Jock Semple even said he didn't mind if women ran, "if they were well-trained—like the Gibb girl." They were angry; felt Kathy had cheated and I hadn't. I hadn't jeopardized their accreditation. So they were fine with my running.

Of course, my goal as always was to inspire people—and sure enough, that year there were reputedly five women running, including me. I didn't see any of them, but I saw some photographs—Marjorie Fish and Elaine Pederson, and two others who it's not clear finished the entire race. Again, I finished first of the women among the unofficial women's division, in 3:30.

In 1969, I decided not to go back to Boston. I had to take care of business. I was graduating from the UC and applying to medical schools. I was taking a real hard biochemistry course and setting up medical-school appointments and interviews.

Besides, I thought I had made my point. I had done what I set out to do. I had demonstrated three times that a woman could run and run well. And now it was up to the officials to change the rules.

I was so happy when women were legalized at Boston in 1972.

[In the seventies, Gibb divorced, remarried, had a child, was rejected from medical school, and began night law school. All the while, she kept running an hour or more a day, often running figure-8s in an open field around her stroller-bound son.]

THE STOLEN LEGACY

Now we can talk about Switzer.

The spring of 1979, when my son was 3, I went down to my cousin's in Chapel Hill, North Carolina. He was a professor at UNC. There was a big running community there. It was wonderful—people to run with. I'd never had that before. That spring, we were watching the Boston Marathon on TV, and the announcer came on and said, "In a moment, we'll have a little piece about the first woman to run the Boston Marathon. And my cousin said, "oh great, you're going to be on TV." I said, "Oh, wow, that's neat."

And the next thing you know, Kathy Switzer is coming on the TV. "Here's the first woman to run the Boston Marathon," they announce. "Oh, hi—hi," she says. And she's got all these pictures and stories about Jock Semple trying to get off her illegal number and everything.

We were outraged. We were stunned. "What is this?" we screamed. We started writing letters to the TV station, calling them. Turns out Kathy was a public relations person, she studied PR. And she's promoting herself as the first woman to run the Boston Marathon!

It was all over the place: in magazines, in books, on TV. And she was a sports announcer, so she was part of the press—and she could say, "On yeah, I'm the first woman to run the Boston Marathon." I didn't have any access to the press, and none of my friends did. Every year, it became a nightmare. This lie!

We'd write, we'd call. Finally, some people in the press picked up the story. "Hey, wait a minute, there's this Gibb girl, and she really did run the year before." And I sent 'em all the photographs and the headlines—"Hub Bride, First Girl to Run Boston ..." and all this. Then they started to correct themselves and say, "Kathy was actually the second woman, there was this other woman ..." But still, 99% of the promotional activity was Switzer saying she was the first woman to run the Boston Marathon. And then, if you asked her directly, she'd say, "Oh no, Bobbi ran the

year before me." But then she'd go on TV and be introduced as the first woman to run the Boston Marathon.

In the early 80s, there was an article in Ms. magazine about Kathy being the first woman, and I wrote a letter to them. Marlene Simmons, the author, called me. I said, "Marlene, didn't you know?" She said. "Yes, I knew you were the first, but they asked me to ignore that."

I said, "That's outrageous!"

She said, "I'm going to make it up to you. I'm going to write an article about the real story." And she did—and it all started coming out, all these articles: "Now the real story can be told, the real first woman to run the Boston Marathon," and all this. I started to get a little better recognition.

Then, on the 20th anniversary of my run, in 1986, I ran the Boston Marathon again in support of world peace. I don't remember what my time was. It wasn't very good because I had torn my hamstring a couple weeks before the race while carrying my kid up the stairs piggyback. There was a little window there where people saw the truth.

I couldn't devote too much effort to this, as I was basically trying to earn a living and raise my kid. I'd gotten divorced from his father and started practicing law part-time. I moved back to San Diego in the early nineties when my son went to UCSD.

In 1996, the 30th anniversary of my first run, and the 100th anniversary of the Boston Marathon, the Boston Athletic Association gave Sarah Mae Berman, who won Boston in '69, '70, and '71, and me each a medal, officially recognizing our wins during what they called "the pre-sanctioned era." I thought that made it pretty clear to everyone that I was the first woman to run the Boston Marathon.

SWEEPING THE COURSE IN 2001

In 2001, I ran Boston again to raise money for research on Lou Gehrig's Disease—ALS. My running now is for charity—Amyotrophic Lateral Sclerosis, children with cancer, and helping shelters for women and children and families in distress. My best friend, the coproducer on the Amony Lovins film, had come down with ALS.

Unfortunately, I came down with bronchitis a week before the 2001 race, and I had to go on all these TV shows and do promotional activities for ALS. But there was no way I couldn't run. I'd been on TV and everyone was expecting me to run.

I ran it with Ed Rice, a writer who had written some really nice articles about me and was also enraged about the Switzer thing. I was really slow. By the time we got to Wellesley, we were going from tree to tree—we'd sight a tree up 100 yards, and run to it, then pick another tree, or a signpost, and run to that. I was running so slowly that he could have walked beside me. But he is a true gentleman— I will always love him for this—instead of walking beside me, he jogged. It was so sweet. I went so slowly that he was freezing. I think we got to the top of Heartbreak Hill, about five miles from Boston, and I really couldn't breathe. I said, "Ed, you go on, you're freezing—you go on to Boston. You get your time. I'm going to go to the medical bus."

So he went on ahead and I got on the bus. We were picking up straggling runners, taking them back to Boston. The driver was driving back out to Wellesley; we picked up race dropouts and water station workers. We came back on the same route, stopped at the exact same point where I got on the bus, somewhere at the top of Heartbreak 40 minutes earlier. I was feeling better. So I said, "Stop the bus. I want to finish the race."

When I got out, this woman, Rebecca Wolf, jumped off the bus behind me. She was dressed in jeans and running shoes. She'd been manning a water station. She surmised my condition and realized that I was going to need a witness—and some help. She ran to Boston with me.

It was cold, the wind blowing. We were running in and out of people on the sidewalk—you know, the race was pretty much over—we were running up and down the curb, by all the bars, where people were drinking. We got all the way to Boston. We turned on to Boylston Street, where 35 years earlier I'd been the first woman and the grandstands were full, and the crowds were cheering, and it was front-page headlines. This year, there were no crowds, everybody was gone, 6 hours had elapsed. The clock that was timing the race was dark, it was off. We were over six

hours. Nobody was there. There were paper cups all over the street, and trash.

And just as we rounded the corner, two big, enormous street sweepers started up, and came down the street beside us. It cracked me up. I just rolled over laughing. "This is so hysterical. What a fitting end. The first shall be last and the last shall be first."

And we cracked up as these two street sweepers came down the street along beside us as we crossed the non-existent finish line together. We straggled into the very end of the awards ceremony. (laughs)

But at least I finished the race, by George. And the group I was running with raised over $100,000 for ALS.

After 2001, and being officially recognized in 1996, I figured it was hard for Kathy to go around making her false claim anymore. But then she started going around saying she was the "First OFFICIAL woman" to run the Boston Marathon, which she wasn't. But by saying so, she could still obscure the fact that I'd run the year before and its importance. She could always say, "what's really important is that I was official, and I had a number, and Bobbi Gibb's run didn't count because she didn't have a number."

What hogwash. I didn't count because I didn't have an illegal number, like hers? This is some sort of Orwellian doublethink.

I demonstrated three times that women could do this. Thirty years later, I was officially recognized and given a medal, with my name officially inscribed on the marathon memorial along with the others. And yet still. . . .

You go to her website. "The official website of the first official woman entrant to run Boston." It's all over. It's on Oprah Winfrey, on ESPN . . ."The woman who will always be known for breaking the gender barrier at Boston, the great Katherine. . . ."

People don't know who to believe. I don't know what to do. I'd like to write a book about it.

On the other hand, fame isn't all that great. I try not to tell writers where I live; I leave it at San Diego. After one article, it got to where I couldn't even run on the beach.

RUN FOR LIFE

People would recognize me, follow me, and stuff. It was a little mess.

FOREVER YOUNG

I feel about 39 and holding—like I'm just starting my life. About ten years ago I finally figured out what I ought to be doing with the rest of my life. I stopped practicing law about 10, 15 years ago to sculpt part-time. Now I've been writing philosophy and a lot of science.

Spent last seven years studying ALS and writing papers. For a living, I'm a professional sculptor, and I do commissioned bronzed portraits for people—and figures of athletes. In fact, there are four of my bronze pieces in the National Art Museum of Sport, in Indianapolis—marathoners, actually. Just generic runners. A man and woman finishing with arms up in the air.

I'm studying, writing, questioning. I'm doing what I want to do when I grow up.

I wake up, I turn on the computer and work on the ALS research. I work on my philosophy book, about the extraordinary miracle of every minute, every molecule, a tree, a piece of dust, sand on the beach, yet we take it all for granted. I've been studying science and philosophy for 10 years, and I've written a lot of books. I haven't published anything. You can always do that after I'm dead. The main thing is to write it down now.

I'm very healthy. I don't belong to a gym—I like to be outside. Running all those years in the sun with no protection did not help my skin. But my hair didn't turn gray. It's good genes. My father is 91 years old, almost 92.

I carry groceries—that's my upper body workout. I don't eat red meat, fat, coffee, alcohol, cigarettes, marijuana, drugs, any of that crap. I drink herb tea. A typical meal: rice, tofu, and salad. I'll have lentil soup, occasional fish or turkey. Nuts I love—almond, pecans, walnuts. Chocolate is the worst thing I do.

I run on the beach, on the hills, on campus, up in Torrey Pines Park, down in Balboa Park, whatever. I just run for an hour, however many miles I do. I don't really time the miles. I love the celebration of running, but I'm not competitive. Besides Boston, I've only run three other marathons—New York, Foxboro, and San Diego—and the Bonne Bell 10k. I'm sure I used to probably run 9, 10 miles an hour, and probably half that now. But it still feels the same, you know?

I go out, and I feel good, and I work up a sweat, and I get on the sand. Suddenly I feel this energy inside of me, and I feel the same joy I did when I was a kid. And the sun is sparkling on the water, and I pick up my pace. And I go splashing along the surf, and the rainbows appear through the droplets of the water. And I just feel happy, and warm, and that the world is really beautiful. And that the ordinary is truly extraordinary.

RUN LIKE A KENYAN

Say "Kenyan" and every athlete in the world thinks the same thing: *Great runners.*

It's not a recent phenomenon. I remember watching Kip Keino on TV winning the 1500 meters at the Mexico City Olympics in 1968, beating the great American miler Jim Ryun. Thirty-six years later, I became a 12-year-old again for a few minutes when I got to meet Keino himself in his homeland at the Fila Discovery Races, sort of an unofficial mini-Olympics for grade-school kids in the heart of Kenya's western highlands running mecca. By now, of course, the Kenyans were known as the world's greatest marathoners, and one by one, I got to meet them, break bread with their coach, even run with them. It was a fantastic opportunity: One week to examine this unique running culture close-up. Could I discover some of their secrets?

CHAPTER 24

THEY'VE BEEN TO THE MOUNTAINTOP

Kenyans were already great runners.
Then an Italian remade them into great marathoners.

They keep coming. Old women in vibrant tribal caftans and warm sweaters, teens in school-uniform dresses, young, freshly circumcised warriors carrying spears. Like an ebony river defying gravity, thousands of them flow uphill—endlessly, inexorably, slowly. They're all on foot; some have plodded as much as 20 miles along the single dirt road that arcs over the verdant hillsides that reach to the horizon, drawn onward, upward by word of an event occurring on a desolate mountaintop nearly 10,000 feet high. Once up there at last, they breathe deep of the thin air and gape at the sight of the Malthusian multitudes who preceded them, a visage they might have seen before only on TV—that is, if anyone had actually possessed one or the electricity to run it. There's no room to sit down, but somehow they do sit, packed so tightly that the mountain seems no longer made of plants and rock and dirt, but of silhouetted skulls, glinting like mahogany marbles in the early afternoon sunlight. Many don't understand the forces that compelled them to leave their scrawny cows and goats and fields untended for a day to trek here, to this 2-mile-high village in the middle of nowhere, Kapsait, population 50, home of a butcher shop, a tearoom, and a one-room store mainly selling maize, salt, Pepsi, and farm implements. But they know that this is one of the biggest things to ever happen in this remote part of Kenya. They know it's important to them as a people, something that might even change all their lives for the better, although they really don't know how.

Facing the masses, looking up from a natural amphitheater pit on a makeshift dais constructed that morning, sit business-suit-clad tribal administrators and others important enough to merit shade and serenade. Following the national anthem, successive groups of dancers, some clad all in pink, some in purple, some in blue, take turns performing. They sing in Swahili, the lingua franca of East Africa, but a Western name abruptly jumps out of their mouths again and again.

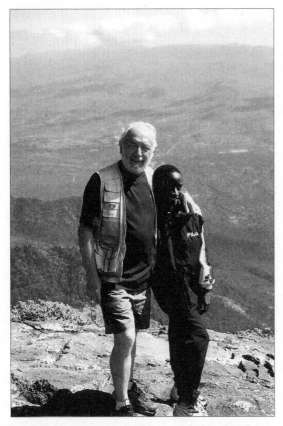

Rosa and star student Margaret Okayo overlooking the Rift Valley.

"Dr. Rosa," later says a featured speaker, "thank you for all you've done for Kenya. Your investment is working. Please, a few words."

Sixty-one-year-old Gabriele Rosa stands. His balding, pink head, fringed in snowy white hair and beard, is a stark contrast to the 5,000 jet-black faces trained on him. The sheer massiveness of the outpouring has surprised him. There's a glint in his eye; for a stoic man, rather reserved for an Italian, it may be as close as he'll come to a tear. He adjusts his matching black sash and woven beanie— kooky court-jester-ish affairs, festooned with dangling white, red, and yellow yarn balls whose meaning is unknown to the Kenyan dignitaries who also wear them, other than that it signifies a momentous occasion—and goes to the microphone. The crowd is hushed.

"This is the greatest moment of my life," Rosa says in Italian-accented English, a language that Kenyans of all ethnicities have studied as a second tongue from the time of the British colonial era. "My dream, ten years in the making, is now real. The only thing that will be greater is if we win both marathon gold medals at the Olympics. Get that, and I can die happy." The crowd erupts in joyous adulation.

Rosa is a medical doctor-turned-sports physiologist-turned-coach who adopted a country, and found that it is adopting him. The ceremony in Kapsait in January 2004 was the grand opening of a new and improved version of a unique year-round, live-in training camp for Kenyan runners that he founded nearly a decade before. Kapsait and four similar high-altitude camps like it that he runs in Kenya's western highlands, all of them funded by sportswear and shoe maker Fila, have one purpose: train the Kenyans, arguably already the greatest runners in history, to win every single marathon on Earth.

The plan is working. In the previous two years, Kenyans coached by Rosa won 54 major marathons around the world, far more than any other nationality. His athletes—half of the Kenyan marathoners competing internationally—are the cream of the crop: 2003 Boston Marathon winners Robert Cheriot and Margaret Okayo (who also won in 2001); Martin Lel, who, with Okayo, led a sweep of the top three male and female spots at the 2003 New York City Marathon; Paul Tergat, who set a new world record of 2:04:55 at the 2003 Berlin Marathon, and second all-time-fastest Sammy Korir, who came in one second behind in the same race. At second-tier events, like the 2003 Los Angeles Marathon, 2nd-string Kenyans won the first 13 male finishing places. All told, Kenyan men won Boston 12 of the previous 13 times, New York 5 of the 7, Berlin 7 of the last 9, and Amsterdam 6 of the last 9. Aside from a few Moroccans and Ethiopians, the Kenyans rule. Go to any marathon around the world offering prize money—Chicago, the Rock 'n' Roll

Marathon in San Diego, the Country Music Marathon in Nashville, the Ximen Marathon in China—and Kenyans will be there. The only blight on their record is that they have never won a gold medal in the Olympic Marathon.

THE BEGINNING

Kenyans can't forget Mexico City. It changed them into runners.

In a much-anticipated metric-mile face-off, Kenya's Kip Keino, one of the first great African distance runners, won gold in the 1500 meters over U.S. legend Jim Ryun at the 1968 Olympics. He took silver the next day in the 5000, then, 4 years later, won silver and gold, respectively in the 1500 and the 3000 steeplechase at the 1972 Munich Games. Spurred by his example, running in Kenya boomed. In seven Olympics through Sydney 2000 (Kenya boycotted the '76 Montreal and '80 Moscow games), the country raked in more medals than any other country—40, including 14 gold—in track events ranging from the 800 to the 10,000 meters.

Kenyans were in such demand at U.S. universities that many non-running Kenyans scammed their way into track scholarships. But the marathon wasn't on the radar screen yet, and results were meager: just three Olympic marathon medals and no gold. Until 1987, when Douglas Wakiihuri won the marathon at the World Championships and Ibrahim Hussein won at New York, no Kenyan had ever won a major international marathon. Their impact on Kenyans was minimized, however, because each lived abroad at the time. Kenya did not get serious about the marathon until an Italian literally brought it to them.

Rosa had cut his sports-medicine teeth working with pro basketball players, bike racers, swimmers, and an Olympic judo champion. In 1981, he was introduced to the running world by Italian marathoner Gianni Poli, who became a guinea pig for Rosa's then-radical theory: To get faster, you need huge miles—up to 150 a week—and you must train together with a large group of similar-ability athletes.

Quickly, the talented Poli outran his partners. He then outran a team of relay runners. In the end, Rosa had him running alongside bicyclists. It paid off. In 1986, Poli won the New York City Marathon. And Rosa was suddenly recognized as a coaching genius.

Rosa's Kenya connection began in late 1990, when Moses Tanui, a Kenyan who finished 8th in the 10,000 meters at the 1988 Seoul Olympics, walked through the door of Rosa's Marathon Medical Center clinic in Brescia, Italy, complaining of knee pain. Eight months later, when Tanui won the 10k gold medal at the world championships in Tokyo, his coach made a proposition: Run marathons.

"Not only is there a lot more prize money in marathons than in track events," Rosa told Tanui, "but you have the physical and psychological characteristics necessary to become a great marathoner."

"Tanui displayed a unique ability to recover and thrive with hard training," Rosa told me. "That indicated he had better running 'economy'—sort of like 'gas mileage' for humans—than Europeans and other Africans I'd seen."

Tanui liked what he heard. "There are thousands more just like me back home in my tribe," he responded. "They just need someone like you to train them."

A lot of Kenyans had been saying that for years. But Rosa was the first one to act. At the end of 1991, he and Tanui flew to Nairobi, then drove 311 kilometers northwest on the Trans-Africa Highway. They crossed the Rift Valley, a gash 30 miles wide and 2,000 feet deep that runs north-south the length of Kenya. Now in the country's far west, they arrived at Tanui's hometown and began meeting runners training in the green highlands that range in elevation from 6,000 to 10,000 feet. What Rosa saw made him feel like he'd won the lottery.

MORE THAN GENETICS

The Rift Valley Province is Kenya's largest. Tanui grew up here in a tiny farming village of mud huts called Sugoi, located 20 miles from the bustling city of Eldoret, 50,000 strong. Like Keino, the legendary "Running Policeman" who grew up in the famous Nandi tea fields just outside of town, Tanui is a member of the Nandi tribe, one of seven subgroups of a larger cultural-linguistic umbrella tribe called the Kalenjin. In the last couple decades, the Kalenjin have earned a nickname that strikes fear into runners everywhere: "The Running Tribe."

The name is well earned. Although they make up only 10% of Kenya's population, the Kalengin today account for 75% of its best runners. "In fact, 50 percent of the best runners in the world today are Kalenjin—amazing since there are only 3 million of them," says John Manners, a Swahili-speaking runner and author who spent four years with the Peace Corps in the Rift Valley and is known as the leading American authority on the Kenyan running scene. "And it's not just running. The Kalenjin have always been among Kenya's best in soccer and cricket, the two most popular sports."

What makes the Kalenjin such great athletes? Besides the genetics that Tanui had so impressed Rosa with, the conditions for athletic prowess seemed textbook: Training and living at elevations between 6,000 to 10,000 feet, which develops a keen oxygen-processing lung capacity; ideal weather (hot, sunny days, low humidity, and chilly nights) for hard workouts and sound sleep; rich farmland and widespread land ownership promote a good diet; low income ($1,200 annual per capita) and lack of career opportunity beyond subsistence farming, which keep motivation high, precludes the purchase of PlayStations and bikes, and keeps everybody walking. Driving into Eldoret, I saw thousands walking along the highway. Kalenjin children often go barefoot into the teenage years, building foot strength and "proprioception"—muscular feel and coordination key to fast running.

Of course, this doesn't explain why the Kalengin make better runners than Peruvians and Nepalese living in similar high-altitude and socioeconomic conditions. One theory is "body type": "They run efficiently and smoothly because they are very light, skinny, not too tall, not too short," said Rosa. "We don't know exactly why they are more economical—they just are."

A Danish study provided a clue, finding that Kalenjin had similar aerobic capacity to Danes, but narrower, lighter appendages. So, compared to Kenyans, Danes (and other nationalities) are running with ankle weights.

John Manners likes the "cattle rustling" theory. Kalenjin were "the foremost practitioners of cattle theft," he says, for centuries trekking over 100 miles to capture and drive livestock home before the former owners could catch up. "The fast raider would accumulate lots of cattle, allowing him to buy more wives and make more children," Manners guesses that "this reproductive advantage might cause a significant shift in a group's genetic makeup over the course of a few centuries."

Some suggest that the ritual of circumcision, a rite of manhood and prerequisite of marriage performed on 13- to 15-year-olds during Christmas vacation without anesthetic, gives the Kalenjin a high pain threshold that allows them to tolerate hard training better. A Kalenjin runner told Toby Tanser, author of *Train Hard, Win Easy: The Kenyan Way*, that "I could face any pain with my eyes open after that ceremony."

The circumcision, the cattle rustling, the skinny legs, the barefoot childhoods, the high altitude, the sunny days and cold nights. All of them help make the Kalenjin great. But putting it all together required a special X-factor that Rosa discovered himself.

IT TAKES A COMMUNITY TO RAISE A RUNNER

Gabriele Rosa speaks the same way that Kenyans run: Softly, economically, no wasted motion. He leans back in a dining room chair in the 8-room gated compound he rents 2 months a year in Eldoret, and answers the question he's heard a thousand times.

"My secret for turning Kenyans into great runners?" he says. "There's no secret. They have the right genetics, right culture. From there, it is just training—hard, hard training." Training 150 to 175 miles per week in altitudes of one to two miles high. Running uphill for 2-, 3-, 4,000 feet at a time, often two or three times a day. A workload never seen before in the running world.

The workload even awes Rosa, who says it came about through simple communication. One day, he asked the Kenyans how they felt after a day's hard run, and wondered if they could push a little faster. When they could, he asked them to do more. And more.

"I was surprised—they happily took everything I could throw at them," said Rosa, his normally even-toned voice spiking with wonder and admiration. "They never complain, they hardly get injured. They are a people whose culture, temperament, genetics, and motivation are better suited to the marathon than any people I've ever seen—and I've trained whites, Mexicans, you name it."

"But there is one key that stands out," he says. "They have the ability to be trained as a group."

"Basically, it's psychological. Running with partners lets you run further and harder because the athletes have the illusion that they are saving energy—even as their inherent competitiveness pushes the intensity higher."

The trick is finding fast training partners, something hard to do in individualistic Western societies. Poli, Rosa's first great project, eventually ran out of them.

But the Kenyans had something that made them a perfect fit with Rosa's group-training philosophy: Community.

"The Kenyans are very kind, correct, and traditional," said Rosa. "They are respectful of their neighbors; they like to help the community. I saw many cases—like Tanui—of Kenyans getting rich and coming back to share with the community. They are the way that people should be."

They are very much the way Rosa sees himself.

THE CAMPS

"Kaza mu Zungu!" they say. "Go white man!"

It is 7 A.M. on the dirt road to Kapsait, the little village where the new training camp is located. Thirty-eight Kenyans, most of whom live at the camp 3,000 feet above where they are right now, thunder past a middle-aged Italian runner three kilometers into a 21k run. Each time the tightly packed herd passes one of the dozen

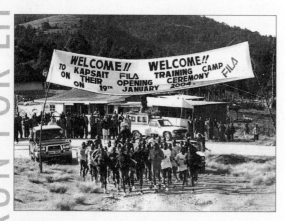
Kapsait camp runners head up the mountain.

members of the Terramia Running club of Milan, Italy, who started ten minutes before them, they say "Kaza mu Zungu."

They love to say that. They say it with laughter and affection and admiration and encouragement. They say it with a slightly paternalistic tinge, reminiscent of the way you might talk to a little brother who tries hard, but who you both know is incapable of keeping up. There's nothing racist or ageist about it. Some of the Italians are twice the age of the Kenyans. But even if they weren't, how could anyone in the world hope to keep up with people who live together and train together for 11 months out of the year, who push each other as relentlessly on a Monday-morning training run as they do on a Sunday at a prestigious international marathon with thousands of dollars on the line?

The Kenyans start slow and gradually pick up speed, just as Rosa had trained them. They run within inches of each other, as if they are a single 76-leg organism feeding off a sole energy source. They run so closely and smoothly and fast that they seem like cyclists riding five deep in an amoeba-shaped paceline, the front-runners blocking the wind for those in back.

Their form, while not identical, is elegant and flowing, their footfalls soft and muffled, as if they don't want to wake the neighbors up this early. They fly past the flat-topped acacia trees that scream "this is Africa." They turn corners that open to breathtaking, *Sound of Music* vistas of the magnificent green hills and valleys, yet they see nothing. They say nothing, except for "Kaza mu zungu" when they pass Aldo Rock, a Milano concert promoter/extreme runner who runs alone. Unlike the Kenyans, the Italians make no effort to run together, to share energy; the second they left the start line, they atomized, the fast ones giving no thought to the slow.

At 9,000 feet, with the run two-thirds complete, the Kenyans accelerate, just as they've been taught. "Kaza mu zungo!"— they swallow up the fastest Italian, a 35-year-old accountant named Luigi, whose jerky, pounding style seems antithetical to Kenyan grace. The pace pushes faster. Luigi gamely hangs in for 15 seconds, then is spit out the back along with 3 Kenyans. Now it's a war of attrition. Bodies drop off the pack like space ice from a meteor. Running uphill, the top three finish at Kapsait at 5-minute-mile pace—astounding after a 13-mile uphill run at high altitude. More astounding: One minute later, their breathing is relaxed and they appear to be perfectly recovered.

Aldo Rock's heart rate didn't drop so quickly. When he comes in an hour later, he describes breathing at 10,000 feet as "running with a gorilla clamped around your neck." Like the others, he paid $2,500 for this one-week "running vacation," and he's getting his money's worth. The club gets the chance to run with athletes at the five training camps Dr. Rosa has set up in Kalenjin country since 1994.

In 1993, determined to test his mass-training marathon theory on the smooth, economical Kenyan supermen, Rosa rented rooms at a Kaptagat hotel for seven runners. The next year, following the New York City Marathon victory of another of his athletes, German Silva of Mexico, he presented Fila with a proposition: Give me $500,000 a year to finance five camps where I'll train 100 of the best potential Kenyan marathoners day and night. They will leave their families and their jobs to live together, eat together, sleep together. Free of distractions, they will push each other in the thin air of the Kalengin highlands, running on mountain roads at 6,000 to 10,000 feet, honing their genetic advantage. Unleashed upon the running world, these Kenyan supermen will bring national pride and piles of prize money to the country. In exchange, you get the greatest possible advertising: the Fila logo emblazoned across the chest of the winners of the world's most photographed marathons, including New York, Boston, Amsterdam, Berlin, and London.

Rosa did not invent the group training camp. Many had existed in Kenya before, the most renowned being St. Patrick's High School in Iten, 20 miles from Eldoret, and some military-affiliated camps. But applying the group concept to large numbers, and to the marathon, was new—and successful. The victories came quickly: In 1996, Kenyans finished in 7 of the top 8 positions in Boston, including winner Moses Tanui, who won again in '98. Joseph Chebet won in '99. Simon Biwott, trained at Kapsait, won Berlin in 2000. At the 2000 Boston Marathon, Kenyan men took 7 of the 10 ten positions; four were Rosa's men, including winner Elijah Lagat and third-place finisher Tanui. As the winners began bringing home paychecks, track racers began to clamor to get in.

Those who make the cut are rewarded with more work than they've ever done in their lives: 3 workouts a day in the early season and 2 in-season, starting at 6 A.M., up to 175 miles per week, with endless hill training. "Multiday workouts is the Kenyan mentality," says Mike Chesire, the 1993 and '95 5000-meter world champion who is now a coach under Rosa. "If you only train once a day, you can't compete." The camps are spartan affairs—cinderblock buildings, 4 or 5 sleeping to a room, no whirlpools, zero creature comforts. Even an ice pack is a rarity because the refrigerator and the electricity needed to freeze it isn't a given.

When the Kenyans and the Italians finally finished their 13-mile run at Kapsait, they first went to the old camp, a rathole consisting of concrete blocks, a spigot, and a nostril-curdling rancidity borne of years of sweat-drenched clothing drying on bedposts. Aldo and Luigi the accountant sit in the small courtyard and greedily slurp down ugali, a maize porridge regarded by some Kenyans as having magic powers of rejuvenation. They eat chapati, a thick, tasty corn tortilla that is a dietary staple; and wash it down with chai, tea leaves boiled with milk and sugar. "Sowa sowa," says Luigi to the smiling Kenyans, eager hosts. That's "very good"—the second bit of Swahili most people learn after "jambo"—"hello."

The new Kapsait camp, to be dedicated that afternoon, was described earlier as "luxurious"—and it is to the Kenyan athletes, who had watched its construction for several months. They were awed when the gates opened that day. Contiguous concrete blockhouses with corrugated aluminum roofs stairstep down a hill, opening to a Mt. Olympus view of the green hills in the distance. The camp has running water and the system will be extended to the entire Kapait town, ending the practice of carrying jugs of water atop heads. There'll be a library, a computer, and a generator to supply electricity for four hours a day, meaning warm showers and TV for the first time. Just 2 men sleep to a room. Eventually, the building will house the area's first hospital. Most significant, perhaps, were the white-lettered words painted on each of the green doors: each spelled out the name of the runners' reason for being, a significant marathon or Olympics: "Amsterdam," "Berlin," "Sydney," they start, continuing to the "New York" dining room and the

"Boston" conference room. One room to note: "Brescia," the home of Dr. Rosa, where all the best eventually pilgrimage. Finally, on the wall of the dining hall: Our Motto: DISCIPLINE AND HARD WORK FOR SUCCESS.

Incidentally, Rosa's program in Kenya was so successful that Fila wanted him to replicate it in California with American runners. The company desperately wanted to break into the American shoe market, and figured having successful Americans would help promote their shoes better than unknown Kenyans. But the program, held at 6,000 feet on Mt. Laguna, California, failed after two years (1999–2000). Turns out that Americans are too individualistic and too used to creature comforts to live huddled together 11 months of the year, running three times a day. "Even if they could handle it, they don't have the genetics of the Kenyans," said Manners. Or the memory of the circumcisions.

THE DISCOVERY GAMES

Kids are running everywhere. A barefooted 5-year-old whose number covers his entire chest runs the 100-meter dash. Twelve-year-old girls in dresses do a 5k. Several 15-year-olds run the 10k fast enough to make the U.S. national team. Hundreds of kids are running every moment, crisscrossing the huge field of the Eldoret Athletic Club in so many opposing lines and angles that it reminds me of the laser etchings on a silicon computer chip.

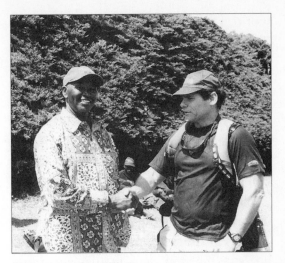

Kip Kieno greets fans at the Discovery Races.

In all, 1,653 school-age runners—probably a third of them barefooted—competed at the 10th annual Discovery Kenya races in January, an unofficial national championship for youngsters. For the kiddies, it's all fun; for some of the teens, it's more: Preparation for the Eldoret Half-Marathon the following weekend, where Rosa and other talent scouts would be out in force, looking for the next Moses Tanui.

The Discovery Races are the result of Rosa's idea, Fila's money, and Tanui's organizational ability. Now retired, the two-time Boston winner now supervises the camp at Kapatagat and coordinates Discovery. Among thousands of spectators that day, I saw plenty of stars: Kip Keino, the godfather, now head of the Kenya Olympic Committee; Martin Lel, the 2003 New York Marathon winner; Paul Tergat, who'd just set a marathon

259

world record in Berlin by running a 2:04:55, an average of 4:46 per mile (since beaten by Ethiopian Haile Gebrselassie's 2:04:26 in 2007). Just named the African representative for the Food for Peace program, Tergat conspicuously wore a Nike Air baseball cap (after years with Fila, he signed a huge contract with its rival, yet still trains with Rosa).

Sammy Korir, who put himself on the map by finishing one second behind Tergat in Berlin (and in 2008 would become the first man in history to run ten sub-2:09 marathons) showed up at Discovery driving the Suzuki Samurai he won at the Rock 'n' Roll Marathon in San Diego in June 2002. Shy but known for his class—Korir waited for a fallen Kenyan rival to get up off slippery cobblestones at the 2004 London Marathon after he tripped over him, then lost the race by 30 seconds—he shakes hands with Rosa and others he'd hosted the day before at his new two-story mansion. Traditional Kenyan culture attaches great importance to inviting guests over to meet family and friends, and the runners consider it a deep honor to be visited by Rosa, who has been to 200 lunches and dinners over the years. "It shows you respect them," Rosa explains. "And it's free food." As expected, he doesn't smile at the joke.

"It's a big change from living five to a smelly room in Kapsait for three years," said Korir when he opened the wrought-iron gates of his two-acre grounds in the exclusive northwest sector of Eldoret, which is protected by two armed guards and surrounded by a 10-foot wall with broken glass protruding from the top.

Rosa's three Range Rovers full of coaches and running club members entered a living room with a large trophy case on one side and plain walls decorated with Christmas cards and a calendar showing Jesus in beatific poses. We were greeted by the home's 12 residents: Korir's wife and their 3 young children, his parents, a maid, a cook, and 4 young runners. The latter give Korir the benefits of daily group training without living at a camp, and this day served as waiters and hand-washers. Carrying a two-foot wide plastic tub and an oversized tea kettle, they stopped to pour warm water over the hands of each seated guest, a hand-washing habit acquired from years of living in a mud hut without running water. Then, one by one, they served traditional Kenyan foods: bright-orange sweet potatoes, ribs with dipping salt, sliced onions, tomatoes and green peppers, lamb chunks and salt, and the main dish: lamb stew with ugali, a glob of white cornmeal the consistency of firm polenta.

Rosa's Italian entourage was unusually quiet during the two-hour lunch, respectfully consuming all the courses, unaccustomed to being treated like royalty, and out of breath after climbing up the stairs to find the bathroom (at 7,000 feet, even one story gets to you). We were fascinated by Korir's "Wall of Fame." The wall-to-wall case was jammed with trophies, plaques, photos, and newspaper articles, with faux gold records of the San Diego Rock 'n' Roll Marathon—a first and a third—calling to mind Elvis's gold record room at Graceland.

Korir revealed that he was teaching himself to play the guitar he also won in San Diego, and at the next day's Discovery races joked with Margaret Okayo that they'd have to start a band. Okayo, a two-time New York and one-time Boston winner who had flown in from her home in Brescia for the occasion, had won Rock 'N' Roll twice. Named to the '04 Olympic team along with Korir and Tergat, she could easily afford music lessons, having won $165,000 at New York in 2003.

David Okaya, general secretary of the Kenyan Athletic federation, says 2,000 Kenyans run professionally around the world. Few rate CEO compensation yet. John Manners estimates a dozen have shoe contracts worth $100,000 each. Fifty make $50,000. The rest might make $15,000, still a fortune by Kenyan standards. Including winnings and appearance fees (Tergat made $300,000 in his first marathon), excluding commissions (Kenya and Rosa get a cut), it's a sizeable injection to the Kenyan economy.

"Way more people are running now due to Rosa. He's had an enormous impact. Now, running is a realistic career in Kalenjin country," said Tom Ratcliff, of KIM International Management, which manages many Kenyan runners.

Of course, there's a downside. The influx of marathon money has "eviscerated" the schools' running programs, says Ratcliff, a frequent critic of Rosa. Like many, he suggests without substantiation that Rosa must be drugging his athletes, and frets that marathon mania has caused Kenyans to abandon the shorter distances. In Spring 2003, Kenya lost the world cross-country championship for the first time in 18 years, a shocking development akin to the United States'

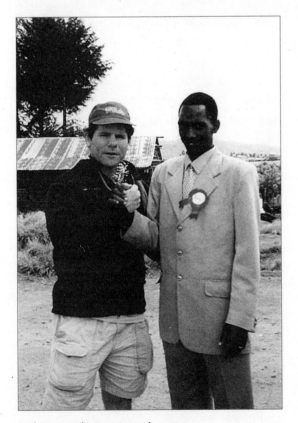

Paul Tergat at the Kapsait grand opening.

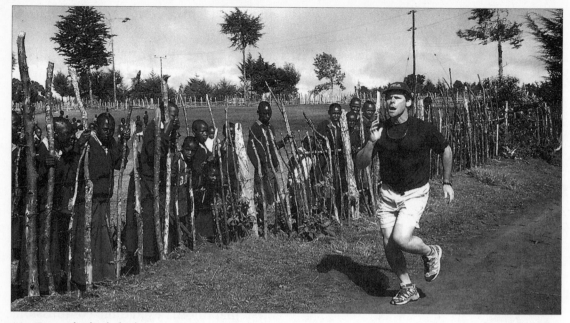

Mu Zungu dazzles the locals.

losing the Olympic basketball medal. "When it comes to running," says Rosa, "it's like black Americans and basketball. The Kalengin own running. It is a matter of pride. They shouldn't lose."

That confidence is permeating young and old in Kenyan society. Fifteen years ago, a doctor told non-runner Elijah Lagut, 27, that he was grossly overweight at 72 kilograms for his height of 5-foot-5. "So at an age when everyone else was retiring, I started running," said Lagut. After six months he'd lost 20 kilograms (44 pounds). And after six years, in 2000, he won the Boston Marathon.

But more importantly, three years later he ran for public office—an Eldoret city council seat. "I lost, but that doesn't matter," he told me. "I will run again—and win. Through my success in running, I have learned about hard work and goal-setting. I have learned what it takes to be great. Thousands are learning that lesson in Kenya every day."

"We are not just creating marathoners here, but creating the future," said Gabriele Rosa in his speech at Kapsait. The cheers were thunderous, deafening. They knew he spoke the truth—truth worth walking 20 miles up a mountain to hear.

Note: In 2008, Kenya finally won its first marathon gold medal with Samuel Kamau Wanjiru's Olympic-record 2:06:32 in Beijing.

CHAPTER 25

HOW TO RUN THE KENYAN WAY

Ten Training Secrets from the homeland of the world's best endurance runners

Two or three runs a day, clawing tooth and nail against hungry competitors, at elevations up to 10,000 feet. Do you really want to work out like this?

If you want to improve your marathon time, what works for the Kenyans will work for any runner, says Dr. Gabriele Rosa, the mastermind behind much of Kenya's marathon running success. Megamiles are not exactly part of the *Run for Life* prescription for running to age 100, but several of the tips below—particularly the calls for off-road and hill running, fat-burning morning workouts, and social running with friends—mesh nicely with the thrust of this book. And a little extra speed once in a while wouldn't hurt.

1. Multiple-run training days: To get in shape quickly in the early season, the Kenyans run 3 times a day. While that may sound daunting, dividing the daily mileage into more shorter, faster workouts rather than fewer, slower, longer workouts is better for building the kind of speed that the Kenyans need to win races. Running the 12k three times, with complete rest/recovery in between, allows the Kenyans to run faster than they would while running 36k all at once. Rosa admits that multiple-run training days are hard on the body. "There's a risk, but it's the only way to run under 2:08 in the marathon," he says, "and the Kenyans have become accustomed to training this way for a long time."

Once the season is under way, the Kenyans run 2 times per day. They drop to once per day in the off-season. The Kenyans build up to 3 or 4 big races per year, often racing half marathons a month before an important marathon.

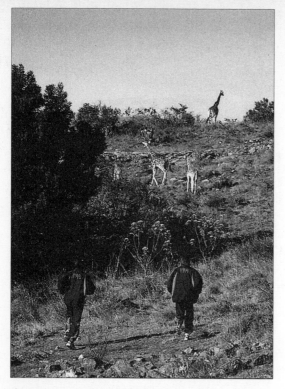
The Kenyans' top secret revealed: chasing giraffes.

The average working person, of course, doesn't have time to run three times a day. But a similar morning-and-night scenario might achieve a similar rapid increase in fitness. For the record, the Rosas do not advocate a multiday schedule for average people, saying that once-a-day workouts 3 to 6 days a week is appropriate for fitness. But they can be useful for serious age-group athletes.

2. Run early in the morning, before breakfast: The Kenyans run at 6 A.M. for three reasons: 1) The temperature is cooler; 2) It helps switch muscle fibers from slow-twitch to fast-twitch, the fibers that literally help you move faster; 3) With a minimum of easy-to-access fuels like muscle glycogen or bloodstream sugar in the system (your body utilizes a good amount of glycogen during the night, especially if you stopped eating dinner at 7:30 P.M.), the body must learn to optimize the use of "intermuscle" fat—the plentiful but hard-to-access fat within the muscle.

Regular folk will enjoy similar training benefits and get a bonus they won't see in later-day training: Weight-loss. The love handles that won't go away with regular-hour exercise will be eaten away by their empty body's energy requirements in the early morning. Also, by training your body to run on fat, you're less liable to bonk during a race. Just don't start out fast (see Tip #3). "Of course, you should run at low intensity/heart rate, because you wouldn't be able to run fast for a long time with so little glycogen" says Rosa's son Marco, who runs the family's Marathon Center sports medicine clinic in Brescia, Italy.

3. Start slow, do intervals, finish fast: The Kenyans use what the Rosas call "a metabolic mix" to build their world-class speed: They start off the first 20 to 30% of a run (12 to 18 minutes in an one-hour run) at an easy jog, followed by intervals, then finish the last third at race pace. Metabolic mix means that in the same workout they work in lipid power, aerobic power, and anaerobic power. (In the first part of the workout, you use fats as fuel, to produce energy. In the second part you

RUN LIKE A KENYAN

go on using fats, plus a minimal amount of glycogen—sugar. In the third part, you only use glycogen.)

Warning: Don't cheat on the jogging. "The jogging period improves your ability to use lipids (fats) for fuel," says Marco Rosa. "Those who need to lose weight should increase the jogging period to 50–60% of the whole." Intervals, those faster-than-race-pace sprints that are essential to building speed, should be done for a full minute, followed by a minute of jogging. Repeat this one minute-on, one minute-off sequence from 8 to 15 times depending on your individual level of fitness. Now properly loosened up, you finish your run at race pace.

4. Run up hills at least once a week, but skip the descents: Running up hills is the best way to improve general leg strength and specific strength for running long distances, to get your body used to higher heart rate frequencies, and to prevent end-of-race fade. It is not important to go fast. Hills give you a huge advantage in the last kilometers of a race. "We consider it no surprise that Martin Lel (who won New York in 2003) and Paul Tergat and Sammy Korir in Berlin (the former set a world record in 2:04:55 and the latter was 2nd in 2:04:56) all ran fastest in their last two kilometers," says Rosa. Do no more than 8 to 10 kilometers of uphill running (40 minutes to 1 hour) at once.

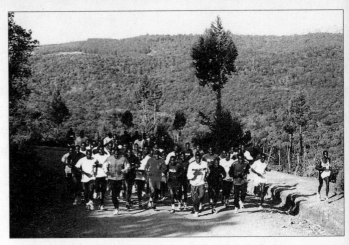
Run with a group at 10,000 feet.

Warning: While short downhills are good for muscles (3 to 4 minutes maximum) long downhills can be very dangerous for them. The Rosas say it's better to return by car after extremely long climbs. Use 2 cars—before your run, drive both to the top, leave one there, and descend with the other.

5. Don't run on asphalt: The Kenyans never pound pavement. Running off-road strengthens ankles, babys tendons, lessens injuries, provides fresher air, and generally makes you feel good. Importantly, dirt roads allow you to run MORE. Kenyans train for 14 to 15 hours a week, and they could never run the same mileage on asphalt.

When Margaret Okayo, winner of the 2002 Boston and 2001 and 2003 New York Marathons, trains at her home in Italy, she alternates between the two kinds of surfaces. It's not as easy to find ten kilometers of dirt road in Italy or the U.S. as it is in Kenya.

RUN FOR LIFE

Ironically, although̶ ̶
great marathons are hel̶d̶
the off-road-bred Kenyan̶s̶
no trouble with the hard su̶
because, at most, a top Kenya̶n̶
on the road only about 2 hours
minutes," explained Marco Rosa. I̶
long enough to get hurt.

6. Don't bob up and down: Bobbing
is not economical—it's a waste of energy.
You are actually pushing backward. To
cure bobbing, says Rosa, run hills. You
automatically run smoother. It teaches
you how to run on the flats.

7. Train with a group: Running with
partners who'll push you—one or 25, no
matter—is a key to getting faster, even
if you follow none of the other tips. It's
why the Kenyans live and train together
for 11 months out of the year. And why
Margaret Okayo runs with men—because
no other woman can keep up with her.
Running with someone at your level or
above on a set schedule keeps you from
skipping sessions and forces you to turn
it up a notch.

"Basically it's a psychological matter,"
says Rosa. "Running with partners during
training gives the athletes the illusion

s̶u̶
marath̶
compromise ̶y̶
that your toes won't̶ ̶

9. Train at high altitude: Kenyans
live and train almost exclusively at 5,000
to 9,000 feet of elevation. Training in
thin air (the partial pressure of oxygen is
20–30% lower in highland Kenya than at
sea level) confers hypoxia-linked benefits:
an increased production of red cells and
consequently of hemoglobin. This leads
to greater oxygen-carrying capacity in the
muscle cells when you run at sea level.

10. Run huge quantities: Kenyan
marathoners train 150 miles per week.
The Rosas are famous for pushing quantity. Whether you do 8 miles or 80, they
suggest you do more. (Note: *Run for Life*
suggests you don't.)

TOM OSLER

The Historian

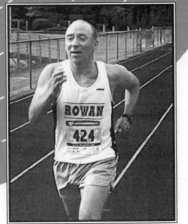

RUN FOR LIFE

Tom Osler is a numbers guy by profession—a New Jersey university mathematics professor who has published 100 papers on the subject—but when it comes to running, he's more like an historian. Starting off as a 13-year-old enthralled with the sport two decades before the running boom, he met and worked with the modern pioneers of running, quietly helping them to shape the sport. As he did, running helped shape his own life. He's run over 2,000 races since he ran a 4.7-mile race in Camden, New Jersey on December 4, 1954, and has gone on to race nearly three out of every four weekends for more than 50 years—every event dutifully logged in his immense race diary. The muscular, opera-loving father of two grown sons is not only a link with the sport's early days but also a champion with three national championships in the 1960s (25k, 30k, and 50-mile). He's authored three important running books, been an early running organizer and founder of several running clubs, and been inducted into the Hall of Fames of the Road Runners Club of America and the National Road Running Club.

Modest and self-effacing, Osler was three months shy of age 68 when he spoke to me on January 22, 2008 about his life, his unique body-weight/racing times formula, his fitness and running regimen (which includes 5k races almost every weekend), and his love for a sport that he says literally saved his life.

I've run practically every day of my life since February 1954, when I was 13. Mostly because I like it. I like the way it makes me feel. The periods of time when I could run well were a bonus.

I had a wonderful boyhood growing up in Camden, New Jersey. I tried the usual popular sports like football, baseball, basketball; couldn't do any of them well. Tired of my nerd status, I went out for the track team to gain some self-respect.

In running, usually you first try 100 yards or 200 yards—I couldn't do those well—then keep going up until you're at the end, which in those days was the mile. So that's where I wound up.

On April 26, I got a stopwatch for my 14th birthday. So I started running a timed mile every day as hard as I could, hoping to someday be the first man under four minutes.

I trained harder than most people, and became a mediocre high school miler. In April of '55 I got my first win in the mile in a dual meet between Camden and Atlantic City High Schools, in a time of 5:10.2. The best I would do was 4:54—good enough to win one out of three or four high school track meets. Couldn't win any championships with it. There was still the occasional kid who could run 4:40 or 4:30. But it was all right. It made me the best miler on my team.

I realized at that time that I wasn't going to be a great runner. I didn't have the speed. If I was in a ten-mile run and there were 30 people, I'd finish about 10th or 15th. I said to myself, "Well, hell, I love doing this—it's really fun. Okay, so what if I never become a great runner? I like it, so I'm going to keep doing it."

Part of the fun was being involved with the local running scene and meeting people—sometimes the best runners in the country.

When I was 14, I'd read in the newspaper about the Shanahan Marathon in Philadelphia, so I went over there. There were less than 20 people in the race. I wound up running 11 miles and had to quit. Before the race, I had a chance to sit down and talk with this great runner, Ted Corbitt, who'd been a marathoner on the 1952 Olympic team. Later in life, he did ultramarathons. Naturally, I wanted to hear what Ted had to say. He told me to be careful about all this enthusiasm for running, and be sure I did well at school. He would have a powerful effect on me.

(Corbitt, who died at 88 in 2007, once held American records in the marathon and the 100-mile run and is considered America's ultramarathoning pioneer. A black man in a era of racial discrimination, he earned a master's degree in physical therapy at NYU in 1950, ran his first marathon in Boston in 1951, and, as the president of the New York RRC in 1959, organized the U.S.' first ultramarathon event. Known to run 200 miles or more a week, Corbitt was one of the first to champion running for exercise, and remained a full-time physical therapist into his 80s).

You really had to know Ted to appreciate the man. He was very quiet, didn't say a lot. And there was something about him that was just different from everyone else. When you were with him, he very much motivated you, impressed you with the fact that you could do all kinds of things that you thought were beyond you, that you thought were difficult. He had a way of making it seem easy. He's the only person I ever met like that. He had a way of doing difficult things like going out and running for 70 miles. He lived in the Bronx, and in training for his ultras, he'd run around Manhattan Island, carrying change so that he could ride the subway back if he got in trouble. Around Manhattan is 35 miles; occasionally, he'd do it twice.

This sort of thing was mind-boggling, especially in those days.

Corbitt wasn't very communicative verbally. He liked to write me letters. Probably most of the letters were about course measurement. I was part of a committee that he formed to propagate proper course measurement techniques.

We were friends, but because he lived in New York City, and I lived in the Philadelphia area, we never got that close. Not close like I got with Browning Ross, who lived about 15 miles from me.

Ross and I were friends. Ross was to running as George Washington was to the United States. He was on the Olympic team in '48 and '52 in the steeplechase. He was national champion at practically everything with regard to distance running—except the marathon. He founded the Road Runners Club of America in 1957 in Philadelphia. That's what really got running going. Before that, there were only a handful of races to run in this area. When he started that, we suddenly had races every week.

He started this magazine, the Long Distance Log, which he typed up and mailed out himself. That started in 1956 and went all the way to 1973. Came out once a month, had about 25 pages, and every race in the

RUN FOR LIFE

country was in there. There were so few races then that you could do that. If Browning had had the business mentality, that could have become Runner's World. He was a mentor to me, about 15 years older. It was hard to run with him; he always wanted to run fast, and it made me very uncomfortable. Every time I ran with him, I said, "I'm not going to do this again." (laughs) Even when there came a point when I was much better runner than him as he grew older, I didn't like to train with him. He trained too fast for my taste.

GOING SLOWER TO GET FASTER

Like I said, I was a mediocre runner, and I stayed that way for a long time after high school. My college, now Drexel University, was an engineering school with no track or cross-country team. So I never competed in collegiate events. But I did run all that time in the open races. After the Road Runners Club had formed, and I was running 5-milers, 10-milers, I ran every day and raced almost every weekend—without distinction.

That started to change when I was 22, in grad school, and read the book, Run to the Top, which described how Arthur Lydiard, a brilliant New Zealand coach [who died in 2004 at 87], trained his Olympic champions.

Lydiard had this idea that you should do long, slow runs that build your base. Now, this was an idea that was always pooh-poohed by everyone I'd talked to. We'd always done interval training. Everyone said that slow running was worthless jogging, and would get you nowhere. Slow running would make you slow. And here was this great coach saying that slow running would not make you slow; it would make you strong.

So I tried it, and found I loved it. I just loved running slow. It was very comfortable and enjoyable. And very much to my surprise, in a few years I was running much, much better.

By the time I was 24, I was no longer finishing in the middle of the pack. Now I was finishing near the front—if not occasionally first.

I thought, "Okay, I tried the long, slow stuff. Now let's add the second half of Lydiard's formula: sharpening

(speed work), and see what that does." And when I tried that, I won my first national championship. (Osler won the 1965 national AAU title in the 25k in 1:27:09. In 1967, he won national championships in the 30k (in 1:40:40.8) and 50-mile (in 5:52:33) and ran his best marathon, 2:29:04, at Boston.)

In 1967, I privately published "The Conditioning of Distance Runners," probably the best thing I ever wrote on running. It's only 32 pages and still circulating underground. What caused me to write it was Lydiard's book. I wasn't Olympic champion material, so I really couldn't do the kind of schedules he had in the book. I reduced them, modified them for a less-gifted runner, more ordinary, like myself—and it worked.

ARRESTED FOR RUNNING

The championships gave me respect, you know: "Oh yeah, he's a good runner." But when I was doing my best running, the public didn't even know what a marathon was. At that time, running was nothing (compared to other sports). It did not become anything the ordinary person noticed until the very late sixties, early seventies. When I'd go out and train and run on the road, they'd usually ask, "Are you a boxer? I thought you were a fighter out doing roadwork."

They had no idea. Nobody was out running on the road. "I'm a distance runner," I'd say. They'd say, "What's that?" I'd say, "We have these 10-mile races, and I do those." They'd say, "Geez, I never heard of that."

People were more formal in those days. When you had a race, there was usually a clubhouse or a YMCA or something associated with it. People didn't show up at a race in their sweat clothes; they showed up in their street clothes with a gym bag and their running stuff in it. So you expected to have a locker room, a shower, et cetera. After the race, you'd go back and take a shower. The reason you could do this is that running was so small; there were just very few people running. Even at the Boston Marathon you had these things, although logistics made it a bit different. When I first ran it in 1963 or 1964, I took the train up there. Everybody stayed at the Lenox Hotel near the finish line in those days. Buses drove you down to a high school in Hopkinton, where the race started. Boston only drew about 200 runners.

So few people were out running that you felt real weird out there. It took a long time before I felt all right putting a pair of shorts on and running down the street. Even in warm weather, you just didn't do that—until the running boom came. "What's wrong with that guy?" they'd say. You didn't do that in public.

Loads of times, if I went out running at night, I'd often have a policeman come up and follow me in his car. "What the hell's this guy doing?" he'd think.

In 1964, when I was a graduate student, I was once tackled by a policeman. Tackled me, put me in his car. He didn't say "stop." He just opened his door and tackled me. It was wintertime. There had just been a light snowfall. I was doing this long, 17-mile loop of mine, and at that point was running through a park. Just me on this road, nobody out, and I see this cop car coming right towards me, directly at me. I'm running on the left side of the road, and the cop's on the left side of the road. I wave at him to give me some room, get out of the way. He doesn't get out of the way. He comes right up, slams on his brake, and stops right in front of me. So I ran around the side of his car, and as soon as I got along the side, the door flipped open and he sprung out like a jack-in-the-box, tackled me, and pulled me into the car.

I'm in the car, utterly startled, thinking, "What the heck is going on?" He picks up the radio, and says, "I got him."

I was really mad. I looked at him and said, "You know what you got? You got a lot of trouble, that's what you got!"

He was kind of startled at my, uh, arrogance. I explained what I was doing. I said, "Look, drive me over to the park police station. The park police here know me. I come through here very frequently. They'll tell you who I am." So he believed me, and took my name, address and phone number, and he let me go. But I was just steaming mad.

When I got home, I called the police to complain. They then told me what had happened. At the time I was

running, a bunch of kids had stolen a car, and had driven into the park, abandoned the car, and ran off in that very direction. Naturally, he thought I was one of those kids. Like I said, no one was running in those days.

It's interesting. Back in those days, myself and most people who ran felt very uneasy about this. We felt guilty that we were doing this. My parents didn't like it. They said, "You're wasting your time. You should be studying, or developing your career. Why are you wasting all that energy running?"

Everybody told you that. I was one of those few people who did it because I liked it. I didn't care whether or not I made the Olympic team.

I came close, actually. The only event I could have possibly made the Olympic team in was the marathon. In 1967, I finished 4th in the national AAU championship marathon. That sort of made me the dark horse for the Olympic Trials in '68. What put a complete damper on that was, because the games were going to be in Mexico City, they were going to hold the trials in high altitude—Alamosa, Colorado, which is something like 6,000 feet. The AAU set up a three-month training camp that anyone could go to prepare for this.

I didn't want to spend the summer in Alamosa, Colorado training—since it wasn't likely I'd make it anyway. So I didn't try.

In 1968, I was working full-time as a math professor at St. Joseph's College in Philadelphia, and I'd just gotten married. My wife Kathy would have thought I'd lost my mind if I'd gone, because I wasn't that kind of person. Like I said, I always felt guilty about running, and the idea of giving up three months of my life just to run sounded insane. That was just too much. I never felt sorry for myself that I didn't go to that camp. I think I would have been miserable. I'd been doing 50-mile runs, but I never wanted to spend all day running. It was bad enough that I was spending a couple hours a day running. There were always other things that I wanted to do. I didn't want to just run. And that's what you do at one of these camps; you were just immersed in running 24 hours a day. Running's a nice complement to the other things I do in my life. But it's not everything.

ANTI-AGING PLAN: WEIGHTS, CROSS-TRAIN, RACE, AND CONVERSATION

At 40, I began to lift light weights. Funny story: I'm a college professor, and I noticed that my right arm began to get tired from writing on the blackboard. It was really annoying in class; I was really getting a lot of pain in my shoulder. So I went out and bought a 110-pound York dumbbell set. I started playing with them, and it worked. The pain went away.

And I had read that when a man turned 35, he loses about a half a pound of muscle a year. So I thought, "Jeez, this not good. I should work against that." I swing 5- to 20-pound dumbbells around in the morning, and have a weight bench in the basement where I press 100 pounds, 8 reps. Just recently, I started weight training my legs. I should have done it earlier, I think. I do some mild squats with 20-pound dumbbells.

I think cross-training is terrific. In fact, for six years beginning in 1987, when I was 47, I did some 39 triathlons and biathlons. But I reluctantly retired from multisport events because I had two bad bicycle accidents, and I figured that was it—it was too dangerous. I got hurt pretty bad, broke bones both times. Now, if I get hurt running—that hasn't happened in a while—I'll swim.

The social component of life is a key element in happiness. That's why I teach—I have my students, my colleagues; it gives me somebody to talk to. It's a big, big part of why I enjoy my work. I'm 67 and have no plans to retire—working or running.

I love racing, because every time you race, it's like a reunion. It's very motivating too, right? Most of my daily running is by myself, although again I enjoy running with people.

My wife does not run. My boys did not run—even through the running boom was on as they were growing up. They were not interested. And I had no interest in encouraging them to do it. Oh, I asked them, but they always said "No." I'm not the kind of dad to push them into doing things; I tended to let them do what they wanted to do. That's how my father was. He didn't push me into

running; he didn't push me out of it, although he certainly never encouraged it.

Once a week for the last 20 years, I've run with Marge Morris, a librarian at Brown University. I saw her running down the street one day, and we just started running together. She's a very good conversationalist. We had a lot in common—children and so on, the same problems raising them. Marge is now the only runner who will train with me because I use such a slow pace—usually slower than 10 minutes per mile.

Running with someone is a personal thing. Most people I don't enjoy running with—because I don't enjoy their conversation. If you enjoy their conversation, fine. Otherwise, I'd rather talk to myself.

RUNNING STRATEGY & FORM: WALK—AND SIT ON THE "COUCH"

Jeff Galloway has done a very good job of popularizing walking while running, but it's nothing new. It's a technique that has been used for going extralong distance—distances longer than you could go with straight running, like if you can run a half marathon, but aren't in shape to do a full marathon. It's very effective. Who knows who invented it?—it's ancient. I used it in my 24-hour ultramarathon in 1976, when I went 114 miles, things like that. It's not new, but it had been forgotten. That's because ultramarathoning had kind of disappeared. There had been a lot of it in the late 1800s. They mainly walked. They didn't call it "ultramarathoning." They called it "pedestrianism." It was professional. They had a lot of races, usually done indoors. They had a lot of gambling on it: 6-day pedestrian races. In fact, it preceded the famous 6-day bike races.

You can read about it in my third running book, Ultramarathoning, the Next Challenge, which was cowritten in 1979 with Ed Dodd, who started researching the performance of old-time pedestrians with me six years before. (Osler's second book, the Serious Runner's Handbook, was published in 1978.) The first half of Ultramarathoning, which Ed wrote, is about these 19th-century 6-day races. The second half, which I wrote, is about ultramarathoning.

TOM OSLER

In my training section, I wrote about using walking, which depends on the distance and how strong you are. When I won a 100-mile race at Fort Meade in 16:11:15 in 1978, I got through it by walking every 2 miles; I ran either 7 laps and walked 1 lap or ran 7½ laps and walked a half lap. That got me through the 100 miles. Galloway is doing a very good thing by reviving it.

I do use walking on shorter distances as I get older. Even in races if I need to.

I don't use heart-rate monitors or energy foods. I used to use iced tea in the heat or warm tea in the cold—with a lot of sugar. I would show up with these insulated Coleman jugs.

I've never tinkered with my form, but I always tried to use my mind to get me into a very efficient running gait. I would do this by trying to relax, and just think about if any muscles seemed a little tight or uncomfortable. I used to try to imagine, while I was running, that I was just sitting on the couch—that I didn't feel anything. My legs just went out and did it.

That worked when I was young, and for many miles during a marathon. "I'm just sitting on the couch," I'd say over and over. I would occasionally give a thought to whether my arm swing or stride length was excessive. I would try to imitate runners that I thought were very relaxed, smooth, and efficient. Probably the person I most visualized was Abebe Bikila, the Ethiopian gold medalist in the 1960 Olympic Games. When I saw Bikila run the marathon, it was so amazing. Here was a man running 5-minute miles in his bare feet, and he was so efficient, so smooth, it just looked like he was jogging. I always held that picture of him in my mind, that seemingly effortless stride. "Be like Bekila," I say in my mind.

I've heard of Chi Running and the Pose Method, but they don't impress me very much because I think running is a very natural motion. We were born to run—it comes naturally. You can overstride and understride. But if you just leave your body alone, concentrate on moving quickly but effortlessly, then it will just figure out the right way to do it. I've tried to concentrate on being completely relaxed. That seemed to be the key.

The injuries come, of course, near the end of any race. You're going to be tired, which lays the seeds for the injury. That's where the trouble comes from. That last steps where you're really pushing and tired, that's where you break down.

Unfortunately, despite all my running, I've had a weight problem all my life. Because of all the eating. (laughs)

When I tell people I have an eating disorder—meaning I like to eat a lot—they laugh at me, because they've never seen me fat. Well, I don't get that fat, but it's very easy for me to gain weight. Typically, my best running weight was around 143. Typically, I'd get that weight in the late summer, then pick up 20 pounds in the winter, Naturally, I'd run slower. So after going through several of these cycles, up and down, up and down, I started to wonder exactly what was going on here.

I started looking at the diaries of all my races. And that's how I came up with my formula: that you gain 2 to 2½ seconds per mile per pound. Of course, it's only valid for data from over 2,000 of my races. Since my training is very consistent, I could predict what would happen to me if I gained 10 pounds—or if I lost 10 pounds. It worked pretty well. (See more about Osler's weight-to-speed formula and easy ways to drop weight in a sidebar at the end of Chapter 26.)

GROWING HIS OWN BYPASS

Can someone run to 100? Yes, but it won't be me. The reason: Genetics.

At least 20 years ago, there was a guy named Larry from San Francisco, aged 104, who appeared on the Johnny Carson Show. He was a waiter. He didn't seem to have a long history of running, but actually ran marathons. He looked good, talked well. My impression was that he was fortunate genetically.

My genetic history isn't that good. If my people made it to 80, that was pretty good. My father had a stroke at 75 and he died at 80. My mother died at 70 from colon cancer. So I seriously doubt that running to 100 is in the cards for me. I don't think I'll live that long. I was happy to wake up today. (laughs)

But I do know that running—and running a lot—will help me live longer than my genetic programming. I've been a runner for 54 years, doing considerably more than half an hour a day. I still do 30 to 40 miles a week. I know it's done me well. I'm probably alive because of it.

I have had two coronary episodes and high cholesterol all my life. When I was in my 20s, David Costill at Ball State did a study of marathon runners that I was part of. I had very, very high cholesterol. I ignored it, figuring that running would protect me from anything. Then, later in life, I found out it didn't.

I had a stroke in early 2003 when I was 63, and fortunately I recovered completely from that. In the middle of the night, I got dizzy and collapsed, then returned to bed and awoke feeling okay. Not knowing I had a stroke, I ran a 5k race that day, in my usual time. Two days later, after another dizzy spell with vomiting, I went to the hospital and was diagnosed with a stroke, caused by a blood clot. In two months, I started working and running at a reduced level again and began racing in May.

Then two years later, I had an arrhythmia, where your heart goes into a very rapid beat, so rapid that it's really not pumping any blood. This happened twice, right after finishing a race. I was very fortunate; the first time, I came out of it immediately when I fell over and hit my head. That brought me back. The second time, I wasn't as lucky. They tried to revive me. Fortunately, there was an ambulance there; they quickly got an external defibrillator out and that got me going. Now I carry my own embedded defibrillator.

After the arrhythmia, I went to the hospital and got a catheterization, where they look inside the heart. And they saw that one of the main arteries, the LAD, was completely blocked. They told me that they could tell by looking at it that it had been blocked for a long time. It hadn't happened recently. That's because there were extensive collateral vessels.

I had essentially grown my own bypass.

They told me that something like that doesn't happen unless you are doing something like running. My cardiologist told me that in most cases, when that artery closes,

people are lying on the floor feeling like an elephant is standing on their chest. When it happened to me, I didn't even know it happened.

I had no idea when it closed. I was going about my ordinary business. If I hadn't been a runner, I might have died.

I don't have high cholesterol now because I take some of these statins, Vytorin. The defibrillator is there in case of emergency. If my heart goes in to rapid beats, it sends an electric shock to it, which should bring it back to normal. It's a computer that watches what the heart is doing. It's not a pacemaker. It's like a cop—waiting for trouble. It doesn't affect the way my heart beats.

HELLO OLD AGE, GOOD-BYE HARD RUNNING

I have made one change in my running because of my heart. I've always enjoyed running a lot of races, and I still do 50, 60, 70 a year. But previous to the arrhythmia, I'd run hard in those races. During the last few miles of any race like that, it's uncomfortable—you're pushing yourself. That's the part I don't do anymore. I don't allow myself to press at the end of a race. I haven't run the marathon recently, but if I do, I'll run 9 minutes a mile. I just run easy, I stay comfortable, I don't breathe hard, I don't do anything stressful.

A good side effect to not pressing it is less injuries. Over the years, I'd injured everything. Usually, it's something like a sciatic nerve. I've been lucky with knees—no trouble. Sometimes foot trouble, plantar fasciitis. To heal up, I'd take it easy, go swimming, something. But I haven't had an injury for years. In fact, I haven't had an injury since I stopped running hard after the arrhythmia.

In that sense, maybe that arrhythmia is a silver lining to the cloud.

One thing I wanted to mention is I think that running and longevity is not all that common. If you look at some of these big races—the marathons and half marathons with 20,000 runners, and you look at the age-group listings, and interesting drop-off pattern tends to arise. If you look at the guys in the 50–55, and the 56–60, and the 61–65, very roughly speaking, the number of participants in each group drops by about a third or half each time. For example, if there are 60 in the 55–59, there'll be 20, maybe 30 in the 60–65. And it keeps cutting. That means, since I'm now 67, my changes of running into the next age-group are 50%. That's pretty sobering. That means you have to be careful to avoid hurting yourself.

Most of that is caused by mechanical injuries. It's not something major—a heart problem, like I have. It's knee problems, foot problems, hip problems. I know a lot of older runners who want to run but can't—they've messed themselves up mechanically.

The trouble is: You run into trouble when you're running fast and you're tired—like what happens in the last stages of a race. You do damage to your mechanical parts, ligaments, what have you. If you avoid doing that, you'll last a lot longer. Of course, that works against you in a race. But when you run hard at the end, you'll pay the price if you keep doing it. So, if you want to keep running for years and years and years, then the best thing to do is don't run hard when you're tired.

Ironically, a warning about going fast appears in my own book, The Serious Runner's Handbook, written 40 years ago when I was 27. It says that "sharpening is necessary, but puts you at risk." The concern there was mostly trying to get to a peak, a best performance. The idea was that you couldn't run at your best year-round. Your body couldn't take it. If you want to do your best, you have to time it for a particular event and time—the Olympic Trials, Olympic Games. The way to do is to train at a relatively slow level prior to this. And about six weeks before this, you begin running harder. The idea: Don't waste the peak too soon. I didn't invent this idea. It came from Arthur Lydiard. I read his book. He was the first one I knew who espoused the idea of building the base and sharpening.

Bottom line: The math (of the age-group attrition rate) is sobering. It makes you aware if you want to keep doing this, you better take it easy. Because you can easily wear yourself out. And that means no more fun.

I love running; it's the most fun I can think of. I'll do whatever it takes to keep doing it.

RUN TRAINED

This last section of *Run for Life* recognizes reality: What's running without doing a race once in a while?

After all, while this book is not an enthusiastic advocate of relentless steady-state running, which often generates a nagging litany of injuries and can possibly lead to systemic hormonal and structure problems over the long run, the goal of running to age 100 can seem like, well, a hundred years away. It is so distant that most of us instinctively need regular short-term shots of 5k/10k/marathon adrenaline to stay motivated. I've had days where the fear or anticipation of a race is the only thing urgent enough to get me out of my chair. The weights, intervals, cross-training, and water running advocated throughout this book will keep you extremely fit, but true race-shape requires more specificity. To race at the best of your ability, and do it with the least amount of stress on your body and mind, nothing beats Periodization, a near-foolproof stairstep training plan that ramps you up safely and leaves you primed to fly.

But keep in mind, however, that training alone isn't enough to get you to your best on race day. That's why, after Periodization, you'll find a world-class warm-up, courtesy of the legendary runner and coach Laszlo Tabori, that he says gets you into your "Second Wind" before the race starts. And since a bigger mass doesn't move as fast (it's a mathematical fact, according to a formula developed by Laszlo's fellow *Run for Life* interviewee Tom Osler), this section concludes with a remarkably easy diet-and-exercise strategy for painlessly dropping weight. So you'll not only get the chance to set a new PR, but you'll look pretty sleek in the race photos, too.

CHAPTER 26

PERIODIZATION

Intervals and weights keep you fast and healthy for the long run. But ramping up for a race requires a classic base-building, strengthening, and peaking plan.

Do races fit in a running longevity plan—and, if so, do the strength-training and interval-intensive workouts advocated in Sections 2 and 4 and prepare you for racing?

Yes and somewhat. The somewhat first: Armoring your body for running longevity with the good form, good posture, strength training, and intervals advocated in *Run for Life* will make you superfit, and certainly allow you to start any training plan at a high level. But short workouts of 20 or 25 minutes at any speed generally can't condition you for anything longer than a 5k. To get conditioned to do your best at a 10k, you need more training time.

The "Yes" answer, of course, is no mystery at this point. Motivation is the reason why races do fit into a longevity plan in a big way, even though the training for them is not as good for you as shorter, sprint-laced workouts. You don't need to race every weekend, like Tom Osler. But even if it's 6 months away, a race gives your daily workouts purpose, urgency, and excitement. I actually think the healthiest way to stay motivated is to schedule a whole series of goals: a big annual race, several smaller "booster shot" races, and long-term meta-goals—like 50 marathons by age 70, or 100 by age 100. You might even have a speed goal, like running a 10k at the same speed at age 60 as you did at age 50, to keep you focused. Take advantage of the age-group format and look forward to "aging up" to, say, the 60–65 age-group, where you'll be the young stud for a couple of years.

So, from a pure motivational point of view, races—and the training for them—are an important lever in the anti-aging toolbox. But no haphazard training will do. You have to train in a way that is good for your body, that speeds it up efficiently with "positive stress" that does not injure you. That way is called Periodization.

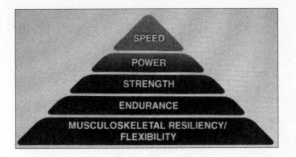

Goals of Periodization: Courtesy of Phase IV

WORK, BUILD, REST, THEN REPEAT A LITTLE HARDER

The foundation of all modern training, Periodization was developed in 1963 by Tudor O. Bompa, a former Olympic rower and faculty member of the Romanian Institute of Sport who trained 11 Olympic and world championship medalists in track and field and rowing. A virtually foolproof method used with great success by Communist athletes, Periodization builds the athlete up to optimal performance with a stairstep series of methodical, progressive challenges and recoveries that strengthen your body and keep your mind fresh. Similar in concept but a bit more involved than Arthur Lydiard's base-and-sharpening discussed in the Osler interview, it starts with a goal—say a 10k race in four months—and builds a workout schedule that breaks those 17 weeks of training into several "periods" or "phases" that vary the volume, timing, and intensity of workouts. Many call it "planned variation."

Why the need for variation? Researchers predating Bompa found that doing the same thing over and over eventually causes the body to stop improving, a process known as the "General Adaptation Syndrome." Turns out that the body is a very efficient adaptive learning machine; it improves in response to incrementally increasing stress for a while, but at a certain point will adapt and plateau. Over time, your body actually "learns" how to run more efficiently, but after a while your muscles don't get stronger. What they get is more efficient in building the neural pathways that let you do that same work with less muscle.

Solution? Stress your body, rest it, then stress it again at a higher level. That's Periodization. By altering your workouts (add more hills to your run, add ten pounds to your bench press, or use a different hand position), you force your muscles to grow in new ways, recruiting new fibers in a different order and adding to overall strength.

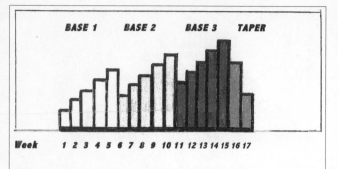

In Periodization, deliberate rest and recovery is planned, too. That's because your body actually consolidates the gains of your workouts during downtime. Hard workouts in particular must be followed by rest and easy "recovery" workouts. Technically, the body doesn't get stronger during a workout; it gets broken down. It is during rest when it repairs and rebuilds itself stronger.

What exactly gets stronger? Periodization simultaneously develops two types of fitness: aerobic and structural. Aerobic, or metabolic, fitness builds your cardiovascular system (heart, veins, and capillaries), the pulmonary system (the lungs), the endocrine systems (hormones), the nervous system, and the energy production in the muscles themselves. Structural fitness includes strengthening muscles, tendons, ligaments, and bone.

Summary: If you run the same miles at the same speed all the time, you'll plateau. Your body responds to Periodization's escalating variety of chal-

lenges and subsequent rest by getting fitter and better able to handle hard work safely and gradually making gains in strength, speed, power, and endurance. The changing variation also alters motor coordination and gives muscles balanced shape and size.

4 PERIODIZATION PHASES: BASE, STRENGTH, PEAK/TAPER, AND TRANSITION

Periodization uses four periods, or phases, to prepare you for your goal. Each phase has a specific conditioning purpose, and can last anywhere from four weeks to several months, depending on your objective and time frame, whether it be a 5k, 10k, a marathon. In Periodization, every workout in a months-long agenda is performed with this objective in mind.

Goal: The examples below will refer to training for a 10k that is 17 weeks away, hence the accompanying chart depicts 17 weeks.

Phase 1: Base Building

Type: Long, slow runs
Duration: 10 weeks
Intensity: 55% to 75% of maximum heart rate (Maximum HR = 220 minus your age)

A 10-week Base Building Phase might contain two 5-week subphases—Base One and Base Two—in which training volume (duration and frequency) slowly increases in stairstep fashion. When you begin a new subphase, you start at a higher level than the old one ended at. Each subphase does not have to be 5 weeks long; it could be 4 or 3 weeks. No matter how long you make the subphases, you have to have a rest week in between them.

A key to success: Go slow. Gradually ramp up the miles and pace with no more than a 10% increase per week. Be patient. Hold back. Fight the urge to pick up the pace, to sharply increase intensity. Mark Allen, maybe the best runner in the sport of triathlon, successfully demonstrated the benefit of this in the early nineties with low-heart-rate training, a then-unique training method in which he deliberately kept his heart rate below 150 at all times, slowly building his base on his way to the last of his 6 Hawaii Ironman championships. Base training is all about low-intensity workouts at maximum volume—long, slow, distance runs, or LSD for short.

The purpose of these gradual, stepwise increases in training time or mileage is to prepare your body and gain confidence for the harder work to follow. Physiologically, you are building up the components of your aerobic foundation: stronger heart and leg muscles, thicker tendons and bones, and miles of capillaries. The latter, the tiniest pipes in the vascular system, serve to distribute and remove fuel and waste products from all parts of your muscles. They are much slower to respond to stimuli than muscles and lungs—all the more reason to throttle up very slowly.

Another purpose in ramping up very slowly during base training is to teach the body how to burn your body's most abundant fuel: fat. You do this by slowly increasing the density of the muscle cells' mitochondria, the tiny aerobic energy production factories that use fats and oxygen to make energy. Before you are trained, intense exercise will outrun your ability to process enough oxygen to burn fat, and you go "anaerobic" (without oxygen): your body, trying to keep going, then reaches for a quicker-burning fuel—your precious, limited stores of carbohydrates. More mitochondria help you meet the muscles' demand for more oxygen and allow you to stay longer in fat-burning mode.

Rest is key: Both 5-week subphases are followed with a rest-and-recovery week. Five weeks on, one week off. The latter is the all-important recovery week—a vastly reduced workload that refreshes your mind and body, letting all your systems consolidate the stresses of training and come back even stronger. Warning: Don't train hard through your recovery week. You'll exhaust your body, stall your progress, and maybe get injured.

But recovery is not limited to this one week. A recovery day should follow any hard workout, no matter the week or the phase.

Recovery doesn't necessarily mean sitting on the couch, although a day of that won't hurt. You can go out for shorter, lower-intensity runs. Here, cross-training comes in handy: swim, do the elliptical machine, play tennis. Stay aerobically active, but lower the burners. A recovery workout doesn't produce additional stress; its low intensity is rejuvenating—like a massage. Recovery permits body (and mind) to test the limits of athletic potential without falling over the edge into over-training/underrecovery.

By the end of our ten-week base training period, a prospective runner should have built his body up to the

LOSE WEIGHT AND FLY

If you want more speed but don't want to periodize your training, remember two words: Lose weight.

"The extra fat load lowers your strength-to-weight ratio without adding more force-producing capacity," says Tom Osler, author of *The Serious Runner's Handbook*, and developer of a formula widely used by runners to calculate the effect of weight changes on speed. Analyzing over 2,000 of his own races over 50 years, from 5ks to ultramarathons, he arrived at his ratio: For every extra pound of body fat, add 2.5 seconds to run one mile. It doesn't sound like much, but it adds up: over a minute in a marathon and 15 seconds in a 10k. Lose ten pounds, and you should be able to knock close to 11 minutes off a marathon with no extra training.

Fine, you're saying. Now, just one little detail: How do I lose the weight?

Below, several ways to cut the fat slowly, permanently, and, best of all, painlessly. But first, advice: Don't combine weight loss and rigorous training. "That can cause a sizeable breakdown of muscle protein, leading to a decline in strength and speed," says David Costill, director emeritus of the Ball State human performance lab. "To train properly, be at a desired race weight no later than two months before your target event." Next, don't lose over a pound or two a week; that can jeopardize muscle mass, says Dr. Arny Ferrando, director of the University of Texas performance lab at Galveston. And if you're thin already, beware; Costill once measured Frank Shorter at 4% body fat and felt he was quite healthy, but says minimal levels for good health are normally 5% for males and 12% for females. Below this, athletes often see decreased performance and increased illness, injury, and development of eating disorders.

The dietary and lifestyle changes here are so easy to incorporate into a daily routine that you may forget you're doing them—until you cross the finish line several minutes ahead of schedule.

1. *Eat more dairy:* Three or four servings of yogurt or milk a day can help you lose an average of 15 pounds a year, according to Robert P. Heaney, professor of medicine at Creighton University in Omaha. Naturally occurring calcium, not supplements, induces the body to metabolize fat more efficiently.

point where it can survive a 10k (6.2 miles). Now it's time to add the strength and speed that will allow you to run it faster.

Phase 2: Strength/Speed Building

Type: Shorter, faster runs with more hill climbing

Duration: 5 weeks

Intensity: 75%, with progressive intervals ranging from 85% to 92% of maximum heart rate

Having built your metabolic and structural foundation, you enter the Strength/Speed Building Phase, where you maintain volume and further increase

2. *Light pre-breakfast aerobics:* With a dearth of easy-access fuels like muscle glycogen or bloodstream sugar in the system, an early workout jump-starts the metabolism and forces the body to reach for "intermuscle" fat, plentiful but hard-to-access fat within the muscle, says Dr. Gabriele Rosa, coach of many top Kenyan marathoners.

3. *Avoid liquid calories:* A sugar-saturated Coke won't make you feel as full as an orange. Studies show that your body doesn't register a feeling of fullness from liquid calories, and they help you gain weight by causing you to overeat and drink later. Stick to water.

4. *Graze:* Eat numerous small meals throughout the day. Long non-food stretches—i.e., a noon lunch to a 7 P.M. dinner—kick the body into survival mode, encouraging fat storage. Digesting lots of small meals "prevents blood sugar spikes and costs lots more energy," says Dr. Arny Ferrando of the University of Texas.

5. *Eat low-GI carbs:* Get most daily carbs from low-glycemic Index foods like yogurt, fruit, nuts, and bananas, which break down slowly, They provide an appetite-curbing feeling of fullness that fast-burning, high-GI bagels, cereals, and rice cakes don't.

6. *Read before you eat:* Look at a 99-cent bag of corn chips. One serving is 150 calories. Read further: There's five servings in a bag, or 750 calories—a third of an adult's RDA.

7. *Walk after dinner:* "A brisk 20-minute stroll after dessert burns up to 100 calories and raises metabolism, so you'll burn more later," says Carl Foster, Ph.D., of the department of Exercise and Sports Science at the University of Wisconsin—La Crosse.

8. *Snack on meat at night:* If you must eat after 8 P.M., make it protein, like turkey, not an orange, toast, or cake. "Those turn into sugar, stimulating insulin, which switches your metabolism from an overnight muscle builder to a processor of carbs, which get stored as fat," says nutritionist Betty Kamen, PhD, author of 1001 Health Secrets.

RUN FOR LIFE

aerobic capacity and build speed and power. One objective of this period is to raise your body's ability to tolerate the kind of hard work your time goal requires without slowing down.

Your tools: hill climbing, sustained hard efforts, and shorter, higher intensity training sessions than the previous phase.

Technically, in the Strength/Speed Phase you are trying to raise your "lactate threshold" (or LT), the point at which a metabolic waste product called lactic acid starts flooding your body and cramping your muscles. The only way to get true LT readings is to ride a stationary bike in a lab and have the technicians prick your fingertips and do a blood analysis. Fortunately, you can approximate LT by looking at your heart rate. Roughly, it's when your breathing's heavy and your working muscles are close to feeling a burn. This means that you are going anaerobic—so hard that you are outstripping your body's ability to bring in enough oxygen for its needs. That's often somewhere in a range around 85 to 92 of approaching maximum heart rate, which you can only sustain for a short period, or "interval" of time. Therefore, your Strength/Speed training sessions might be mainly at 75 of maximum heart rate, with occasional interval sessions at 85, 88, and 92. Try to push the intervals a bit higher each time.

Since what isn't trained gets detrained, long efforts are still part of the Strength/Speed Phase. Every second week, run a distance close to your longest day of the Base Phase, and follow it with recovery time, to prevent overtraining.

Phase 3: Peak and Taper

Type: Continued fast runs, but for less time
Duration: Two weeks—to race day
Intensity: 75 with intervals to 85% to 92% of maximum heart rate

Relax—but only a little. With the Strength/Speed Phase over, you're at peak fitness, but not well rested. For that, you must "taper"—back off on the volume. You'll work out just enough to stay sharp, but gain a deep recovery that will leave you fresh. Work out too much and you'll be fatigued on race day. It's a fine line that plenty of elite athletes botch from time to time. You can walk the line successfully if you follow two rules:

Rule #1: Avoid the urge to go for one last long run. You cannot develop any more fitness, but you can tire yourself out and sabotage the event you've been training for for months. The stress levied on your body must now be unloaded for your top-level fitness to show up with you at the start line.

Rule #2: Maintain intensity, but cut training volume by 30%. Then the next week reduce it another 30%. Shave duration from longer efforts. Maintain frequency, if possible. You may be able to hold a peak for a month, but not much longer, so when targeting several events keep them close together on the calendar.

Phase 4: Transition

Type: Easy running and cross-training
Duration: At least a week, depending on your next event
Intensity: 55 to 75% of maximum heart rate

After the 10k is over, especially if it's a tough, hilly one, spend the next week recovering. Swim or row for aerobic fitness; give your legs a break. Jog a bit on Wednesday and Thursday if another event is planned in a week. If you have an event planned for a month away, recover for a week, do strength/speed for a week, and recover for two.

THE EVIL 5th PHASE: OVERTRAINING

Is Periodization fail-safe? In theory, applying stressor forces to the body in a progressive manner, broken up by rest and variation, will always compel muscles to adapt by getting stronger. But what happens when you apply too severe a stressor for too long? After all, the endorphin high can encourage runners to run too much. And an average load for you one year may be too much the next, when personal circumstances have changed.

The answer: When the body lacks the energy source and/or recovery time to continue adapting, it gets overwhelmed and simply capitulates. This is the dreaded Exhaustion Stage, most commonly known as "Overtraining." For lab rats, overtraining often means death. For humans, it could manifest as tendonitis, frequent colds, unexplained edginess, or worse, poor race performance. It behooves you to be aware of its causes and symptoms, so that you can make adjustments before a crisis occurs.

Common Causes and signs of Overtraining

According to Andy Pruitt, director of the Boulder Center of Sports Medicine, the most frequent overtraining mistakes include:

1. Nonstop hard running: Too much training and racing without adequate rest and recovery.
2. Runny-nose running: Exercising through sickness and injury.
3. Too much, too soon: Intense training without a sufficient mileage base.
4. Empty gas tank: Poor nutrition, particularly a failure to eat enough carbohydrates and protein soon after a run to replenish glycogen stores.

Dr. Cooper's 20 Symptoms of Overtraining

At the American College of Sports Medicine meeting on May 27, 1992, Australian sports scientist Ian Gilliam reported that the overtraining syndrome may include a decline in testosterone, a rise in cortisol (a steroid from the adrenal glands), hemolysis (destruction of red blood cells), reduced performances, and amenorrhea (failure to menstruate). A practical 20-point checklist, compiled by Dr. Neil F. Gordon of the Cooper Institute for Aerobics Research, Dallas, Texas, should help you identify overtraining symptoms:

1. Changes in sleep patterns, especially insomnia
2. Extended periods of healing for minor cuts and scratches
3. Fall in blood pressure and dizziness when getting up from a prone or seated position
4. Gastrointestinal disturbances, especially diarrhea
5. Gradual loss of weight in the absence of dieting or increased physical activity
6. Greater than usual increase in heart rate during a standard exercise session
7. Leaden or sluggish feeling in legs during exercise
8. Impaired mental acuity and performance or inability to concentrate
9. Inability to complete regular exercise sessions that are usually no special challenge
10. Increase in resting heart rate (in early A.M.) by more than 10 beats per minute
11. Excessive thirst or fluid consumption at night
12. Greater susceptibility to infections, allergies, headaches, and injuries
13. Loss of appetite
14. Listlessness/tiredness
15. Loss of libido or interest in sex
16. General loss of enthusiasm, drive, and motivation (including sports you enjoy)
17. Muscle and joint pains
18. Swelling of the lymph nodes
19. Irregular or no menstruation in premenopausal women
20. Sluggishness that persists more than 24 hours after a workout

Overtraining can be exacerbated by poor nutrition, which can impair immune responsiveness and increase probability of illness. Cooper recommends the following:

1. Antioxidants—Vitamins E, C, and the carotenoids, which stabilize highly active free radicals that cause cellular damage in the body. Fruits and vegetables are high in antioxidants; research indicates large consumption can cut cancer rates
2. Adequate recovery time (8–9 hours sleep)

LASZLO'S "SECOND WIND" RACE-DAY WARM-UP

Acclaimed coach Laszlo Tabori, the third man to break the 4-minute mile (see his *Run for Life* interview following Chapter 11), trains his athletes with techniques that readers of this book should be familiar with by now: lots of intervals, a classic running posture that synchronizes a "pendulum" arm swing, a flat foot strike under the body, vertical torso posture, and high strides with elevated knees and heels. But Tabori says it's all for naught if you toe the starting line without being properly warmed up. In fact, he says the great miler Jim Ryun could have been even greater if he'd only learned how to warm up. Here's the 45-minute race-day warm-up he says gets you into your "second wind" before the race begins.

1. 15-minute warm-up jog—at least 50% of race pace
2. Stretch 5 minutes only
3. 10 x 100 yds. back and forth—6 medium pace, 4 hard (85–95%)
4. Walk 50 yds.
5. 165 yd. build-up, starting at 50% and building to 100%
6. Walk 50 yds.
7. 265 yd. pickup—back and forth—pick it up, like shifting gears. Last 100 yds., blow it—total sprint
8. Walk 50 yds.
9. Repeat 165 yds.
10. Walk 100 yds.
11. Six 100s—3 x (1 blast, 1 medium)
12. 15-minute rest period: go to the bathroom, put on race clothes, change shoes, lay down, and play dead for 2 or 3 minutes
13. Do three or four 15-to-20-yard sprints immediately before the race, then go to the start line

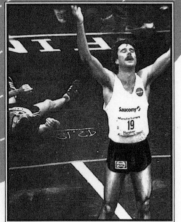

INTERVIEW 10

ROD DIXON

Mr. Versatility

I instantly recognized 56-year-old Rod Dixon at the 2006 L.A. Marathon pre-race press conference, because it looked as if he hadn't aged a day in decades. *Oh, there's that great miler from the early 1970s—what's he doing here?* I thought. It turns out that "miler" barely scratched the surface. In addition to his sub-4 miles (PR of 3:53.6), Dixon was also a great 5k, 10k, and *marathon* runner deep into the eighties, often beating the best of his era and displaying a range and longevity at world-class levels that is nothing short of astounding. At the top of most of running's "Most Versatile" lists, the New Zealander won bronze in the 1972 Olympic 1500, was third at the cross-country worlds in 1973 and 1982, was nearly unbeatable at the 5k in 1975, and became a virtual running celebrity with a come-from-behind win of the 1983 New York Marathon so dramatic that some have compared it to an Alfred Hitchcock thriller.

Tall for a runner and Hollywood handsome with an engaging, upbeat, storytelling personality, the 4-time Olympian with a penchant for flamboyant outfits became the first and maybe only "rock-star" runner. Dixon mingled with CEOs, presidents, and movie stars as he jet-setted between bases in the U.S. and New Zealand. He rang up lucrative sponsorship deals, battled his own national federation over the legality of prize-money trust funds and amateur status, and organized running events, many for kids. He has four of his own through several marriages. An inveterate cross-trainer long before the word existed, the enthusiast mountain biker, kayaker, mountain climber, and weight trainer excitedly talked about his accomplishments and age-defying fitness (he still runs a sub-5 mile) in a *Run for Life* interview by phone from his Studio City, California, office on April 1, 2008.

Sometimes, I think I was born in the wrong country.

I'd throw my arms in the air and blow kisses to the crowd—and Peter Heidenstrom, our athletic historian, was quite critical of me for that. He didn't like my showmanship. New Zealand wasn't like that. It has this incredible history of running that probably came from the running clubs in England—I went to a club there in 1970 that was 110 years old. Jack Lovelock of New Zealand set the 1500-meter world record of 3:47.8 in the 1936 Olympics, beating Glenn Cunningham, the great U.S. miler. That was the beginning. And we were very fortunate to have a coach named Arthur Lydiard who in the forties and fifties experimented and developed the principles of aerobic and anaerobic training. He inspired Bill Bowerman, the great University of Oregon coach, who brought jogging to the U.S. Nike was born from that. And we did get people into the stadium in England, Australia, and New Zealand. But the athletes were never expressive.

We are a rugby nation—the All-Blacks. They set the tone; they'd score this brilliant tri, and then the guy would pick the ball up and he'd hang his head back and say, in a very low-key, almost apologetic way, "I'm very sorry, I didn't mean to score a tri." We were very humbled by the whole thing. We didn't show a lot of excitement, a lot of expression.

But in Europe in the seventies, that's what was expected of you. I'm a passionate person; as a young boy, all my passion and love for life was expressed through my running. And when I went to Europe, and ran in the great stadiums of Scandinavia and Italy, with twenty thousand people going to see track and field, it was unbelievable. Bislet Stadium in Oslo, right in the center of the city—tickets would sell out in an hour, like a rock concert. 20,000 people right on top of you. In winter, they used it as a speed-skating stadium. They would beat the fence, and you would run faster and faster. More world records were set there than anywhere. I set a world record in the four-by-1500 relay and missed three world records by less than a second—the 2-mile twice and the 5000-meter, although I did beat the great Henry Rono, 4-time world record holder, in that race.

In Europe, the crowd would be on their feet. It was a lot different from the environment I grew up with in New Zealand.

At least Heidenstrom did name me the "most versatile" runner that New Zealand's ever produced, although he would have liked me to focus more. I think that's what he was referring to when he'd say: "If Dixon wasn't so easily distracted . . ."

Actually, that was kind of like a prophecy from my school days in Nelson, my hometown on the South Island. It was totally true. The teachers would never put me near the window, because I would be out looking at the mountains. I'd be looking at this ridge line, planning, thinking, "I could go up there, and get across there, on top and there'd be a 2-hour run . . ."

All the kids used to laugh because I could beat the school bus home. As soon as the school bell rung, I'd race. I'd have put on my T-shirt and shorts at the lunch break. As the bell went off, I'd whip my school uniform off, put it in my bag, give it and my homework to my mates to take home on the bus. And I'd throw my running shoes on, be out the gate and beat the bus home. I was 14.

As early as I can remember, I was running. I was fast at 5 or 6. People in New Zealand build fences around their property to keep the world out. My parents had to put up a gate to keep me from running away. At four years old, I got out and I ran to my brother's school, 2 miles away, because I missed him. My mother said a neighbor told her that she saw me running down the road; she thought I'd be just a few dozen yards away. But she had to go back and get a car, because she figured out that I went to the school. I knew the route because we used to walk with him in the morning. And when she got there, there I was.

My brother John was a great runner, too. John was my hero. He was four years older. He could do everything—swim across a river, climb a tree, run for miles. He would say, if you want to be like me, then you have to do what I do. So I did.

ROD DIXON

KEINO ON THE WALL—AND IN THE LEFT LANE

I loved to compete, to run, to train, the world of an athlete. I'm still like that. I always loved the rough runs. The day I turned 12, July 13, 1962, I had a ten-shilling note and used it to join a running club, the Nelson Amateur Athletic Harrier and Cycling Club. It had 300–400 members.

The running club was like a second family. We'd travel across the country. Every Sunday, training. A party and a keg of beer every Saturday night.

But we did more than run. We were always in the mountains, hiking, tramping, skiing. I could shoot a deer at 300 yards.

In 1963, when I was 13, Bowerman came to New Zealand. He'd read about Lydiard. He brought his team to challenge our record 4-by-1-mile team. I found out where they were staying and biked 6 miles into the city to get autographs. A few years later, my mates had Beatles posters on the wall; I had Jim Ryun and Kip Keino on mine.

I had the passion. In high school, I became the New Zealand under-18 mile champion. I'd been doing 4:24, 4:19, 4:12, and then 4:06.8, the fastest ever at that age in the country.

A critical moment came in 1968. I listened to the Mexico City Olympics on the radio, when Kip Keino beat Jim Ryun in the 1500. It turned me on. I was 18—my mates were scattering around the world—a last hurrah, a last crazy year before they settled down. But I realized now that I wanted to be a great athlete. I wanted to get that 4-minute mile.

So I talked to my brother John. He started to coach me.

John was a great coach and motivator, and he had a long-term plan: Build a foundation. It was the Lydiard principle, which you take 2 to 3 years to build an aerobic base.

Aerobic training has to be like a big bank account, so I'd do 2½-, 3- and 4-hour runs. The Japanese women go hiking before starting their running program—it builds sinew, connective tissue.

By 1970–1971, I was showing good times in long distances. John said to me, "You're stuck on the idea of the 1500 meter, but everything points to the 5000 for you. So you decide what you want to do."

I finished 10th in the 1971 world cross-country championships, and everyone said, "You've got to focus on the 5000."

I said, "No, I'll be doing the 1500." I would not be influenced by others. And slowly but surely, I got the mile time down, 4:02, 4:01, 4:00.1.

In Wellington (N.Z.) in January 1972, I ran the mile in 3:59.3. It was a big day psychologically.

At the '72 Olympics, I went into the Munich 1500 heats ranked 43rd in the world. I'd listened to Ryun and Keino race each other in this race four years earlier. Now, I look down the aisle: Ryun and Keino are in my heat! Guys I've looked at on my wall all these years. Shit!

Kip is a world champion and commonwealth champion. He's won the steeplechase in these Olympics already. Ryun was not in the Top 10 anymore, but he'd won the U.S. Olympic Trials.

Ryun trained completely different than me; he was naturally fast. I wasn't; my speed came from strength. My 800-meter time was the slowest of all the runners. But once I got wound up, I was away.

I had a great kick off a fast pace—not off a slow race. A lot of runners knew that, and tried to keep the pace very slow. That's what's fascinating about the mile: so much strategy. It's the perfect event—tactics, speed, strength.

They call the runners to the line. On my left, Jim Ryun. My right, Kip Keino.

At two laps to go, Keino sits at the back. Then he swings out wide and at 800 meters pours it on. All right! That suited me perfectly. My brother and I had talked about this. Kip Keino is the perfect pacer for me!

I knew I had to be within striking distance. As Keino came around, everyone tried to follow him.

Then I hear the clashing of metal spikes. I suddenly feel a hand go down my right calf muscle. Then the race settled down and we chased Keino.

To my side there was Franco Arese of Italia, the European champion. Ryun has to be coming around the back straight, I'm thinking. Keino is putting on the pace on nicely. And here it is, I'm in second!

It's a bloody good race—perfect for me as a strength runner. I ran a 3:40, a personal best. I took a glace back at the finish. No Ryun!

It was Ryun who fell. He got up and chased us, but he was 10–15 meters behind.

We were informed that there was an appeal. Would we agree for him to go on to the next round? I said okay. But no one else did.

The next day was Heat 2, the semifinals. I ran 3:37.9, a tie for second. In the final, I ran a 3:37.5. That broke Peter Snell's New Zealand national record. It was good for third behind the Finn (winner Pekka Vasala) and Keino.

Third place in the Olympics! I just couldn't believe it. I was so happy. I was suddenly world famous. There was a comment by Ron Picking, the great BBC announcer, that he'd never seen a happier bronze medalist.

Earlier that week, I ran into the New Zealand rowers. Those boys could drink beer. They were natural athletes. I came up to Athol Earl. He took his gold medal out of his pocket and put it around my neck. "How does that feel, mate?" he said. "I want to see one of these on you, too."

And 3 or 4 days later, I am holding my own medal—just a different color. The dream was real.

In 1968, I'd dreamed of it. I'd held onto the goal. That night, I went to the Hofbrau House. I woke up with a huge hangover.

I flew to London for a meet a week later and beat Steve Prefontaine, who took 4th in the 5000 in Munich, in the 3000, the 2-mile. He was the perfect pacemaker. He'd try to run you into the ground. I just sat on his heels, and sprinted by him on the last lap. Set the world and commonwealth record.

Then I flew back to New Zealand, back to normality, I thought.

FROM NATIONAL HERO TO 1976 DISAPPOINTMENT

Several TV reporters interviewed me when I arrived in Wellington, New Zealand's capital. Since my parents weren't home in Nelson, a ferry ride across the strait, I stayed an extra day in a hotel.

In the morning, I looked out the window and thought, what's going on here? There were thousands of people!

It didn't stop when I got off the plane in Nelson. Jeepers creepers—my mates from the running club carried me off in the king's chair. I had morning tea with the mayor. Then they put me in a sports car, and drove me down the city's main street to the cathedral at the end. The street was lined with 30,000 people—everyone in Nelson! And the Prime Minister of New Zealand was there.

This day opened up the rest of my life.

The planning began for the 1976 Olympic Games in Canada. We planned a European tour; I identified 20 races. I needed to get hardened in more races.

I had to fund it all myself. I'd saved quite a bit of money and had bought a car, but now I had to sell it—a real heartbreaker.

A friend, Dick Taylor, wanted to go to Europe, too. And John Walker decided to come with us. He hadn't qualified for the '72 Olympics. We became friends when I came home. He was an 800-meter runner who began to experiment in the 1,500. At our first race, he flew by me in a flash—in 3:38 or 3:39, equivalent to a 4-minute mile. Holy hell, this guy Walker is good, I thought. I beat Walker a lot in Europe, but I knew he'd be very good very soon.

My brother targeted my training for the 1974 Commonwealth Games, to be held in New Zealand in Christchurch. Walker would do the 800 and 1500.

Unfortunately, six weeks before the meet, I was training in the bush when I leapt over a tree, fell, and could hardly get up. My back popped. It took me an hour to struggle back to the parking lot. A chiropractor worked on me for two weeks. I missed the opening ceremonies, and went down to Christchurch two days before the finals.

The 1500 was shaping up to be a great race. Walker had won silver in the 800, behind Filbert Bayi of Tanzania and Ben Jipcho of Kenya. They were all in the 1500 and it turned out to be one of the greatest of all time.

Bayi beat Ryun's world record in 3:32.2. Walker also broke it in 3:32.5, Jipcho did 3:33.2, and I was 3:33.89. I ran the 5th-fastest time in history—and took 4th place!

And I came to a realization: I had to go longer. Bayi and Walker were far better in the 1500 than I could hope to be. For the '76 Olympics, I had to do what my brother and others had told me years before: I had to step up to the 5000.

In 1975, I ran 26 or 27 races, all specifically selected by John to build me up. It worked. By the end of the year, I was ranked number-one in the world in the 5k.

And ironically, as I got better in the 5k, I got better in the 800—doing 1:48–1:49. I realized that you had to keep feeding God-given speed. So I did the 4-by-100-meter relay on my club team.

I was absolutely ready for the 5,000 in Montreal. Unfortunately, I ran a stupid race, finishing fourth behind Lasse Viren of Finland. Four of us, all within .74 of a second of each other. The German Hildebrand dove across the line and beat me for third. I was devastated. It was the most disappointing race of my athletic life. In addition, there was known blood doping going on—immoral but not illegal then. I wouldn't do it under any circumstances, but knowing others did left me so frustrated. I had never been so well prepared for a gold medal.

I halfheartedly trained after that, still doing well on the European circuit—won two British championships, including running away from Sebastian Coe in the 1500. But I needed a shot of adrenaline before I went home.

I got it in Dublin in the 5000, July 1977. The day before the race, after I'd gone out for a light jog with Walker, I got a call. My wife gave birth to my daughter Kate 10 days early. When I was interviewed on TV, the Irish crowds went wild at the announcement. At the race, 300 meters to go, I surged to the front and they went ballistic. It was a special moment—a 5000-meter win and my daughter's birth in 24 hours.

At the bar of the Donnybrook Hotel, a guy called out, "See here laddie—all for you." There were 23 pints of Guinness on the bar. I left at 5:30 A.M. They poured me into a taxi to the airport to London, and 54 hours later I met my first child.

THE NEW YORK MARATHON TRAINING PLAN

To go from the mile and the 5000 meters to the marathon is rare. Haile Gebreselassie is the only one to do it, I think. It'd be like asking Carl Lewis to run the mile. It's no surprise that decathletes are very uncomfortable running 1,500 meters. I was uncomfortable with the idea of doing the marathon, but events sort of forced it. And to be honest, I've always loved new challenges. I once ran a steeplechase on a dare from Walker. That I ended up a marathoner was logical given the circumstances.

In the late seventies, I was focused on the 1980 Olympics—running the 5k and 10k in Moscow. When the boycott came on (over the USSR invasion of Afghanistan) I was training in Pennsylvania for the Diet Pepsi 10k in Philadelphia and other local races. "You've got to be kidding," I said. I was devastated.

By then, I had built myself up into being one of the world's best 10k runners, although the public didn't really know it. I was beating great guys—Craig Virgin, Greg Meyer. The plan: I've got to race them, win the big ones. And the biggest one was the Falmouth Road Race (7.06 miles) on Cape Cod. For that race, I was unknown and didn't wear a sponsor's name. I didn't qualify for assistance, so I stayed with a family. And I won the race. That was the beginning of a huge wave of interest in me in the U.S.

I also won the Philadelphia Half-Marathon. I was unbeaten in 1980.

Now, with the Olympics gone, I decided to try new distances. But when Runner's World magazine called me up (after Philadelphia) and said, "This sets you up for the marathon," I said, "Hell no!" I was afraid of it.

I was afraid of the distance. I thought it would change me—wreck my speed for shorter races. Of course, that was a myth. You can run a marathon and come back, just don't only do marathons. Do short races, too, to keep your speed, agility, and elasticity.

But I had to face the facts. I was now 31 years old, and noticing that I was losing my strength and speed. I could still run a 4-minute mile, but it was getting harder and harder. So I realized that I had to get back into cross-country, get back to basics. And I won a bronze in the 1982 world championships in Rome behind Mohamed Kedir of Ethiopia and Alberto Salazar.

The day before that, I'd sat down at a table with Fred Lebow, the director of the New York Marathon. He was so stimulating. He'd say, "When are you going to run it?" I said I had no interest in running the marathon, but he wouldn't stop. "You're not known in the U.S. yet. To do that, you've got to run the marathon."

So we agreed: If I finished in the top ten, I'd consider it. And If I won a medal, I'd definitely do New York.

The next day, I had barely recovered my breath walking through the gate and Fred was on me. "See you in New York," he said.

I told him I'd be there as a spectator that fall. I wanted to see if the marathon was for me. If it was, I'd do the 1983 race.

I ran Bay to Breakers (in San Francisco), then flew back to New Zealand in May to run the Children's Hospital City of Auckland Marathon as a trial. It was a favor to the organizers. "Rod, you're a national hero, and we need a sponsor," they told me. So I said I'd RUN it—not RACE it. I needed to put myself through the process, to build my data bank, learn what it takes.

A marathon runner thinks different from a 10k runner. For a 10k, I normally run two or three miles beforehand as a warm-up. But why do that if I've got 26.2 miles to go?

Jack Foster, one of New Zealand's all-time greats, paced me. He wanted to be the first 50-year-old to run under 2:20 [Note: He barely missed it in 2:20:18]. He said the first mile you ease yourself into it—like a Sunday run, get into the flow.

So we ran a 6½-minute first mile—and the leaders were gone. By mile five, our pace was down to 5:45–5:50. Jack wanted me to win. So about then, he looked at me and said, "If you're serious, get going now."

So away I went.

As I picked runners off, I was picking up information. I noticed errors—runners staying on one side of the street. That's inefficient given the camber of the road. You had to stay in the middle.

It all started to unfold for me. I realized that the marathon is an economy run—and you're like an economy car. Pretend that there's an egg under the accelerator. No surging. Get a cadence. Monitor yourself. Am I over-striding? This is a thinking game, a game of chess.

After 12 or 13 miles, I got up with the leaders. Soon, it was me and the favorite, Kevin Ryan.

He kept looking at me. "You wanna push the pace?" he said, getting a little stroppy (agitated). "If you can, wise-ass, do it."

It's a picturesque course in Auckland—way out to Heliers, and then coming back into the city. I got about 50, 60 yards ahead, and then decided to put on a good show, boy. I picked up the pace, then asked myself, "Can you hold this comfortably?" I'd pick it up again, and ask again. Soon, I put minutes on Ryan.

My time: 2:11:21.

I jogged up and back the course, waved to everybody, then jumped in the water and took a 10-minute swim around the bay. Then I went on a bike ride around the waterfront to get the cobwebs out.

I knew from that point that I was on the way to figuring out what the marathon—this amazing event—was all about.

I had a run Sunday morning, then flew to Philadelphia the next weekend and raced a 10k in 29 minutes. I ran six races in the next six weeks, all faster than 31 minutes. I wasn't overdrawing from the bank.

Fred kept calling. "You running New York this year?"

I stuck with my plan of monitoring the race in '82, and running it in '83. I attended the press conference, the expo, the breakfast run, then watched an incredible race—Alberto Salazar and Rodolfo Gomez running side by side. Alberto won by 4 seconds in 2:09:29. On the cab ride to the airport, I said out loud, "I will return next year and win." I sat down with my sponsors—Pepsi and Pan American Airlines—and told them I wanted to run New York.

I knew I needed six months to train. Training for New York was the most intensely focused time of my life. Every day I would ask, what am I learning from all this?

I ran Bay to Breakers, set a course record. I ran Lynchburg, Virginia. Ran the Freedom Trail in Boston—a 10-miler—to see where I was. Looking back in my diary in December of '82, I see that I was doing light weights with high reps, no big-chain-ring cycling, water running in the pool with a vest to get my heart rate up, and working with Jerry Attaway, the strength and nutrition coach of the San Francisco 49ers. We were dialing in my nutrition; while running, we'd carry plastic bags full of different foods. You gotta find out what's good for you. It turns out that Gerber Baby Food worked for me at the race.

In the fall of '83, as I was doing my long runs through the hilly forest near Reading, Pennsylvania, my home base, I was happy. Everything was going exactly as planned for the first time in my life. It was the first time I realized that I was the best prepared for any event I'd ever been. It was an overwhelming feeling of satisfaction. All I had to do was go to New York to get the medal.

I didn't go to the expo and the press conference. My masseuse told me that I was in the best shape of my life.

I'd done a profile of the New York course. I knew the elevation, the bridges. I wrote my time splits on my hands—for 5 miles, 7, half marathon, 18 miles, 23 miles.

I wrote down 2:09 as my finishing time.

COMING FROM BEHIND IN MANHATTAN

As the race got under way, one thing I didn't plan on was the leaders getting so far ahead of me so early. Geoff Smith, an Englishman, and a Tanzanian, Gidamis Shahanga, went out faster than Salazar's record pace in 1981. I hung with the second group, told myself to concentrate and remain patient, figuring I'd reel them in later.

They were doing 4:45 miles, while I was going 4:57, 4:58 pace. I got a little desperate, began overstriding in Central Park, and slightly slipped at 5 miles, stressing my hamstring. Part of it was that New York was raining; I had custom shoes made by Saucony, a new sponsor, and I

chose the wrong shoe—a slick. So from then on, I kept away from the white lines.

I knew that a 4:40 pace would blow my hamstring, so I stayed with my pace. At the 17-mile mark, coming off the Queensboro Bridge and onto First Avenue, I looked up to see the two leaders a half-mile ahead.

My first thought was, "Oh my God, that's a big margin!" But I looked at the clock, did the calculations, and knew I had 47 minutes to make up the gap.

The Tanzanian faded. I had to hope and believe that Smith would slow down, too, and I could reel him in at 22 or 23 miles.

With three miles to go, heading down Fifth Avenue and turning into Central Park, he was slowing down, but I was still 22 seconds behind. Now I'm running 5:08–5:09, but he's 7 or 8 seconds slower than that. I could see him getting wobbly—being cautious by staying in the center of the road while I'm more risky, running the tangents, closest to the crowds. I'm furiously calculating the numbers. The marathon seemed like a big chess game. At this rate, we'd tie. I'd catch him right at the finish line!

But luckily, I forgot about the extra 385 yards.

I was watching him. I said to myself, "I'm not going to give him anything—no warning, no motivation." So I snuck up on him—waited for a more open stretch where we would be in a straight line. Then I ran straight behind him, staying in his blind spot, just as I learned to do in 10ks. I caught him right on the 26-mile mark.

And before he had a chance to react, to attach himself to me, I just ran as hard as I could. I shocked him—and myself. After two hours behind, I'm actually leading this race! I didn't think it was mine until the last 10 yards. I put 8 seconds on him by the finish.

2:08:59! Incredible! One second off my plan!

When I crossed the line, a million emotions flooded me—redemption from the '76 Olympics, from the stolen shoes [his athletic bag was stolen just before a much-anticipated 5,000 meters at the 1978 Edmonton Commonwealth Games], the boycott … I had worked so hard. I was at peace with myself. It was the icing on the

RUN FOR LIFE

cake. The culmination of my career. The defining moment of everything I've done in running.

I looked at the heavens because I believed someone was looking after me, and then thanked the earth, wind, and sky. I dropped to my knees, kissed the wet asphalt, raised my arms, and put my hands to my head as Smith tumbled across the line, lay on his back on the concrete, utterly exhausted. There's a famous picture of me at the finish, which was made into a poster. Roone Arledge of ABC called it "The agony of victory." This was my moment. This is what it was all about. I thought to myself, "I have earned the right to slow down." I went over to Tavern on the Green. While I was sitting there about the 4-hour mark, I looked up at all the runners streaming through, all of them high-fiving.

And I thought, "Damn—I'm not the only winner here today. This is what I'm all about. This is where I'm meant to be."

LIFESTYLE OF THE RICH AND FAMOUS

I went to the L.A. Olympics in '84. But there was a big problem by then: I got too drawn into the celebrity thing.

After my New York Marathon win, everyone wanted me. I met President Reagan. He used to breed horses on his ranch—Appaloosas. We were in the middle of a big Washington gathering talking about horses.

Saucony made a Dixon Trainer shoe, and I got royalties.

Pepsi flew me out to meet the CEO, Roger Enrico. He gave me an envelope with a fat check inside.

Pan Am named a 747 plane after me and gave me a first-class ticket anywhere, anytime. I'd fly first-class all over the world! I was treated like royalty. They'd announce me on the plane.

So after all this, I went back to New Zealand in 1984 to train. It's an Olympic year. I should be training. I should be focusing. But I fell short of preparation.

And so I went off to Los Angeles. I met (the composer) Burt Bacharach on the plane. He said I could stay at his house. So here I am in L.A., sleeping in his bed!

I told my brother John, "I'm short of training. I need more time. I'm 3 to 4% off. They need to delay the Olympics 3, 4 weeks for me to be 100%." I knew that I didn't have the Eye of the Tiger.

I ran a good race, actually. But when we hit the freeway, my legs went dead. I slipped to 24th place before climbing back to 10th. I ran a 2:12—1.3% over my previous best, in New York.

I lost it because I became a celebrity. "Come to Sydney for a banquet—we'll pay you $7,000." That was two days of no training. At the time, I thought I could handle it. Make hay while the sun shines, they say. But too many 3-hour runs in the forest were missing.

I was 34. Pepsi signed me again. I could still win 70% of my 10k races, although I couldn't keep up with the 22-year-olds anymore.

I won the 1987 New Zealand cross-country trials—at age 37. I could still win, but it became more and more inconsistent.

In 1988, I didn't make my fifth Olympic team. I had to qualify at the L.A. Marathon, but only ran a 2:14:30. I needed a 2:14:15. It was quite disappointing.

I turned 40 in 1990, and my competitive career was over. I started my Rod Dixon Family Fun Runs. I wanted to be the first 40-year-old to run a sub-4 mile, but I caught viral pneumonia from some air conditioning in Erie, Pennsylvania. It took me almost a year to get over that. (In 1994, 41-year-old Irish legend Eamonn Coghlan became the first—and, as of 2008, only—masters runner to post a sub-4 mile.)

CROSS-TRAIN FOR LIFE

While I was competing, I trained all year round. I never took off between seasons. I had two summers a year in the '80s, splitting time between the U.S. and New Zealand.

I always ran 34 minutes a day, at least, but I also did a lot of cross-training. So sometimes instead of an easy run, I'd do an easy bike ride. I'd bike in the forest after running. I'd go hiking, hunting, fishing. I'd do some boxing—hit the heavy bag for 15 rounds of 3 minutes each. Get my heart rate up to 190–200. I saw it all as a complement to my training.

No other runners were doing this. Some of that is due to being a New Zealander, where we all modeled ourselves after Sir Edmond Hillary, the first man to climb Mt. Everest. He influenced us all. He was our giant—and he could do everything.

I see runners whose life is governed by a watch. I never ran with a watch. But I always kept a diary. I got done with my workout, then I wrote in my diary—what I did, how I felt, where I went, simple pulse-checking. A diary is so necessary. My athletic world had to be a balance of four quarters: emotional, physical, mental, spiritual. I had to be balanced every day—you can't train at 100% if you're emotionally upset.

In the early eighties, as triathlon arose, I was fascinated with triathletes. Scott Tinley, Dave Scott—the common sense and intelligence of training for three sports at once. You must know what you're about.

In my forties, I added more cross-training. I did a lot of multisport. I did the Coastal Challenge on a team every year—a big New Zealand event where you run, bike, mountain climb, and kayak for several days—and we'd win it every year.

Today, I'm still a competitive age-group runner. I've even gone back to the mile and can still run a 4:34. Biome-

chanically, I'm okay—no injuries. I attribute it to my cross-training. Here's my schedule:

- 35 to 40 minutes running every other day
- Kundalini yoga once a week
- Hiking 2½ or 3 hours once a week
- The gym once a week. Low weights and high reps. No squats. Chin-ups and dips, 15 at a time, 5 sets. Push-ups, 50 at a time, 2 sets. Inverted crunches, twists. On bike rides, I stop at the old Muscle Beach equipment south of the pier in Santa Monica and climb rope and do the rings.
- Bike 4 times a week, with 2 rides of at least 2 hours, often going from the Palisades to Hermosa Beach and back.

Bottom line: Don't even think about just running. If I only had one hour to train, I'd run for 40 minutes and strength-train for 20.

I feel 30 or 35, maybe. I just don't do the extreme stuff that I used to do. No more pig hunting—because you're always going to fall in a river. I don't hang-glide anymore. Now I walk my mountain bike across the creek.

I've always said, "It's the long run of life." I was the hare, and now I'm the tortoise. But it doesn't matter, because I still just love to run.

Acknowledgments

Before I run off, special thanks to four people who've played important roles in helping me get this book to the finish line: 1. Santa Monica physical therapist Robert Forster, who has given me invaluable information and advice that I have used in countless articles over the years, and allowed me to make use of his PHASE IV training facility (www.phase-iv.net) and specialists during the writing of *Run for Life*; 2. The relentlessly creative and brilliant Bill Katovsky, the founder of *Triathlete* magazine, coauthor of my previous book, *Bike for Life*, and my connection to Skyhorse Publishing; 3. Bob Babbitt, the ubiquitous, always-enthusiastic editor-publisher of *Competitor* magazine, who over the years has provided me with dozens of running-oriented assignments and a platform for writing about my various adventures; and finally, 4. Bernard Lyles, founder of the Tri-Masters Club of Chicago and tireless promoter of bringing thousands of minority adults and kids into the sport of triathlon, who I profiled in a 1998 Triathlete magazine story, "The Rainbow Coalition." I hope he's pleasantly surprised to find that his invitation to join him and his friends at the 1999 Boston Marathon led to my interest in running form and ultimately, to this book.

About the Author

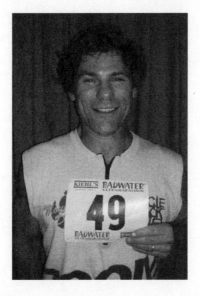

Roy M. Wallack is a *Los Angeles Times* health-and-fitness columnist and a contributor to many publications, including *Outside*, *Men's Journal*, *Runner's World*, *Competitor*, *Bicycling*, and *Mountain Bike*. A former editor of *Bicycle Guide* and *Triathlete* magazines, he is the author of *Bike for Life: How to Ride to 100* and *The Traveling Cyclist: 20 Worldwide Tours of Discovery*. Along with competing in innumerable running, cycling, and triathlon races, Roy has participated in some of the world's toughest endurance events, including the Eco-Challenge and Primal Quest adventure races, the Paris-Brest-Paris, TransAlp Challenge, La Ruta de los Conquistadores road and mountain-bike races, and the TransRockies Run. He lives in Irvine, California with his tandem bike partners, wife Elsa and son Joey, and his running partner, Bruce the dog.

JAN   2010
Northport-East Northport Public Library

To view your patron record from a computer, click on
the Library's homepage: **www.nenpl.org**

You may:
- request an item be placed on hold
- renew an item that is overdue
- view titles and due dates checked out on your card
- view your own outstanding fines

**151 Laurel Avenue
Northport, NY 11768
631-261-6930**